Select Topics in Dermatology

Editor

PETER G. FISHER

VETERINARY CLINICS
OF NORTH AMERICA:
EXOTIC ANIMAL PRACTICE

www.vetexotic.theclinics.com

Consulting Editor
AGNES E. RUPLEY

September 2013 • Volume 16 • Number 3

ELSEVIER

1600 John F. Kennedy Boulevard • Suite 1800 • Philadelphia, Pennsylvania, 19103-2899
http://www.theclinics.com

VETERINARY CLINICS OF NORTH AMERICA: EXOTIC ANIMAL PRACTICE Volume 16, Number 3
September 2013 ISSN 1094-9194, ISBN-13: 978-0-323-18876-0

Editor: John Vassallo; j.vassallo@elsevier.com
Developmental Editor: Susan Showalter

Veterinary Clinics of North America: Exotic Animal Practice (ISSN 1094-9194) is published in January, May, and September by Elsevier, Inc., 360 Park Avenue South, New York, NY 10010-1710. Subscription prices are $243.00 per year for US individuals, $389.00 per year for US institutions, $124.00 per year for US students and residents, $289.00 per year for Canadian individuals, $457.00 per year for Canadian institutions, $326.00 per year for international individuals, $457.00 per year for international institutions and $159.00 per year for Canadian and foreign students/residents. To receive student/resident rate, orders must be accompanied by name of affiliated institution, date of term, and the *signature* of program/residency coordinator on institution letterhead. Orders will be billed at individual rate until proof of status is received. Foreign air speed delivery is included in all *Clinics* subscription prices. All prices are subject to change without notice. **POSTMASTER:** Send address changes to *Veterinary Clinics of North America: Exotic Animal Practice*, Elsevier Health Sciences Division, Subscription Customer Service, 3251 Riverport Lane, Maryland Heights, MO 63043. **Customer Service: Telephone: 1-800-654-2452** (U.S. and Canada); **1-314-447-8871** (outside U.S. and Canada). **Fax: 1-314-447-8029. E-mail:journalscustomerservice-usa@elsevier.com** (for print support); **journalsonlinesupport-usa@elsevier.com** (for online support).

Reprints. For copies of 100 or more of articles in this publication, please contact the Commercial Reprints Department, Elsevier Inc., 360 Park Avenue South, New York, New York 10010-1710. Tel.: 212-633-3874; Fax: 212-633-3820; E-mail: reprints@elsevier.com.

Veterinary Clinics of North America: Exotic Animal Practice is covered in *MEDLINE/PubMed (Index Medicus)*.

Printed and bound by CPI Group (UK) Ltd, Croydon, CR0 4YY

Transferred to digital print 2012

Contributors

CONSULTING EDITOR

AGNES E. RUPLEY, DVM
Diplomate, American Board of Veterinary Practitioners–Avian Practice; Director and Chief Veterinarian, All Pets Medical & Laser Surgical Center, College Station, Texas

EDITOR

PETER G. FISHER, DVM
Diplomate, American Board of Veterinary Practitioners–Exotic Companion Mammal; President, Pet Care Veterinary Hospital, Virginia Beach, Virginia

AUTHORS

ERIC J. BAITCHMAN, DVM
Diplomate of the American College of Zoological Medicine; Director of Veterinary Services, Zoo New England, Boston, Massachusetts

ANDREW D. BEAN, DVM
Pet Care Veterinary Hospital, Virginia Beach, Virginia

JENNIFER BLAIR, DVM
Private Practitioner, St Francis Animal and Bird Hospital, Roseville, Minnesota

MICHAEL FEHR, PhD, DVM
Diplomate, European College of Zoological Medicine–Small Mammals; Clinic for Exotic Pets, Reptiles and Birds, University of Veterinary Medicine Hannover, Hannover, Germany

PETER G. FISHER, DVM
Diplomate, American Board of Veterinary Practitioners–Exotic Companion Mammal; President, Pet Care Veterinary Hospital, Virginia Beach, Virginia

SARI KANFER, DVM
Exotic Animal Care Center, Pasadena, California

SASKIA KOESTLINGER, DVM
Clinic for Exotic Pets, Reptiles and Birds, University of Veterinary Medicine Hannover, Hannover, Germany

ADOLF K. MAAS III, DVM
Diplomate, American Board of Veterinary Practitioners–Reptile and Amphibian Practice; Center for Bird and Exotic Animal Medicine, Bothell, Washington; ZooVet Consulting, PLLC, Bothell, Washington

ANNA L. MEREDITH, MA, VetMB, PhD, CertLAS, DzooMed, MRCVS
Professor of Zoological and Conservation Medicine, Head of Exotic Animal Service, Royal (Dick) School of Veterinary Studies and The Roslin Institute, Easter Bush Veterinary Centre, University of Edinburgh, Roslin, Midlothian, Scotland, United Kingdom

MARK A. MITCHELL, DVM, MS, PhD
Diplomate, European College of Zoological Medicine–Herpetology; Professor, Department of Veterinary Clinical Medicine, University of Illinois, College of Veterinary Medicine, Urbana, Illinois

BRIAN S. PALMEIRO, VMD
Diplomate, American College of Veterinary Dermatology; Lehigh Valley Veterinary Dermatology and Fish Hospital, Allentown, Pennsylvania

ALLAN P. PESSIER, DVM
Diplomate, American College of Veterinary Pathologists; Senior Scientist, Amphibian Disease Laboratory, Wildlife Disease Laboratories, Institute for Conservation Research, San Diego Zoo Global, San Diego, California

DRURY R. REAVILL, DVM
Diplomate, American Board of Veterinary Practitioners-Avian Practice; Diplomate, American College of Veterinary Pathologists; Zoo/Exotic Pathology Service, West Sacramento, California

HELEN ROBERTS, DVM
Aquatic Veterinary Services of WNY and 5 Corners Animal Hospital, Orchard Park, New York

VALARIE V. TYNES, DVM
Diplomate, American College of Veterinary Behaviorists; Premier Veterinary Behavior Consulting, Sweetwater, Texas

MICHAEL R. WALDEN, MS, DVM, PhD
USDA-FSIS, Cargill Meat Solutions, Waco, Texas

E.P. SCOTT WEBER III, VMD, MSc
Associate Professor of Clinical Aquatic Animal Health, VM: Medicine and Epidemiology, University of California, Davis, Davis, California

AMY BETH WORELL, DVM
Diplomate, American Board of Veterinary Practitioners–Avian Practice; Avian Veterinary Services, West Hills, California

Contents

understood. A significant amount of research exists on barbering in mice that suggests it is an impulse control disorder and may represent a good animal model for trichotillomania in humans. Stress seems to play a complex role in the development and maintenance of some behavioral dermatopathies, but genetics and experiences, especially during development, also likely play a role. Pain or discomfort may underlie the development of many of these problems.

VETERINARY CLINICS OF NORTH AMERICA: EXOTIC ANIMAL PRACTICE

Preface

Select Topics in Dermatology

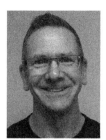

Peter G. Fisher, DVM, Dipl. ABVP–Exotic Companion Mammal
Editor

When the Consulting Editor of *Veterinary Clinics of North America: Exotic Animal Practice*, Agnes Rupley, asked me what topic I would like to cover as editor, I pondered for around 30 seconds and answered with affirmation, "Dermatology." Agnes asked, "Are you sure you don't want to think about it?" I said, "No, that's my topic. Dermatology." In that 30 seconds I had quickly thought about the kinds of cases I commonly see on a daily basis in my private companion animal practice and the obvious answer was dermatologic. I also knew that it had been awhile since the last dermatology issue (10 years to be exact) and it was time for an update. Having made my decision, I began digging around in my journal and text library for ideas on how to cover this topic. Being in private practice for 33 years, I wanted this issue to be practitioner-friendly and useful. After some research, I decided on "Select Topics in Dermatology," with the goal of covering the most commonly seen exotic species and the varied spectrum of underlying etiologies for skin disease. My goal was to expose readers to state-of-the-art information on emerging diseases, delve into the pathophysiology of select dermatoses, update the standards of care for common syndromes, and find better ways to diagnosis and treat challenging dermatopathies. This issue begins with an overview of exotic species dermatologic disease and diagnostic techniques and then looks at dermatitis resulting from infectious agents (bacterial, fungal, viral, parasitic), neoplasia, endocrine problems, autoimmune disease, behavioral causes, and underlying anatomical and environmental influences.

I want to thank all the authors for lending their time and expertise in making this a great issue. This group is as varied as the topics covered: national and international academicians, researchers, zoological veterinarians, specialists, seasoned general practitioners, and those new to the field. I would also like to thank John Vassallo, Editor, *Veterinary Clinics of North America: Exotic Animal Practice*, for his thoughtful guidance, sense of humor and patience during the editing process. I hope you enjoy

Vet Clin Exot Anim 16 (2013) xi–xii
http://dx.doi.org/10.1016/j.cvex.2013.05.014
1094-9194/13/$ – see front matter © 2013 Published by Elsevier Inc.

vetexotic.theclinics.com

reading this issue as much as I have enjoyed being editor on this project, and I hope that it will serve as a valuable resource for the latest information on both the common and the uncommon in exotic species dermatology.

Peter G. Fisher, DVM, Dipl. ABVP–Exotic Companion Mammal
Pet Care Veterinary Hospital
5201-A Virginia Beach Boulevard
Virginia Beach, VA 23462, USA

E-mail address:
pfisher@petcarevb.com

Clinical Approach to Dermatologic Disease in Exotic Animals

Brian S. Palmeiro, VMD, DACVD[a],*, Helen Roberts, DVM[b]

KEYWORDS

- Exotic animal dermatology • Reptile dermatology • Avian dermatology
- Fish dermatology • Small mammal dermatology

KEY POINTS

- Skin disease is an extremely common presenting complaint to the exotic animal practitioner.
- Skin disease cases may be challenging because dermatologic diseases are often multifactorial and many have underlying husbandry or environmental deficiencies that must be identified.
- A thorough diagnostic evaluation is critical for successful management of exotic animal cutaneous disease.

INTRODUCTION

Skin disease is an extremely common presenting complaint to the exotic animal practitioner. A systematic diagnostic approach is necessary in these cases to achieve the appropriate diagnosis and formulate an effective treatment plan. In all exotic species, husbandry plays a central role in the pathogenesis of cutaneous disease, so a thorough evaluation of the husbandry is critical for successful management. There are vast differences in the structure and function of the skin in exotic species; an understanding of these unique properties is important when treating skin disease in exotic pets. This article focuses on the clinical approach to skin disease in exotic pets including structure and function of the skin, appropriate diagnostic testing, and differential diagnoses for commonly encountered cutaneous diseases.

REPTILES

Cutaneous disease is common in reptiles, is often multifactorial, and is most often secondary to husbandry and environmental deficiencies. A recent retrospective

Disclosures: The authors have nothing to disclose.
[a] Lehigh Valley Veterinary Dermatology and Fish Hospital, 4580 Crackersport Road, Allentown, PA 18104, USA; [b] Aquatic Veterinary Services of WNY and 5 Corners Animal Hospital, 2799 Southwestern Boulevard 100, Orchard Park, NY 14127, USA
* Corresponding author.
E-mail address: petfishdoctor@gmail.com

study of dermatologic lesions in reptiles found that from 29% to 64% (dependent on institution and reptile group) of the cases had underlying husbandry-related deficiencies.[1]

Skin Structure and Function

Reptile skin is modified into scales and composed of a three-layered epidermis and a dermis that typically is aglandular.[2–4] The three layers of the epidermis are (1) stratum corneum (six to eight cell layers, heavily keratinized); (2) stratum intermedium; and (3) stratum germinativum (deepest).[2–4] Two types of keratins compose the stratum corneum.[4] The softer more flexible α-keratins are elastic and pliable and form the suture/hinges and spaces between scales.[4] The β-keratins (unique to birds and reptiles) compose the hard horny scale.[4] The skin is protected by scales produced by the stratum germinativum; scales are separated by scale pockets.[2] The keratinized layers of chelonians are modified into scutes.[5] The scales or scutes of chelonians and some lizards (plated and girdled lizards, skinks, and crocodilians) are underlain by dermal bony plates referred to as osteoderms or osteoscutes.[2–5] In tortoises, the stratum corneum produces the shell, which consists of the carapace (dorsal) and plastron (ventral); the keratinized scutes cover osteoderms that fuse with the vertebrae and sternebrae.[2–4] Chromatophores (pigment cells) are found in the dermis and melanocytes are present within the stratum germinativum.[3] Reptiles shed their skin at regular intervals in a process called ecdysis. The skin of lizards and chelonians shed in several smaller pieces, whereas snakes typically shed their entire skin as one piece.[4] Chelonians and crocodilians shed their epidermis continuously, whereas lizards and snakes shed their epidermis periodically.[5]

Dermatologic Examination and Diagnostic Testing

A detailed clinical history is important in all cases of reptile skin disease; important husbandry-related questions include those pertaining to diet, substrate and housing, lighting, heating, humidity, and temperature.

Common findings during clinical examination of reptiles with dermatologic disease include abrasions, erosions, ulcers, wounds, swellings, pustules, blisters/vesicles/bullae, crusts, dysecdysis, petechial and ecchymoses, discoloration, macroparasites, and edema. In some cases, cutaneous changes can be secondary to systemic disease; petechia and ecchymoses are commonly seen with septicemia and ventral edema may be seen with renal or liver disease.[3] In one study, 47% of all reptiles with confirmed or suspected cases of sepsis had petechiae, with the highest association seen in chelonians (82%).[1]

Commonly used dermatologic diagnostic tests in reptiles include the following[2–5]:

1. Skin cytology and impression smears
2. Acetate tape impression
   - Press clear tape against skin and evaluate microscopically
   - Useful to diagnose mites
3. Skin scrapings
   - Typically use number 15 scalpel blade to collect epidermal samples
4. Microscopic evaluation of shed skin fragments
   - Findings may include mites
5. Skin biopsies for dermatopathology
6. Skin cultures
   - Bacterial, fungal
7. Fine-needle aspirate

○ Most useful for swellings and growths
8. Clinicopathologic evaluation including complete blood count (CBC) and biochemistry analysis
9. Radiographs are useful when assessing damaged osteoderms and for the presence of bony changes associated with secondary nutritional hyperparathyroidism or other internal disease

Common Differential Diagnoses for Cutaneous Diseases

See **Table 1** for a review of common differential diagnoses for dermatologic diseases in reptiles, including bacterial dermatitis, shell rot, bacterial ulcerative dermatitis, snake mite, and secondary nutritional hyperparathyroidism (**Figs. 1–5**).

AMPHIBIANS

The thin, relatively unprotected skin of amphibians combined with the significant diversity of amphibian habitats and their biphasic life cycles render them particularly susceptible to a wide range of infectious and noninfectious cutaneous diseases.

Skin Structure and Function

Amphibians belong to three distinct Orders: Anura (frogs); Caudata (salamanders); and Gymnophiona (caecilians). The skin of amphibians is clinically the most important organ system of amphibians and varies depending on the life stage (premetamorphosis or postmetamorphosis); habitat (generally divided into aquatic or terrestrial); and the species.[6] The skin functions in osmoregulation, gas respiration, and water absorption.[6,7] Amphibian epidermis is typically thin; keratinized; and consists of the stratum corneum, stratum granulosum, stratum spinosum, and the stratum basale.[7–11] Modifications of amphibian skin include the presence of dermal scales (caecilians); folds and grooves for increased surface area (salamanders); partial ossification of the cranial skin and adherence to the skull (bufonids); a specialized highly vascularized ventral dermal organ for water absorption ("drinking patch" in anurans); and the presence of dermal bones (some anurans).[10,12] The stratum corneum is typically shed in one piece at regular intervals and consumed (dermatophagy) unless the animal is ill.[6,11,13] The skin of anurans is loosely adhered to the body and can become edematous in disease states.[11] Two key features separate adult caecilians and anurans from their larval form: the epidermis is keratinized in adults and the dermis contains a variety of dermal glands.[7,9,11] Mucus, produced by mucous glands and epithelial cells, aids in respiration, prevents evaporative water loss, contains antibacterial and antifungal properties, can be defensive noxious or contain toxic chemicals, may act as pheromones, and can aid in reproduction.[12,14–17]

Dermatologic Examination and Diagnostic Testing

A thorough history and dermatologic examination are important when evaluating any case of amphibian skin disease. Husbandry-related factors often underlie the development of many skin diseases in amphibians. Important questions to consider include recent introductions into the collection; diet; and tank setup including filtration, aeration, water quality, and temperature. During examination, it is important to always handle amphibians with rinsed gloves to avoid damaging their skin and prevent cutaneous absorption of potentially toxic glandular secretions.[18–20] Many amphibian skin diseases can have a similar appearance with cutaneous hyperemia and discoloration, dermal papules and nodules, ulceration, hemorrhages, edema, and excess mucus being the most common findings.[21]

Table 1
Differential diagnoses for cutaneous diseases in reptiles

Disease/Condition	Causes	Clinical Signs/Properties	Diagnosis
Bacterial			
Bacterial dermatitis[a–f] (see **Fig. 1**)	Often secondary to environmental/ husbandry deficiencies or trauma Gram-negative environmental bacteria often act as opportunistic pathogens in these cases Various isolates including *Aeromonas; Pseudomonas; Citrobacter; Escherichia coli; Klebsiella; Proteus; Salmonella; Serratia; Flavobacterium; Staphylococcus; Streptococcus; Morganella; Neisseria; Dermatophilus congolensis; Mycobacterium;* and anaerobes, such as *Bacteroides, Fusobacterium,* and *Clostridium*	Moist, exudative, and erythematous, but may also appear as blisters, crusts, and ulcerations of the integument	Clinical signs, impression cytology, and culture/ sensitivity
Shell rot[a,c,e] (see **Fig. 2**)	Most common isolates include *Beneckea chitinovora, Citrobacter* spp. and *Aeromonas*	Most common bacterial infection in chelonians, ulcers of the shell, often rimmed by areas of hyperpigmentation; loose scutes may be present and lesions can progress to osteomyelitis	Clinical signs, impression cytology, and culture/ sensitivity
Septic cutaneous ulcerative disease[a,d]	Disease syndrome in aquatic turtles maintained in poor-quality water *Citrobacter freundii* is most commonly implicated but other gram-negative bacteria may be isolated	Craterifom ulcers on the shell and skin with septicemia and systemic signs	Clinical signs, impression cytology, and culture/ sensitivity
Blister disease[a–f] (see **Fig. 3**)	Often associated with moist, dirty substrate or inappropriately humid environments *Aeromonas* and *Pseudomonas* are the most common clinical isolates	Lesions typically start on the ventrum as vesicles and pustules that progress to ulceration, necrosis, and abscessation; secondary septicemia is possible; most commonly seen in snakes	Clinical signs, impression cytology, and culture/ sensitivity

Abscesses[a-f]	Common isolates include Pseudomonas spp, Proteus spp, Aeromonas spp, Serratia spp, Providencia spp, E coli, Citrobacter, Proteus, Salmonella, Streptococcus, Corynebacterium pyogenes, and Neisseria	Localized soft to firm, usually nonpainful swellings that have well-defined capsules; because reptile leukocytes lack the isoenzymes to liquefy pus, a thick caseous exudate is often present	Clinical signs, fine-needle aspirate, culture/sensitivity, histopathology
Ectoparasites			
Chiggers[a-f]	Family Trombiculidae	Ingest lymph and dissolved host tissue; zoonotic; skin irritation, pruritus, irregular shedding cycles; mites are most commonly found under scales and around nostrils, eyes, and gular fold (snakes)	Direct observation, microscopic identification
Mites[a-f] (see Fig. 4)	Family Macronyssidae; including Ophionyssus natricis (commonly seen in snakes) and Ophionyssus acertinus (common in lizards)	Feed on blood; skin irritation, pruritus, irregular shedding cycles, and anemia in severe infestations mites are most commonly found under scales and around nostrils, eyes, and gular fold (snakes)	Direct observation, microscopic identification
Leeches[b]	Various species	Skin irritation at site of attachment, anemia with severe infestation	Direct observation
Fungal			
Fungal dermatitis[a-f]	Often secondary to environmental/husbandry deficiencies and immunosuppression Reported isolates are often opportunistic pathogens including Aspergillus, Basidobolus, Geotrichum, Mucor, Saprolegnia and Candida, Fusarium, Trichosporon, Trichoderma, Penicillium, Paecilomyces, Oospora, and Trichophyton	Superficial infections present as moist, exudative erythematous ulcers or blisters, with crusts or hyperkeratotic lesions Deeper infections often present as nodules/swellings, systemic signs may be present with deeper/systemic infections	Impression smears, fungal culture, histopathology

(continued on next page)

Table 1
(continued)

Disease/Condition	Causes	Clinical Signs/Properties	Diagnosis
Yellow fungus disease[e,f]	*Chrysosporium* anamorph of *Nannizziopsis vriesii*	Seen most commonly in lizards (especially the bearded dragon, *Pogona vitticeps*) Deep, granulomatous dermatomycosis that is contagious and progressive, severe yellowish hyperkeratotic skin lesions, often fatal	Fungal culture, histopathology, PCR
Cheilitis in spiny tail lizards (*Uromastyx* sp)[f]	*Devriesea agamarum*	Cheilitis	Fungal culture, histopathology
Viral			
Green turtle fibropapillomas[d,f]	Herpesvirus	Papillomatous growths affected soft tissues	Histopathology
Neoplasia			
Cutaneous neoplasia[a,b]	Reported types include squamous cell carcinoma, fibrosarcoma, myxomatous tumors, lipoma/liposarcoma, melanoma, chromatophoromas	Cutaneous growths	Histopathology
Husbandry-related/multifactorial/miscellaneous			
Dysecdysis[c] (see **Fig. 3**)	Dysecdysis is almost always a result of deficiencies in husbandry and inappropriate environmental conditions including temperature and humidity	More commonly seen in snakes and some lizards than in chelonians; in lizards and turtles, most commonly affects the digits; in snakes, can be localized or generalized; localized dysecdysis commonly affects the spectacles and retention of this scale can result in other ocular abnormalities, such as subspectacular bullae and abscesses	

Condition	Cause	Clinical signs	Diagnosis
Secondary nutritional hyperparathyroidism (see **Fig. 5**)	Multifactorial: severe imbalance of the Ca:P ration in the diet, no access to a full spectrum (ultraviolet B) light source, and a lack of activated vitamin D_3; other inappropriate husbandry-related factors	Seen more commonly in lizards and chelonians abnormal bones and shells and chronic abscesses especially around jaw	History, clinical signs, radiographs, serum phosphorus, ionized calcium levels
Trauma	Injuries from prey-induced trauma, with rodents being responsible for most cases; trauma from other household pets is also not uncommon	Damaged skin, ulcers, erosions	History and clinical signs
Burns	Burns most commonly result from malfunctioning, malpositioned, or inappropriate heating elements or inactivity of the animal	More frequent in lizards and snakes; discolored, ulcerated and sloughed areas of skin	History and clinical signs, histopathology
Hypovitaminosis A[a–d]	Dietary deficiency of vitamin A results in squamous metaplasia and epidermal hyperkeratosis	Abnormal shedding Most commonly affects lizards and chelonians Lizards: dysecdysis, impaction/abscessation of cutaneous glands Chelonians: dysecdysis, chemosis/blepharedema and aural abscessation. most common cutaneous changes include hyperkeratosis, dysecdysis, scute loss, and thickened/lichenified skin	History and clinical signs

[a] Hoppmann E, Barron HW. Dermatology in reptiles. J Exot Pet Med 2007;16(4):210–24.
[b] Goodman G. Dermatology of reptiles. In: Patterson S, editor. Skin diseases of exotic pets. Ames (IA): Blackwell; 2006. p. 73–118.
[c] Johnston MS. Scales and sheds: the ins and outs of reptile skin disease. In: Proceedings North American Veterinary Dermatology Forum. Denver (CO): 2008. p. 62–6.
[d] Mitchell M, Colombini S. Reptiles. In: Foster A, Foil C, editors. BSAVA manual of small animal dermatology. Gloucester (England): BSAVA; 2003. p. 269–75.
[e] Hat JM. Dermatologic problems in reptiles. In: Proceedings of the World Small Animal Veterinary Association World Congress. Geneva (Switzerland): 2010.
[f] Mader D. Reptile dermatology. In: Proceedings of the Atlantic Coast Veterinary Conference. Atlantic City (NJ): 2011.

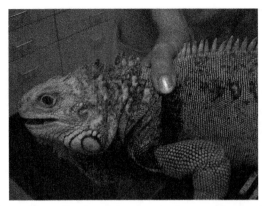

Fig. 1. Bacterial dermatitis on the dorsolateral neck of a green iguana (*Iguana iguana*).

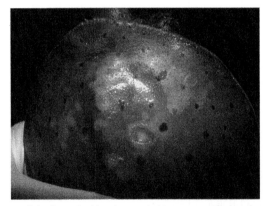

Fig. 2. Shell rot in a softshell turtle (*Apalone* sp). Note crateriform ulcers on the carapace.

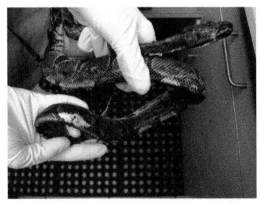

Fig. 3. Ball python (*Python regius*) with bacterial ulcerative dermatitis (blister disease) and dysecdysis. Note ulcerative skin lesions, retained skin, and spectacles.

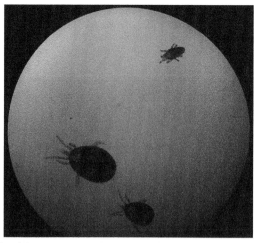

Fig. 4. Snake mite (*Ophionyssus natricis*).

Commonly used dermatologic diagnostic tests in amphibians include the following:

1. Skin scraping[8,10,13]
   - Using a coverslip, blunt scalpel blade, or edge of a glass slide, gently scrape over the surface of the skin
   - Samples taken from lesions may be more diagnostic
   - Place the sample on a slide
   - If needed, wet the slide with physiologic saline for a wet mount preparation
   - Examine immediately using lowest power objective first
   - Shed skin can also be examined as a wet mount preparation
   - Samples can also be dried and stained for later examination
2. Impression or swab smears, fine-needle aspirates[6,8,13]
   - Typically these samples are air dried and stained
   - Less traumatic than skin scrapings
3. Bacterial culture[10,13,22,23]

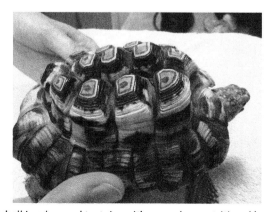

Fig. 5. Abnormal shell in a leopard tortoise with secondary nutritional hyperparathyroidism.

- Gentle irrigation of the lesion with sterile physiologic saline or getting a deep sample can reduce contamination of normal surface microflora and environmental bacteria
- Dermal glandular secretions and normal microflora may inhibit bacterial growth because of antibacterial properties
- Swabs can be moistened with sterile saline or transport media to minimize skin damage and maximize recovery of bacteria
- Optimal temperature for sample growth is 35°C/95°F
- Most isolates are gram-negative bacteria but gram-positive and mycobacterial infections also occur
4. Fungal cultures[24,25]
- Tissue sections can be placed directly onto fungal culture media
- Sabouraud dextrose agar media is a good choice for most fungal isolates
- Culture at room temperature
5. Polymerase chain reaction (PCR) of skin swabs[26–29]
- Consult laboratory for availability; verification of positive results; type of PCR (conventional, Taqman, real-time, and so forth); use of negative and positive controls; sample collection and swab type; and shipping details
- Avoid cross-contamination
- Available test for identifying of subclinical carriers of *Batrachochytrium dendrobatidis*
  - Test of choice for screening new animals, detection of subclinical infections, and confirmation of positive cytologic examinations
  - False-negatives can occur with low-level subclinical infections
  - Skin swabs are preferred sample
  - Three swabs taken at various times over 14 days increases chance of identification
  - Tadpole samples are taken from mouthparts (keratinized area)
  - Can be expensive
- Ranavirus PCR
  - Frozen tissue, biopsy of skin lesion
- Chlamydophilosis PCR
- Flavobacteriosis PCR
- Mycobacteriosis PCR
  - Reliability of results for amphibians is unknown
6. Histopathology

Common Differential Diagnoses for Cutaneous Diseases

See **Table 2** for a review of common differential diagnoses for dermatologic diseases in amphibians.

FISH

Cutaneous disease is an extremely common presenting complaint to the fish veterinarian. Many owners notice abnormalities in the integumentary system as the first sign of disease in their pet fish. In addition, the skin is an extremely common target for many infectious diseases of ornamental fish. The skin of fish provides a protective barrier against infection, osmotic pressure, and injury. Disruptions of the skin can result in osmotic disturbance, disruption of internal homeostasis, morbidity, and mortality.

Table 2
Differential diagnoses for cutaneous diseases in amphibians

Disease/Condition	Causes	Clinical Signs/Properties	Diagnosis	Comments
Parasitic				
Protozoal	*Trichodina* sp, *Epistylis*-like ciliates, *Piscinoodinum*, *Ichthyosporidium*, *Dermocystidium*, *Tetrahymena*, *Vorticella*, *Ichthyobodo*	Increased mucus, discoloration, cloudy skin patches, ulcers, secondary skin infection, pruritus	Skin cytology, skin scrapings, histopathology	Trichodinids are typically associated with poor water quality, low numbers may be commensal/nonpathogenic
Nematodes	*Pseudocapillaroides xenopi*; capillarid nematodes that live in tunnels in epidermis of *Xenopus laevis*	Weight loss, lethargy, skin roughness and ulceration particularly over the dorsum, secondary bacterial and fungal infections	Skin scrapings, histopathology	
Trematodes	*Clinostomum, Cathaemasia*	Cutaneous, yellow nodules	Identification of encysted parasite	Typically not pathogenic
	Neascus sp	Nodular cysts on lateral line (*Xenopus* sp)	Identification of encysted parasite	Typically nonpathogenic, but heavy infestation can be fatal
	Riberia ondatrae	Limb deformities (usually hind limbs but can affect all)	Histopathology	Damage occurs because of disruption of limb formation in larval stage, usually frogs farmed or housed outdoors with exposure to snails (intermediate hosts)
Arthropods	*Argulus* sp	Secondary infections, ulcers	Direct observation	Infest aquatic life stages
	Lernaea sp	Secondary infections, ulcers	Direct observation	Infest aquatic life stages
Leeches	Various species	Secondary infections, open wounds	Direct observation	Can transmit *Ichthyophonus* sp–like organism

(continued on next page)

Table 2
(continued)

Disease/Condition	Causes	Clinical Signs/Properties	Diagnosis	Comments
Trombiculid mites	Various species	Red-orange vesicular lesions, cutaneous cysts	Microscopic identification	Larval stage only; adults live in the environment also known as "chiggers"
Ticks	Various species	Focal irritation, hemorrhage	Direct observation	
Fly larvae (myiasis)	Sarcophagidae, Calliphoridae, Chloropidae species larvae	Ulcers, secondary infections, erythema, deep wounds	Direct observation, histopathology	
Bacterial				
Red leg syndrome (bacterial dermatosepticemia)	Bacterial septicemia in amphibians often presents as reddening of skin on ventrum and hindlegs; can be secondary to environmental stressors; most commonly gram-negative pathogens (*Aeromonas hydrophila*, other) but gram-positive reported	Erythematous hemorrhagic skin, usually ventrally and on extremities, nodules/abscesses, edema, erosions, ulcers, skin sloughing	Clinical signs, culture, histopathology	
Flavobacteriosis ("edema syndrome")	*Flavobacterium* spp	Generalized edema, hydrocoelom, cutaneous hemorrhages	Bacterial culture, PCR	
Mycobacteriosis	*Mycobacterium* spp	Cutaneous nodules	Stained impression smears, histopathology, culture and identification, PCR	
Chlamydophilosis	*Chlamydophila* sp	Reported in *Xenopus laevis* Cutaneous petechia and ulceration with edema	Culture, histopathology	

Viral	Ranavirus (an iridovirus)	Edema, red leg syndrome, pale, raised foci, erythema and swelling near gills and hind limbs, cutaneous erosions and ulcers, secondary bacterial infection; thick mucus, cutaneous white polyps and hemorrhage (salamanders); tadpole edema virus infection in larval stages of anurans	Clinical signs, histopathology, PCR, virus isolation, transmission electron microscopy
Fungal			
Chytrid	*Batrochochytrium dendrobatis* (chytrid)	Systemic signs (lethargy, anorexia); skin sloughing; color changes; ventral edema and petechiae; mortalities related to osmoregulatory stresses	Cytologic examination of skin scrape, shed skin, PCR, histopathology	Colonizes keratinized skin only, the only keratinized area in larval stages are mouthparts so subclinical infections can occur (can break with clinical disease after metamorphosis); more than 400 amphibian species susceptible; higher incidence in winter months in wild populations
Pigmented fungi	Many species including *Phialophora, Fonsecaea, Hormodendrum, Cladosporium*; fungi found in soil, enter through skin lesions, stress predisposes to infection	Papular and ulcerative skin lesions, nodules, systemic signs	Histopathology, culture

(continued on next page)

Table 2
(continued)

Disease/Condition	Causes	Clinical Signs/Properties	Diagnosis	Comments
Water molds	*Saprolegnia, Aphanomyces;* opportunistic, usually secondary to trauma, immunosuppression, severe physical stress, poor water quality	Focal lesions typically, white to tan cottony growth over ulcers or erosions	Stained impression smears, wet mount impression smears or skin scrape, culture, histopathology	
Noninfectious diseases				
Nutritional				
Metabolic bone disease		Subcutaneous edema, scoliosis, mandibular deformity, postural abnormalities, fractures, tetany, bloating, prolapse	History, clinical signs, radiographs	
Husbandry-related				
Gas bubble disease	Water supersaturated with oxygen	Gas bubbles in skin especially toe webbing, eyes; erythema and hemorrhage of the skin, mortality	Direct observation of gas bubbles in tissues	
Acidic or alkaline environment	Increased or decreased pH (water, soil)	Excess mucus production, skin irritation and ulceration, erythema, respiratory and systemic symptoms	Check pH of environment	
Elevated water hardness	Increased water hardness	Skin lesions seen in some species of caecilians	Test water hardness	

	Cause/Source	Clinical Signs	Diagnosis	Comments
Ammonia toxicity	Elevated ammonia	Increased mucus production, color changes, erythema, skin sloughing, dyspnea, neurologic signs, secondary infections	Test ammonia levels	Less toxic at lower pH, caution when changing water to prevent overall pH increases (favors more toxic unionized ammonia)
Lead toxicity	Lead (plumbing fixtures, décor)	Epidermal sloughing, postural abnormalities, muscular twitching, lethargy, death	Lead levels in tissues	
Rostral abrasions	Shipping, jumping in startled animals, iatrogenic handling, cagemate aggression, live prey items, inappropriate cage	Abrasion of the rostrum, color changes, secondary infections, atrophy of rostrum	History, observation	Usually secondary to nervous, easily startled animals. Buffer panels/coating rough surfaces inside enclosure may help reduce incidence
Neoplasia	Many including squamous cell carcinoma, adenomas, papillomas, chondromas	Masses (focal or diffuse), color changes, secondary infections	Histopathology	

Data from Refs.[7,22,26–29,38,39]

Skin Structure and Function

The skin can be divided histologically into the cuticle, epidermis, dermis, and subcutis. The cuticle (outermost layer) is approximately 1 μm thick and contains mucus, sloughed cells, and cellular debris. It has antimicrobial properties mediated by antibodies (IgM), free fatty acids, and lysozymes.[30,31] This layer is commonly referred to as the "slime coat" by aquarium hobbyists because of its high concentration of mucus. This layer is usually lost during routine processing for histopathology. Together with the cuticle, the epidermis produces a waterproof barrier. The epidermis is a nonkeratinizing (most species) stratified squamous epithelium that contains 3 to 20 cell layers.[30,31] It contains many mucus-producing goblet cells and, in some species, club cells that secrete an "alarm substance" when the skin is damaged. Unlike mammals, epidermal cells are not keratinized and are capable of mitotic division in all layers; however, division most commonly occurs in cells adjacent to the basement membrane where the epidermis junctions with the dermis.[30,31] The upper dermis contains collagen and reticulin and forms a supportive network; the deeper dermis contains more compact collagen and provides the main structural strength to the skin.[30,31] Scales are flexible bony plates that develop in scale pockets in the dermis; they are not shed regularly.[30,31] As scales emerge they are covered by a layer of epidermis, and often overlap one another, providing structural support and protection. Two main types (ctenoid and cycloid scales) are described that differ in surface sculpture.[30,31] Ultrastructurally, scales contain collagen fibers interspersed with an organic matrix in which hydroxyapatite crystals are deposited.[30,31] Some fish are scaleless and histologically have a thicker epidermis. Chromatophores (pigment cells) are present in the dermis and include melanophores; xanthophores (yellow); erythrophores (orange-red); leucophores (white); and iridophores (reflective/iridescent/silver). The pigments consist mainly of carotenoids. The subcutis contains connective tissue and fat and is highly vascular; bacterial disease can spread rapidly along this layer.[30,31]

Dermatologic Examination and Diagnostic Testing

The diagnostic approach to a fish with dermatologic disease should include a complete history, direct observation of the fish in its aquarium or pond, dermatologic examination, complete water quality, skin scrapings, and a gill biopsy.

As with other species, historical evaluation is extremely important. Because infectious disease is very common in pet fish, questions pertaining to quarantine protocol, most recent fish introduction, and number of fish affected are extremely important. Husbandry-related questions (water changes, filtration, tank or pond setup, water quality testing, and so forth) are extremely important because many diseases in fish are related to poor husbandry and water quality. The owner should be questioned regarding prior treatments because many fish hobbyists attempt numerous over-the-counter remedies before consulting with a veterinarian.

Direct observation is best performed in the home aquarium or pond. Isolation is often an early indication of disease in schooling fish. Other signs that can be seen during direct observation include piping (gasping for air at the surface) and flashing (a sign of pruritus in which the fish rubs against objects in the aquarium or pond). The skin and fins can also be evaluated for abnormalities.

During the dermatologic examination, the skin, fins, and scales should be evaluated thoroughly. Some fish require sedation for this procedure. Latex gloves should be worn to protect the cuticle. Abnormalities that are commonly seen on the dermatologic examination include skin discolorations; erythema; frayed and irregular fins; erosions and ulcerations; petechial and ecchymoses; edema and raised scales; macroparasites (anchor worm, fish lice); papules and nodules; excess mucus production; scale loss; and white-to-gray irregular patches.[30]

Commonly used dermatologic diagnostic tests in fish include the following:

1. Water quality evaluation
   a. Poor water quality is the most common cause of morbidity and mortality in pet fish
   b. Poor water quality is the most common underlying cause of immunosuppression and opportunistic infections in pet fish
   c. Parameters that should be monitored include temperature, pH, ammonia, salinity, nitrite, nitrate, dissolved oxygen, and alkalinity[3]
2. Skin scrapings and gill biopsy
   a. Skin scrapings
      i. If there are lesions on the skin, a coverslip should be dragged across lesional skin in a head-to-tail direction, collecting mucus on the coverslip. The coverslip is then placed onto a slide with a drop of tank water. Some fish require sedation for this procedure. Sedation may reduce the number of ectoparasites found on skin scrapings.
      ii. When there are no obvious lesions on the skin, sites commonly sampled include just caudal to the pectoral fin, operculum, and the ventrum. Samples should be taken from two to three different sites; when possible, several fish should be sampled.
   b. Gill biopsy
      i. Gill is epithelial tissue and many ectoparasites affect the gills and skin. Occasionally, ectoparasites are found only on the gills.
      ii. Typically requires sedation
      iii. The operculum is lifted and a small snip of distal gill lamellae is taken (usually with iris scissors) and placed onto a slide with a drop of tank or pond water to examine.
   c. Skin scrapings and gill biopsies are examined under the microscope; superior results are obtained with the condenser down. Most parasites can be seen on ×4 or ×10 magnification. However, with some smaller parasites, such as *Ichythobodo*, and bacteria, such as *Flavobacterium columnare*, ×40 magnification is required.
3. Bacterial culture and sensitivity
   a. Tissue biopsy for culture sampling is preferred over superficial swabbing of ulcerative lesions
4. Histopathology
5. Clinical pathology (complete blood count, biochemistry panel)
6. Viral testing
   a. Koi herpes virus serology and PCR
7. Necropsy

Common Differential Diagnoses for Cutaneous Diseases

See **Table 3** for a review of common differential diagnoses for dermatologic diseases in fish, including *Gyrodactylus* and ulcerative bacterial dermatitis (**Figs. 6** and **7**).

AVIAN

Cutaneous disease is extremely common in pet birds; assessing the skin can be difficult given the variation in species presenting to the avian practitioner. Avian

Table 3
Differential diagnoses for cutaneous diseases in fish

Disease/Condition	Causes	Clinical Signs/Properties	Diagnosis
Ectoparasites			
Ciliated protozoans			
"Ich," white-spot disease[a]	*Ichthyophthirius multifiliis* (freshwater), *Cryptocaryon irritans* (marine)	Punctate white nodules (up to 1 mm in size) on the skin/fins caused by the encysted trophont feeding stage, increased mucus, flashing, respiratory symptoms	Skin scrapings, gill biopsy
	Chilodonella (freshwater), *Brookynella* (marine)[a]	Erythema, scale loss, white-to-gray irregular patches, hemorrhages, discolorations, flashing, excessive mucus production, respiratory symptoms	Skin scrapings, gill biopsy
Guppy killer disease[a]	*Tetrahymena* (freshwater), *Uronema* (marine)	Erythema, scale loss, white-to-gray irregular patches, hemorrhages, discolorations, flashing, excessive mucus production, respiratory symptoms; common in guppies (*Poecilia reticulata*)	Skin scrapings, gill biopsy
Sessile ciliates[a]	*Epistylis, Ambiphyra (Scyphidia), Apiosoma (Glossatella)*	Erythema, scale loss, white-to-gray irregular patches, hemorrhages, discolorations, flashing, excessive mucus production, respiratory symptoms	Skin scrapings, gill biopsy
Flagellated protozoans			
	Ichthyobodo (Costia)[a]	Erythema, scale loss, white-to-gray irregular patches, hemorrhages, discolorations, flashing, excessive mucus production, respiratory symptoms	Skin scrapings, gill biopsy
Freshwater and marine velvet[a]	*Piscinoodinium (Oodinium)* (freshwater), *Amyloodinium* (marine)	Amber or gold dust-like sheen to the skin, excess mucus, respiratory symptoms	Skin scrapings, gill biopsy

Flukes[a] (see **Fig. 6**)	Dactylogyrus, Gyrodactylus	Erythema, scale loss, white-to-gray irregular patches, hemorrhages, discolorations, flashing, excessive mucus production, respiratory symptoms	Skin scrapings, gill biopsy
Capsalids[a]	Benedenia, Neobenedenia	Erythema, scale loss, white-to-gray irregular patches, hemorrhages, discolorations, flashing, excessive mucus production, respiratory symptoms	Skin scrapings, gill biopsy
Macroparasites (crustaceans)			
Anchor worm[a]	Laernea	Parasite visible on examination; long, and narrow parasite with anchor at one end and egg sacks at opposite end; erythema and ulceration at site of attachment	Direct observation, microscopic identification
Fish lice[a]	Argulus	Parasite visible on examination, erythema, excess mucus production, flashing	Direct observation, microscopic identification
Bacterial			
Columnaris disease[a,b]	Flavobacterium columnare	Cottony white proliferative lesions on the skin/fins; most commonly affects live bearers	Clinical signs, skin scrapings, bacterial culture
Koi ulcer disease[a,b] (see **Fig. 7**)	Multifactorial, often underlying husbandry issues and environmental stressors, secondary bacterial infection	Koi (Cyprinus carpio) with ulcerative skin lesions, often rimmed by annular hemorrhage	Clinical signs, bacterial culture
Mycobacteriosis[a,b]	Mycobacterium spp	Clinical signs include ulcerative skin lesions, reduced appetite, emaciation, lethargy, exophthalmia, swollen abdomen, and fin/tail rot. Mycobacteriosis is zoonotic and can cause "fish tank granuloma" in people	Clinical signs, identification of bacteria on acid-fast stains of histopathology, culture, PCR

(continued on next page)

Table 3
(continued)

Disease/Condition	Causes	Clinical Signs/Properties	Diagnosis
Bacterial septicemia[a,b] (see **Fig. 6**)	*Aeromonas* and various other gram-negative isolates	Lethargy, anorexia, abnormal swimming patterns/spinning, hemorrhagic lesions on the skin, abdominal distension/ascites, abnormal position in the water column, exophthalmia, external ulcerative lesions, gill necrosis and mortality	Clinical signs, culture
Viral			
Lymphocystis[c]	*Lymphocystivirus*	Iridovirus that infects dermal fibroblasts causing them to swell up to 10,000 times results in whitish nodules, typically on the fins. Common species of fish affected include freshwater glass fish, marine angelfish and clownfish	Wet mounts/skin scrapings with classic swollen dermal fibroblasts that appear like a cluster of grapes, histopathology
Carp pox[c]	Cyprinid herpesvirus 1	Affects koi (*Cyprinus carpio*), causing epidermal hyperplasia; results in papillomatous "candle-wax" appearing lesions that typically occur on the fins and skin in cooler water temperature (<68°F) during the winter and spring. Progression to squamous cell carcinoma reported	Clinical signs, histopathology
Goldfish Herpesvirus[c]	Cyprinid herpesvirus 2	Affects goldfish (*Carassius auratus*), causing mortalities, lethargy, anorexia, and patchy pale areas of gill necrosis and skin lesions including cutaneous ulceration, sloughing of scales, increased mucus production, secondary bacterial/parasitic infections, and petechia/ecchymoses	Clinical signs, histopathology, PCR

Koi herpes virus[c]	Cyprinid herpesvirus 3	Massive mortality (80%–100%) in koi (Cyprinus carpio) Common cutaneous signs include cutaneous ulceration, sloughing of scales, decreased mucus production, secondary bacterial/parasitic infections, and petechia/ecchymoses All affected fish have gill necrosis and typically show respiratory signs, in addition to lethargy, weight loss, enophthalmos, and occasionally a notched appearance to the head between the eyes and nares	Clinical signs, histopathology, PCR, virus isolation
Neoplasia			
Cutaneous neoplasia	Various types including fibromas; fibrosarcoma; pigment cell tumors (melanoma, erythrophoroma) and tumors of neural origin (neurofibroma, neurofibrosarcoma, schwannoma, peripheral nerve sheath tumor); squamous cell carcinoma	Nodular growths	Histopathology
Husbandry-related			
Poor water quality	Various causes including overstocking, overfeeding, inadequate filtration or aeration, infrequent water changes	Skin changes including increased mucus production, erythema, erosions/ulceration, injected fins, flashing; behavioral changes, lethargy, anorexia, poor growth, secondary opportunistic infections, respiratory signs, gill hyperplasia, neurologic abnormalities and mortalities	Water quality evaluation (temperature, pH, ammonia, salinity, nitrite, nitrate, dissolved oxygen, and alkalinity)

(continued on next page)

Table 3
(continued)

Disease/Condition	Causes	Clinical Signs/Properties	Diagnosis
Gas supersaturation, gas bubble disease	Supersaturation of water caused by faulty equipment, sudden elevations in temperature, Venturi effect	Gas emboli formed in circulation and tissues; gas bubbles may be seen in eyes, on fins, gills, and under skin; behavioral abnormalities, positive buoyancy (small fish), death	Clinical signs, linear gas bubbles can be seen on fin clippings and gill biopsies
Idiopathic			
Head and lateral line erosion[d]	Multifactorial: proposed causes include hexamitid parasites; activated carbon/carbon dust; heavy metals, such as copper; stray electrical voltage; ozone; ultraviolet radiation products; poor nutrition; nutrient deficiencies of vitamins A and C and minerals; internal disease; and various other stressors	Freshwater cichlids (*Symphysodon* spp, *Astronotus ocellatus*, other South American cichlids) are commonly affected. Marine fish that are commonly affected include surgeonfishes and tangs (family Acanthuridae) and marine angelfish (family Pomacanthidae). Examination reveals often symmetric, depigmented erosions and ulcerations that coalesce to produce large crateriform lesions and pits on the head; may extend down the lateral line/flanks	Clinical signs, histopathology

[a] Roberts HR, Palmeiro BS, Weber SW. Bacterial and parasitic diseases of fish. Vet Clin North Am Exot Anim Pract 2009;12(3):609–38.

[b] Palmeiro BS. Bacterial diseases. In: Roberts HR, editor. Fundamentals of ornamental fish health. Ames (IA): Wiley-Blackwell; 2010. p. 125–36.

[c] Palmeiro BS, Weber SW. Viral pathogens of fish. In: Roberts HR, editor. Fundamentals of ornamental fish health. Ames (IA): Wiley-Blackwell; 2010. p. 112–24.

[d] Wildgoose W, Palmeiro BS. Specific syndromes and diseases. In: Roberts HR, editor. Fundamentals of ornamental fish health. Ames (IA): Wiley-Blackwell; 2010. p. 214–23.

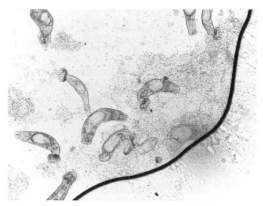

Fig. 6. *Gyrodactylus* sp (fluke) on a skin scraping from a goldfish (*Carassius auratus*).

dermatology cases can be complex and are often multifactorial; nutritional deficiencies, poor management, lack of exercise, and environmental stimulation and behavioral disorders frequently contribute to clinical disease.[32]

Skin Structure and Function

Avian skin is composed of an epidermis and dermis; the skin is thicker in nonfeathered areas. The layers of the epidermis include the stratum germinativum and the stratum corneum.[33] The stratum germinativum (bottom most layer) produces cells that mature to form the keratinized stratum corneum and can be divided into three distinct layers: (1) the stratum basale, (2) the stratum intermedium, and (3) the stratum transitivum. The cells show signs of keratinization in the stratum transitivum.[33] Feathers are formed from feather follicles in the dermis. The dermis is thicker than the epidermis and contains structurally supportive collagen, blood vessels, fat, nerves and neuroreceptors, feather follicles, and associated smooth muscle.[32,33] Avian skin is aglandular with the

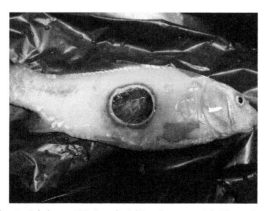

Fig. 7. Ulcerative bacterial dermatitis in a koi (*Cyprinus carpio*). Note deep ulcerative lesion with exposed muscle and peripheral annular rim of hemorrhage. This koi also has secondary septicemia and hemorrhages on the skin and fins.

exception of the uropygial (or preen) glands; the pericloacal glands (secrete mucus); and the sebaceous glands of the ear canal.[32,33] The uropygial gland is a holocrine gland found at the base of the tail that secretes a liposebaceous material important in protecting and waterproofing feathers; it is spread through the feathers in a process called preening that is also necessary for interlocking of feather barbules.[32,33]

Feathers are arranged into tracts known as pterylae that are separated by feather-less areas of skin called apteria.[32–34] **Table 4** illustrates the common feather types and their properties. The calamus is the part of the feather that attaches to the follicle.[32–34] The main shaft of the feather is called the rachis; where the rachis meets the calamus is a pulp cap referred to as the superior umbilicus.[32–34] There may be a smaller feather attached to the superior umbilicus that is referred to as the after feather.[32–34] Projections from the rachis are referred to as barbs, which bear projections called barbules.[32–34] Most barbules contain hooks called barbicels that hold the barbs and barbules together.[32–34] Molting occurs when the growth of a new feather in the follicle forces out the older feather; all feathers of adult birds are replaced regularly during molting. Most species of pet birds molt once to twice yearly.[32,33]

Dermatologic Examination and Diagnostic Testing

A thorough history and dermatologic examination are important when evaluating any case of avian skin disease. Dermatologic examination in birds should include evaluation of feathers, skin, beak and cere, ears, legs and claws, preen gland, and cloaca.

Table 4 Feather types	
Feather Type	**Feather Properties**
Natal down	Initial feather covering usually present at time of hatching
Juvenile feathers	Smaller and narrower than adult feathers, replace natal down feathers
Feather sheath	Cover feathers as they grow from feather follicle. Typically ruptures and releases barbs
Contour feathers	Predominant adult feather; main type present on wings and body
Remiges	Flight feathers of wings; divided into primary remiges (attach to metacarpus) and secondary remiges (attach to ulna) Typically there are 10 primary feathers and up to 14 secondary feathers per wing
Rectrices	Flight feathers on tail
Coverts	Feathers that cover the bases of remiges and rectrices
Down	Fine feathers that lack barbules on the barbs
Filoplume	Close to the follicle of each contour feather, fine hairlike feathers
Bristle	Few or no barbs and very stiff rachis; found at base of beak and around eyes
Powder down	Specialized down feathers that disintegrate to produce fine granules of keratin that waterproof feathers
Semiplume	Large rachis with fluffy vane; present under contour feathers, important in insulation
After feathers (hypopenae)	Smaller feather attached to the superior umbilicus

Data from Refs.[32–34]

Table 5
Differential diagnoses for cutaneous diseases in pet birds

Disease/Condition	Causes	Clinical Signs/Properties	Diagnosis
Parasitic			
Scaly leg/beak mite[a,b]	Cnemidocoptes spp	Hyperkeratosis and crusting (often honey combed) of the cere/beak, face, legs and feet; common in Budgerigars	Skin scraping
Red mite[a,b]	Dermanyssus gallinae	Some cases asymptomatic, papular eruption, anemia, overpreening	Can be difficult because mite lives off host
Ornithonyssus spp[a,b]	Ornithonyssus spp	Feathers matted with gray-black discoloration, skin thickened and scaly, anemia	Skin scraping
Feather mites[a,b]	Various species	Usually asymptomatic, large numbers may cause discoloration of the feathers and self-trauma	Direct microscopy of feather
Quill mites[a,b]	Various species of family Syringophilidae (quill mites), Laminosioptidae and Fainocoptinae (quill wall mites)	Usually asymptomatic, large numbers may cause brittle feathers, hyperkeratosis of quill sheath, pruritus	Direct microscopy of feather or feather preparation with KOH
Giardiasis[a,b]	Giardia spp	Feather plucking over the torso in cockatiels (Nymphicus hollandicus)	Fecal examination
Bacterial			
Bumblefoot bacterial/ulcerative pododermatitis[a,b]	Various bacterial isolates including Staphylococcus and Escherichia coli; hypovitaminosis A; poor perch design (all of same diameter)	Commonly seen in overweight cage birds including buderigars, canaries, and cockatiels; lesions including swelling, hyperkeratosis, and swelling on plantar surface of foot	History, clinical signs, impression smears, and culture/sensitivity
Mycobacterial granuloma[b]	Skin lesions most commonly caused by Mycobacterium tuberculosis, less commonly M avium	Most common in Amazons, blue and gold (Ara ararauna) and green wing (Ara chloropterus) macaws; localized lesions often around the head or face; zoonotic risk	Histopathology, microbiology, PCR

(continued on next page)

Table 5
(continued)

Disease/Condition	Causes	Clinical Signs/Properties	Diagnosis
Fungal			
Aspergillosis[a,b]	Aspergillus spp (fumigatus most common)	May occur secondary to skin trauma, greenish blue or dark gray ulcerated patches on skin	Clinical signs and fungal culture
Candidiasis[a,b]	Candida albicans	In canaries may cause intense head/neck pruritus, also associated with feather picking	Clinical signs, skin cytology and fungal culture
Malassezia[c]	Malassezia spp	No difference in Malassezia levels were found between feather picking and normal psittacines	Skin cytology
Viral			
Psittacine beak and feather disease[a,b]	Psittacine circovirus	Chronic form causes feather dystrophy/abnormalities (clubbing and blunting); feather loss; shiny beak; deformed beak and nails; and immunosuppression. Acute infections may occur in chicks, with systemic symptoms followed by profound changes in the developing feathers and death (similar to polyoma virus)	Clinical signs, PCR of blood sample of feather pulp
Polyoma virus[a,b]	Avian polyoma virus	In budgerigars, may cause French moult, which presents as abdominal distention, subcutaneous hemorrhages, lack of down/contour feathers and deformed feathers; other species often subclinical with rare feather abnormalities; subcutaneous and follicle hemorrhages may be seen	Cloacal swab for PCR
Papillomas[a,b]	Considered to be viral induced; herpesvirus or papillomavirus	Papilloma-like hyperplastic/hyperkeratotic lesions most common around palpebrae, commissure of beak or feet (finches), cloaca or choana of psittacines	Clinical signs, histopathology

Poxvirus[b]	Species-specific poxviruses	Dry form causes nodular lesions on nonfeathered areas around face, cere and feet; wet form affects similar areas plus mouth, pharynx, and viscera; canary pox highly infectious with 20%–100% mortality and three forms (cutaneous, diphtheritic, or septicemic)	Histopathology
Nutritional			
Hypovitaminosis A[a,b]	Most commonly seen in parrots on unsupplemented all seed diets deficient in vitamin A	Skin hyperkeratosis/scaling (worse on feet); white plaques in oral mucosa; rhinitis; blepharitis; sublingual salivary gland abscessation caused by squamous metaplasia	History of inappropriate diet and clinical signs
Neoplasia			
Skin neoplasia[a,b]	Uropygial adenocarcinoma, lipoma, fibrosarcoma, lymphosarcoma, squamous cell carcinoma, melanoma, hemangiosarcoma	Nodular lesions	Histopathology
Idiopathic/multifactorial/miscellaneous			
Feather picking[a,b,d] (see **Fig. 8**)	Many behavioral and nonbehavioral causes Nonbehavioral causes include ectoparasites; endoparasites (*Giardia*); heavy metal toxicity; hypothyroidism; infectious folliculitis (viral, fungal, bacterial); malnutrition; neoplasia; and other systemic diseases	Self-induced feather loss, often sparing the head	Rule out nonbehavioral causes of feather plucking before diagnosing as behavioral
Chronic ulcerative dermatitis[a,b]	Unknown; possibly associated with stressful environment	Small Psittaciformes, such as lovebirds, cockatiels, and parakeets ulcerative skin lesions over wing web or patagium and under wing	Ruling out other potential causes
Xanthomatosis[a,b]	Unknown; possibly caused by high-fat diet, trauma, or disorder of lipid metabolism	Nodular lesions caused by accumulation of lipid-containing macrophages Common in smaller Psittaciformes and present as discrete yellow-brown dermal swellings; most common on wing tips	Histopathology

(continued on next page)

Table 5
(continued)

Disease/Condition	Causes	Clinical Signs/Properties	Diagnosis
Allergic skin disease[a,b,d]	Cutaneous hypersensitivity; IgY seems to be involved in allergic reactions	Presence of true allergic dermatitis is controversial in birds; clinical signs include signs of pruritus (possibly seasonal) including feather plucking and skin mutilation	Rule out other causes of pruritic skin disease, intradermal allergy testing, skin biopsies
Feather follicle cysts[a,b]	Probable hereditary basis, may occur secondary to traumatic damage to feather follicle and nutritional deficiencies	Common in small caged birds, such as budgerigars and canaries; cyst/swelling develops because of inability of growing feather to break through skin, may have caseous exudate or become infected	Ruling out other causes; histopathology
Constricted toe syndrome[a,b]	Fibrous band of tissue constricts one or more digits, possibly caused by decreased humidity	Most common in African greys (*Psittacus erithacus*), macaws, eclectus (*Eclectus roratus*); swollen toes distal to area of fibrosis	Clinical signs
Articular gout[a,b]	Accumulation of urates in the synovial capsules and tendon sheaths of the joints, most commonly secondary to renal pathology	Most common in psittacines; white gritty swellings around the intertarsal or metatarsal joints	Cytologic demonstration of uric acid crystals, elevated serum uric acid
Hypothyroidism[a,b]		Rare disease of parrots, may be overdiagnosed, causes decreased molting, feather discoloration, hyperkeratosis, alopecia, obesity	Thyroid-stimulating hormone stimulation

[a] Girling S. Skin diseases and treatment of caged birds. In: Patterson S, editor. Skin diseases of exotic pets. Ames (IA): Blackwell; 2006. p. 22–47.
[b] Forbes NA. Birds. In: Foster A, Foil C, editors. BSAVA manual of small animal dermatology. Gloucester (England): BSAVA; 2003. p. 256–67.
[c] Preziosi DE, Morris DO, Johnston MS, et al. Distribution of *Malassezia* organisms on the skin of unaffected psittacine birds and psittacine birds with feather-destructive behavior. J Am Vet Med Assoc 2006;2:216–21.
[d] Nett CS, Tully T. Anatomy, clinical presentation and diagnostic approach to the feather picking pet bird. Comp Cont Educ Pract 2003;25(3):206–19.

Common findings during clinical examination of birds with skin disease include feather abnormalities (broken or absent feathers, dystrophic and discolored feathers); scaling; crusting; ulceration; redness; and nodules and masses.

Commonly used dermatologic diagnostic tests in pet birds include the following:

1. Feather pulp cytology[32,33]
   ○ Feather pulp cytology is collected from a freshly plucked feather and used to assess for the presence of folliculitis. The calamus can be removed from the feather and contents smeared onto a microscope slide. Possible findings include bacteria, inflammatory cells, viral inclusion bodies, and dermatophytes.
2. Gross and microscopic examination of feathers[32,33]
   ○ Evaluate for overall condition, ectoparasites, fret marks and stress bars, evidence of self-trauma
3. Feather preparation with potassium hydroxide[33]
   ○ To improve mite identification, the calamus of the feather can be placed into a 10% potassium hydroxide solution, gently heated, and then centrifuged, followed by microscopic examination of the sediment
4. Acetate tape impressions
   ○ Used to detect ectoparasites, yeast, and bacterial infections. Feather dander and keratinaceous debris is very abundant on these samples and in some cases can be difficult to differentiate from bacteria and yeast.
5. Impression smear
   ○ For moist, exudative, or crusted lesions, direct slide impressions are often used
   ○ For drier lesions, direct impressions can be attempted but acetate tape impressions may be preferred. Alternatively, a moistened swab can be used to collect a sample and contents rolled onto a slide.
6. Skin scrapings
7. Culture and sensitivity (bacterial, fungal)
   ○ Calamus and feather plucking, sterile tissue biopsy, or superficial swabs
8. Biopsy
   ○ Avian skin is much thinner than dogs and cats. In some cases, it is easier to biopsy the skin with a scalpel compared with a punch biopsy. If a punch biopsy is

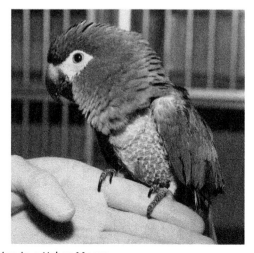

Fig. 8. Feather picking in a Hahns Macaw.

Table 6
Differential diagnoses for cutaneous diseases in rabbits

Disease/Condition	Causes	Clinical Signs/Properties	Diagnosis
Ectoparasites			
Ear mites[a–d]	Psoroptes cuniculi	Pruritic otitis, pinnal crusting, head shaking, canal erythema, thick ceruminous debris in canals, otitis externa and secondary otitis media; lesions rarely reported on face, neck, trunk extremities, and perineum; life cycle 3 wk and adults can live in environment for up to 3 wk	Otoscopic examination, microscopy of aural debris
Scabies[c]	Notoedres cati var cuniculi, Sarcoptes scabei var cuniculi	Crusting, pruritic dermatitis, most often affecting the head	Skin scrapings, trichogram, acetate tape impression
Cheyletiellosis[a–d] (see **Fig. 9**)	Cheyletiella spp (parasitivorax most common)	Scaling, walking dandruff, pruritus, alopecia, some cases asymptomatic, lacks host specificity and is zoonotic; life cycle 3 wk and can live off host for up to 10 d	Skin scrapings, trichogram, acetate tape impression
Fur-clasping mite[a–d]	Listrophorus (Leporacarus) gibbus	Often asymptomatic, scaling, alopecia; coinfestation with Cheyletiella common	Skin scrapings, trichogram, acetate tape impression
Demodicosis			
	Demodex cuniculi[b,c]	Most often aclinical, alopecia	Skin scrapings, trichograms
Fleas[a]	Numerous species including Spilopsyllus cuniculi (rabbit stick-tight flea), Ctenocephalides felis (cat flea), Cediopsylla simplex (Eastern rabbit flea), Odontopsyllus multispinous (giant Eastern rabbit flea), Echidnophaga gallinacea (stick-tight flea)	Often asymptomatic, may have pruritus or poor coat; S cuniculi: flea life cycle tied to reproductive cycle, transmits myxomatosis; C felis most commonly found on pet rabbits	Removal and microscopic identification
Lice[a]	Haemodipsus ventricosus	Anemia, pruritus	Trichograms, scrapings, microscopic identification
Ticks[a,c]	Numerous species including Haemaphysalis leporis-palustris		Removal and microscopic identification

Disease	Organism	Clinical signs	Diagnosis
Myiasis[a,c,d]	Various fly species including *Wohlfahrtia vigil*, *Lucilia*, and *Calliphora* spp	Fly strike common in outdoor environments in warm summer months, typically seen in rabbit with soiled perineum, inguinal/perineal skin most commonly affected	Removal and microscopic identification
Cuterebra[a-d]	*Cuterebra* spp larvae	Subcutaneous nodular swelling with small breathing hole; neurologic and respiratory signs rare; rabbits housed outdoors most commonly affected in summer months	Surgical removal, identification
Fungal			
Dermatophytosis[a-d]	*Trichophyton mentagrophytes* (most common), *Microsporsum gypseum, Microsporum canis*	Crusting, scaling alopecic lesions most common on the face and feet	Trichogram, fungal culture
Viral			
Myxomatosis[a-d]	Myxoma virus (poxvirus)	Swelling of eyelids, genitals, and pinna; fever; lethargy; anorexia; nodular swellings of the face and ears; death typically within 14 d; more mild form of the disease with widespread cutaneous nodules reported in vaccinated rabbits; Insect vectors, such as mosquitoes and rabbit flea; vaccines developed, availability depending on country	Histopathology, virus isolation
Shope papilloma virus[a-d]	Shope papilloma virus (papovavirus)	Multifocal hyperkeratotic papillomas typically around ears and eyelids; can become neoplastic (squamous cell carcinoma) and metastasize to axillary lymph node or resolve over several months; insect vector	Histopathology, virus isolation
Shope fibroma virus[a]	Shope fibroma virus (poxvirus)	Fibroma lesion; single or multiple flat subcutaneous nodules especially on genitals, perineum, ventral abdomen, legs, nose, pinna, eyelid; up to 7 cm in diameter, tumors typically regress over a period of months	Histopathology, virus isolation

(continued on next page)

Table 6
(continued)

Disease/Condition	Causes	Clinical Signs/Properties	Diagnosis
Bacterial			
Rabbit syphilis, venereal spirochaetosis[a–d]	*Treponema paraluiscuniculi*	Venereal transmission and by direct contact Lesions (redness, edema, vesicles, ulcers, hemorrhagic crusts) often limited to mucocutaneous junctions of nares, philtrum, vulva, perineum, eyes Can be subclinical	Dark field microscopic visualization of organism or silver stains on histopathology, serology
Subcutaneous abscesses[c,d]	Dental disease, bite wounds, other injuries; isolates include various anaerobic bacteria, *Pasturella multocida* (may be less common than previously reported), *Staphylococcus* spp, *Streptococcus* spp	Rabbit heterophils cannot liquefy pus so abscesses are caseous with thick capsule; facial abscesses most commonly caused by dental disease	Clinical signs, fine-needle aspirate/cytology, culture/ sensitivity, imaging for dental-associated abscesses
Moist dermatitis "blue fur disease"[a,c,d]	Severe chronic dental disease and excess salivation (slobbers). Overweight animals with large dewlap; constant wetting predisposes to colonization with *Pseudomonas* spp	Moist erythematous dermatitis of chin, neck, and dewlap, blue-green discoloration to fur (from pyocyanin pigment produced by *Pseudomonas*)	Clinical signs, impression cytology, culture/sensitivity
Neoplasia			
Neoplasia[e]	Reported types (in decreasing frequency) trichoblastoma, collagenous hamartoma, shope fibroma, lipoma, squamous cell carcinoma, myxosarcoma, peripheral nerve sheath tumor, malignant melanoma, fibrosarcoma, carcinoma, squamous papilloma, liposarcoma, leiomyosarcoma, trichoepithelioma, apocrine carcinoma, shope papilloma	Cutaneous growths	Histopathology
Husbandry-related/multifactorial/miscellaneous			
Urine scalding	Urinary tract disease (hypercalciuria, urinary calculi, urinary tract infection), wet bedding, obesity, inactivity, neuromuscular disease, and so forth	Moist erythematous dermatitis perineal region, plantar hind limbs	Clinical signs

		Necrosis of pinnal margins	Clinical signs; histopathology
Frostbite[a]	Cold environmental temperatures	Necrosis of pinnal margins	Clinical signs; histopathology
Ulcerative pododermatitis[a,d]	Loss of thick fur on plantar/palmar limbs leads to pressure induced necrosis of skin Overweight, inactive rabbits, wet/soiled bedding, grid wire floors, hereditary factors with Rex rabbits being commonly affected because of lack of protective guard hairs; secondary infection with Staphylococcus aureus common	Alopecia, erythematous, painful ulcerative dermatitis of the metatarsal (less commonly metacarpal) regions; can progress to osteomyelitis	Clinical signs, impression cytology, culture/sensitivity
Barbering[a-d]	Dominant animals in collection; occasionally self-barbering during estrus or with low-fiber diet	Broken hairs, alopecia	History, clinical signs, trichograms showing broken hairs
Sebaceous adenitis[f]	Unknown; immune-mediated attack on sebaceous glands	Nonpruritic scaling and alopecia, follicular casting	Histopathology
Telogen defluxion[a-d]	Systemic stress/illness or after parturition	Widespread hairloss 4–6 wk after systemic stress, nonpruritic, hair easily epilated, patchy alopecia	History, clinical signs, histopathology
Cutaneous asthenia	Heritable collagen defect	Hyperextensible skin, thin atrophic scars, wounds	Electron microscopy, histopathology may be supportive
Thymoma-associated exfoliative dermatitis[g]	Thymoma	Generalized scaling, alopecia	Histopathology, thoracic radiographs

[a] Meredith A. Dermatology of mammals. In: Patterson S, editor. Skin diseases of exotic pets. Ames (IA): Blackwell; 2006. p. 175–312.
[b] Scarff D. Rabbits and rodents. In: Foster A, Foil C, editors. BSAVA manual of small animal dermatology. Gloucester (England): BSAVA; 2003. p. 242–51.
[c] Jenkins JR. Skin disorders of the rabbit. Vet Clin North Am Exotic Anim Pract 2001;4:543–63.
[d] Johnston MS. Small, cute, fluffy and itchy: clinical approach to rabbit and rodent skin diseases. In: Proceedings North American Veterinary Dermatology Forum. Denver (CO): 2008. p. 74–8.
[e] von Bomhard W, Goldschmidt MH, Shofer FS, et al. Cutaneous neoplasms in pet rabbits: a retrospective study. Vet Pathol 2007; 44(5):579–88.
[f] White SD, Linder KE, Schultheiss P, et al. Sebaceous adenitis in four domestic rabbits (Oryctalagus cuniculus). Vet Dermatol 2000;11:53–60.
[g] Florizoone K. Thymoma-associated exfoliative dermatitis in a rabbit. Vet Dermatol 2005;16(4):281–4.

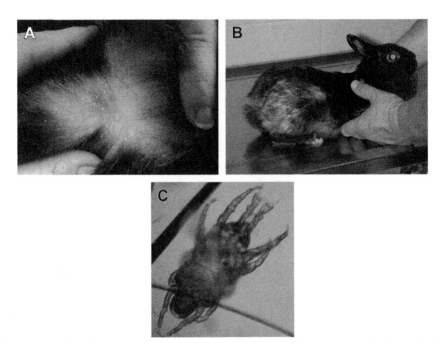

Fig. 9. (*A, B*) Note moderate scaling and self-induced alopecia. (*C*) *Cheyletiella parasitivorax.*

to be performed, a technique has been described where acetate tape is placed over the biopsy site to maintain the structure of the skin.[35]
9. Clinical pathology evaluation including complete blood count and biochemistry panel and heavy metal testing[32,33]
    ○ Systemic diseases can cause cutaneous changes including feather picking
    ○ Testing for lead and zinc levels may be needed in some cases
10. Crop washes[33]
    ○ Can identify *Trichomonas* or *Candida*, which can present in birds that feather pluck over the crop area
11. Fecal examination
    ○ Certain intestinal parasites may result in feather plucking[32,33]
12. Intradermal allergy testing
    ○ Codeine phosphate at 1:100,000 wt/vol preferred over histamine as a positive control in birds[36]
    ○ Further research is needed to evaluate appropriate protocols for intradermal allergy testing in pet birds and establish correct allergen dilutions and thresholds
13. Viral testing including PCR for polyoma virus and psittacine beak and feather disease[32,33]

Common Differential Diagnoses for Cutaneous Diseases

See **Table 5** for a review of common differential diagnoses for dermatologic diseases in pet birds, including feather picking (**Fig. 8**).

Table 7
Differential diagnoses for cutaneous diseases in guinea pigs

Disease/Condition	Causes	Clinical Signs/Properties	Diagnosis	Comments
Infectious				
Bacterial				
Cervical lymphadenitis	Bacterial infection of cervical lymph nodes, coarse feed causes oral trauma	Fluctuant to firm swelling in cervical lymph nodes	History of consumption of coarse feed causing oral trauma, typical clinical signs, culture	Node may rupture, *Streptococcus zooepidemicus* most commonly isolated, stress increases predisposition
Staphylococcal pyoderma	*Staphylococcus aureus*, *Staphylococcus epidermidis*, other; secondary to bites or wounds, self-trauma	Alopecia, erythema, crusts, abscessation, ulcers, folliculitis	Clinical signs, cytology, culture/sensitivity	
Otitis media/interna	Multiple bacterial etiologies	Head tilt, head shaking, circling, purulent discharge, ataxia	Clinical signs, diagnostic imaging of bulla, culture exudate	
Abscesses	Bite wounds, environmental trauma	Fluctuant to firm subcutaneous swelling, drainage	Clinical signs, culture	

(continued on next page)

Table 7
(continued)

Disease/Condition	Causes	Clinical Signs/Properties	Diagnosis	Comments
Ectoparasites				
Lice (see **Fig. 10**)	*Trixacarus caviae*	Pruritus, alopecia, crusts/scales, erythema, excoriations, secondary pyoderma, Pruritus can be intense, resembling seizures	Skin scraping, acetate tape impression, trichogram	Zoonotic but self limiting
	Glirocola porcelli, Gyropus ovalis	Often subclinical, rough coat, scale, alopecia, pruritus in heavy infestations	Skin scraping, acetate tape impression, trichogram, direct visualization	Biting lice; environmental cleaning essential part of treatment
	Chirodiscoides caviae	Subclinical, pruritus, self-induced alopecia	Skin scraping, acetate tape impression, trichogram	
	Demodex caviae	Alopecia, erythema, crusts, affected animals immunosuppressed	Skin scraping	
Fungal				
Dermatophytosis	*Trichophyton mentagrophytes*	Scaling alopecia on face, legs, ears; occasional pruritus; crusts; papules; pustules; secondary bacterial pyoderma	Trichogram, fungal culture, biopsy	
Noninfectious/husbandry-related/miscellaneous				
Hypovitaminosis C	Vitamin C deficiency	Poor wound healing, depression, rough hair coat, pinnal scaling, swollen joints, abnormal gait, petechiae of mucous membranes, lameness, secondary infections		Guinea pigs cannot synthesize vitamin C, condition can be seen in cavies fed rabbit pellets or other ascorbic acid–deficient diet

Condition	Cause	Clinical signs	Diagnosis	
Cystic ovarian disease (see **Fig. 11**)	Cause unknown; estrogenic substances in hay have been implicated	Bilateral, symmetric alopecia (back, flanks, ventrum), nonpruritic	Clinical signs in a female cavy, palpation, diagnostic imaging	
Pregnancy-associated alopecia		Sow with nonpruritic bilateral flank alopecia during late pregnancy	History, ruling out other causes	
Pododermatitis	Poor cage hygiene, wire cage flooring, obesity, sedentary cavy, hypovitaminosis C; Staphylococcus aureus most commonly isolated	Mild swelling of plantar surface of foot progressing to ulcerations and osteomyelitis	Clinical signs, culture lesions, history	Multimodal approach to treatment is required. Prognosis is poor after deep ulceration present
Cheilitis	Oral trauma; feeding acidic and abrasive food stuffs, hypovitaminosis C; Staphylococcus commonly isolated; possible pox virus etiology	Perioral ulceration erythema and crusting	History, clinical signs, impression cytology culture	
Scent gland impaction	Scent glands on rump become impacted	Malodorous dermatitis, matted hairs, secondary infection	History, clinical signs	
Barbering	Barbering in group of animals or self-barbering	Incomplete/traumatic alopecia, chewed whiskers	History, trichogram showing broken hair shafts	
Neoplasia	Trichofolliculoma most common cutaneous neoplasm, others include sebaceous adenoma, lipoma, fibromas, fibrosarcomas, schwannoma, vascular anomaly	Nodules, masses and lumps; trichofolliculomas often have central pore through which keratinaceous debris is discharged	Biopsy, fine-needle aspirate/cytology	

Data from Refs.[37,40,41]

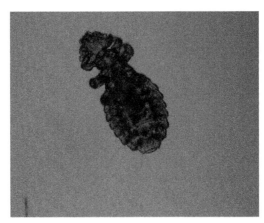

Fig. 10. *Gyropus ovalis* from a guinea pig.

SMALL MAMMALS

The skin is a common site of disease in small mammals and a very common presenting complaint to the exotic animal practitioner. Parasites, bacterial infections, and husbandry- and environmental-related conditions are most commonly seen.

Skin Structure and Function

The basic structure and function of exotic small mammal skin is very similar to that of the dog and cat. Relevant differences are discussed. The skin is divided into a four-layered avascular epidermis (stratum corneum, stratum granulosum, stratum spinosum, stratum basale) and the underlying, structurally supportive, collagenous, and vascular dermis. The subcutis is below the dermis and consists of connective tissue and fat. In rodents, brown fat is located between the scapulae, in the ventral neck, and in the axillary and inguinal regions; it is more prominent in smaller rodents, rabbits, and ferrets and less so in guinea pigs and chinchillas.[37]

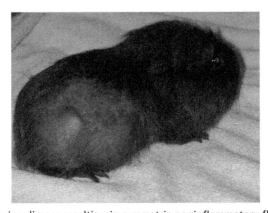

Fig. 11. Cystic ovarian disease resulting in symmetric noninflammatory flank alopecia.

Table 8
Differential diagnoses for cutaneous diseases in gerbils and hamsters

Disease/Condition	Causes	Clinical Signs/Properties	Diagnosis	Comments
Infectious causes				
Bacterial				
Bacterial pyoderma	Secondary to trauma, ectoparasites, or accumulated hardenian gland secretions in nasal dermatitis (gerbils) or dental disease (hamsters) *Staphylococcus* spp most commonly isolated	Erythema, crusting, alopecia	Impression smears, cytology, culture	
Viral				
Hamster polyomavirus (papovavirus)	HaPV	Associated with cutaneous epithelioma/ trichoepithelioma; verrucous mass near eyes, mouth, and perianal region in young hamsters; transmitted by urine	Histopathology	

(continued on next page)

Table 8
(continued)

Disease/Condition	Causes	Clinical Signs/Properties	Diagnosis	Comments
Parasitic		Pruritus, scales, crusts, secondary infections	Skin scraping, impression smear, biopsy	
	Demodex aurati (hamsters) (see **Fig. 12**)	Alopecia, scaling, erythema	Skin scraping	Cigar-shaped, inhabits hair follicles; evaluate for underlying immunosuppressive disease
	Demodex criceti (hamsters) (see **Fig. 12**)	Alopecia, scaling, erythema	Skin scraping	Short- and fat-bodied, superficial, inhabits keratin; evaluation for underlying immunosuppressive disease
	Notoedres notoedres (hamster), *N cati* (hamster)	Yellow crusts, pinnae, tail, paws, muzzle	Skin scraping	
	Demodex meroni (gerbils)	Alopecia, scaling, ulceration, secondary bacterial infection; most commonly affects face, thorax, abdomen, and limbs	Trichogram, skin scrapings	
	Acarus farris (fur mite, gerbils)	Alopecia, scaling, thickening of skin over tail, head, hind end	Trichogram, skin scrapings	
	Trixacarus caviae (hamster)	Pruritus, alopecia	Skin scraping	Transmissible to other animals including humans
Fungal				
Dermatophytosis	*Trichophyton mentagrophytes, Microsporum canis, M gypseum*	Pruritus, alopecia, crusts, scales, erythema, dry skin, secondary bacterial infections	Fungal culture, trichogram	Asymptomatic carriers possible, environmental cleaning essential, can be zoonotic and also spread to other susceptible species

Noninfectious

Condition	Etiology	Clinical signs	Diagnosis	Comments
Hyperadrenocorticism (hamster)	Primary-neoplasia of adrenal gland, secondary-pituitary tumor, iatrogenic	Symmetric alopecia, hyperpigmentation, thin skin, comedones, polyuria/polydipsia, polyphagia, pot-bellied, secondary demodicosis	Clinical signs, adrenal ultrasound. Dynamic function tests like ACTH stimulation test or dexamethasone suppression test, urine cortisol creatinine ratio not well described and difficult because of required blood and urine volumes	Can resemble demodicosis and cutaneous lymphoma. Hyperadrenocorticism with secondary demodicosis is common
Hair coat roughness (hamster, gerbils)	Aging, fighting, high humidity (gerbils, >50%), overall bad health, stress	Rough appearing, greasy coat	History, clinical signs, ruling out other causes	
Facial dermatitis, nasal dermatitis, "sore nose" (gerbils)	Gerbils stressed by overcrowding and high humidity, hypersecretion of gland results in accumulation of porphyrin pigment around nares; may lead to self-trauma and secondary staphylococcus infection	Alopecia, erythema and crusting around the nares, can progress to face, paws, and ventral abdomen, alopecia, secondary moist dermatitis	Clinical signs, impression smears, bacterial culture porphyrins fluoresce under ultraviolet light	
Bald nose	Rubbing on wire cage or feeders or burrowing	Traumatic alopecia on dorsum of nose and muzzle	Clinical signs, history, trichogram	
Barbering	Dominant individual chews hair off of other animals	Traumatic alopecia on dorsal head and tail base	Clinical signs, history, trichogram	
Tail slip (gerbils)	Improper handling of tail	Skin lost from tail exposing muscle and bone	History and clinical signs	

(continued on next page)

Table 8
(continued)

Disease/Condition	Causes	Clinical Signs/Properties	Diagnosis	Comments
Neoplasia				
Hamsters	Epitheliotrophic lymphoma	Alopecia, erythema, scaling, pruritus, secondary infections, ulceration, crusts, plaques, or nodules	Histopathology	Rule outs include demodicosis or hyperadrenocorticism; demodicosis can be secondary to epithelioptrophic lymphoma
	Melanoma, melanocytoma, epithelioma, trichoepithelioma, squamous cell carcinoma, fibrosaroma, basal cell carcinoma, papilloma		Fine-needle aspirate, histopathology	
Gerbils	Melanoma, melanocytoma, neoplasia of ventral scent gland (scent gland carcinoma), squamous cell carcinoma, basal cell carcinoma		Fine-needle aspirate, histopathology	

Data from Refs.[37,42,43]

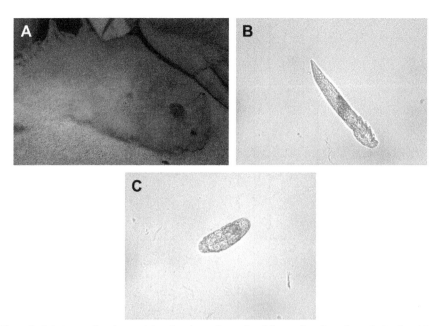

Fig. 12. (*A*) Demodicosis resulting in alopecia and mild crusting in a long-haired golden hamster (*Mesocricetus auratus*). (*B*) *Demodex aurati*: note long cigar shape. (*C*) *Demodex criceti*: note short stubby appearance.

Hairs can be divided into primary (guard) hairs; secondary (undercoat) hairs; and tactile hairs.[37] The number of hairs per follicle varies with the species, breed, age, and other external factors; chinchillas have as many as 60 hairs per follicle, producing the characteristic dense soft coat.[37] The keratinized hair consists of the innermost medulla, pigmented cortex, and outermost cuticle. Primary hairs are associated with sebaceous glands, apocrine sweat glands, and an arrector pili muscle. Rodents and ferrets have no epitrichial (apocrine) sweat glands.[37] Secondary hairs are typically only accompanied by sebaceous glands.[37] The rat and mouse tail is very sparsely haired. In interfollicular regions, there is surface parakeratosis and no stratum granulosum, whereas follicular ostia contain the typical orthokeratosis and stratum granulosum; these changes give the tail its characteristic scaly appearance.[37]

The footpads are areas of specialized thickened epidermis with underlying shock-absorbing fat deposits. Atrichial (eccrine) sweat glands are located only in the footpad. Rabbits lack foot pads, but instead have coarse fur on their distal limbs. Sebaceous scent glands are a common feature in many small mammal species and are important in scent marking and communication. Hamsters have large darkly pigmented glands on their flanks, more prominent in males.[37] Gerbils have large oval-shaped yellowish hairless scent glands on the ventrum.[37] Guinea pigs have a large gland over the rump that can secrete an oily substance, especially in boars.[37] Rabbits have sebaceous scent glands on the chin (mental gland) that is used for territorial marking, anal glands, and androgen-dependent inguinal scent glands.[37] Ferrets have active sebaceous glands throughout their skin that results in their typical musky odor and greasy coat; they also have two prominent perianal scent glands.[37]

Table 9
Differential diagnoses for cutaneous diseases in mice and rats

Disease/Condition	Causes	Clinical Signs/Properties	Diagnosis	Comments
Infectious causes				
Bacterial				
Pyoderma	*Staphylococcus aureus, Streptococcus,* other Can be secondary to ectoparasites, trauma, or salivary gland infection	Pruritus, hairloss, abscessation	Impression smears, culture	
Viral				
Sialodacryoadenitis (rats; rat coronavirus)	*Coronavirus*	Sneezing, oculonasal discharge, swelling near eyes, cervical edema, cervical lymphadenopathy, corneal ulceration/hyphema, secondary infections	Clinical signs, serology, histopathology	
Ectoparasites				
Fur mite (mice, rats)	*Radfordia* spp (fur mite, mice and rats)	Alopecia, pruritus, ulceration, scaling, secondary bacterial dermatitis; asymptomatic	Skin scraping, acetate tape impression, trichograms	

Fur mite (mice, rats) (see **Fig. 13**)	*Myobia musculi*	Alopecia, pruritus, ulceration, scaling, secondary bacterial dermatitis; asymptomatic	Skin scraping, acetate tape impression, trichograms	
	Psorergates muricola (mice)	Small white nodules, especially on the pinnae	Skin scraping, acetate tape impression, trichograms	Burrowing mite, found in stratum corneum
	Demodex musculi (mice), *Demodex ratticola* (rats)	Rare, follicular mite, localized alopecia, secondary infection		
Rat mange mite	*Notoedres muris* (rat)	Most common on pinnae and nose, hyperkeratotic, papules, yellow crusts	Skin scraping, acetate tape impression	
	Myocoptes musculinus	Alopecia, pruritus, ulceration, scaling, secondary bacterial dermatitis; asymptomatic	Skin scraping, acetate tape impression, trichograms	
Lice (see **Fig. 14**)	*Polyplax serrata* (mouse), *Polyplax spinulosa* (rats)	Pruritus, hairloss, restlessness, anemia		Possible vector of tularemia
Pinworms	*Syphacia* sp	Perianal pruritus	Acetate tape impression from perineal region	
Fungal				
Dermatophytosis	*Trichophyton mentagrophytes*, *Microsporum canis*, *M. gypseum*	Alopecia, crusts, scales, erythema, dry skin, secondary bacterial infections; asymptomatic carriers common	Fungal culture, trichogram	Environmental cleaning essential, can be zoonotic and also spread to other susceptible species

(continued on next page)

Table 9
(continued)

Disease/Condition	Causes	Clinical Signs/Properties	Diagnosis	Comments
Noninfectious				
Neoplasia	Mammary gland fibroadenoma (rats); adenocarcinoma; fibrosarcoma (mice); squamous cell carcinoma (mice, rats); fibroma; papillomas; basal cell carcinomas	Clinical signs and typical location, fine-needle aspirate/cytology, biopsy	Histopathology	Mammary masses in rats can get very large
Husbandry-related				
Barbering (mice)	Hair and whiskers of subordinates are chewed by dominant mouse	Incomplete/traumatic alopecia, chewed whiskers, dominant mouse has intact whiskers	History, clinical signs	Typical in group housing, especially males Reducing numbers may help
Ring tail (mice, rats)	Low environmental humidity	Annular constriction at base of tail, secondary edema and necrosis develop	History, clinical signs	Usually young mice/rats, not common in pet rats

Data from Refs.[37,42–44]

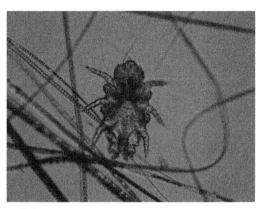

Fig. 13. *Myobia musculi* from a mouse.

Dermatologic Examination and Diagnostic Testing

As with other exotic species, a thorough questioning and evaluation of the husbandry is critical for successful diagnosis and treatment of small mammal dermatoses. Important questions include those pertaining to the environment and husbandry (type of housing, indoor or outdoor, substrate or bedding, diet, and so forth), and more targeted questions pertaining to skin disease. In small mammals, it is important to know whether the condition is pruritic and whether any other animals are affected.

A thorough dermatologic examination is necessary in all patients with skin disease. Common lesions include hairloss, erythema, scaling, crusting, excoriations, erosions, and ulcers. Restraint to obtain quality diagnostic samples from small mammal skin can be challenging in some cases, so anesthesia or sedation may be needed.

Commonly used dermatologic diagnostic tests in small mammals include the following:

1. Impression smear
   ○ For moist, exudative, or crusted lesions, direct slide impressions are often used

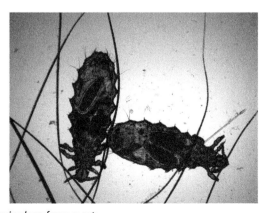

Fig. 14. *Polyplax spinulosa* from a rat.

Table 10
Differential diagnoses for cutaneous diseases in ferrets

Disease/Condition	Causes	Clinical Signs/Properties	Diagnosis	Comments
Infectious				
Viral	Canine distemper virus (paramyxovirus)	Brown crusted lesions on chin, nose, inguinal, and perianal region Hyperkeratosis and swelling of footpads; pyrexia, nasal, and ocular discharge, coughing, anorexia, neurologic signs and death	Clinical signs, fluorescent antibody of conjunctival smears, peripheral blood smear, serum antibody titers, histopathology	Vaccine available
Bacterial				
Bacterial pyoderma	Secondary to trauma, bite wounds, rough playing, ectoparasites; most commonly caused by *Staphylococcus* or *Streptococcus*	Superficial to deep pyoderma, abscesses, cellulitis	Cytology, culture	
Fungal				
Dermatophytosis	*Trichophyton mentagrophytes, Microsporum canis;* uncommon, may be secondary to underlying immunosuppression	Circular alopecia, erythema, scaling, secondary pyoderma	Trichogram, fungal culture	

Parasitic

Ectoparasites	Fleas (*Ctenocephalides felis*)	Pruritus, scaling, crusting, alopecia, excoriations	Observation, clinical signs, flea "dirt" or live fleas on flea combing
	Ear mites (*Otodectes cynotis*)	Otic pruritus, excess dark brown ceruminous debris, head shaking, ectopic sites include feet and tail tip	Otoscopic examination, microscopy of aural debris
	Sarcoptic mange mite (*Sarcoptes scabei*)	General form: focal to diffuse alopecia, pruritus, scaling; Localized form: only toes/feet affected inflammation, swelling, crusts, and pruritus of paws; nails may become deformed and slough	Skin scraping, mites may be difficult to find

Noninfectious

Endocrine

Hyperadrenocorticism (see **Fig. 15**)	Adrenocortical hyperplasia, adenoma or adenocarcinoma; neutering may play role in pathogenesis	Bilateral, symmetric alopecia, pruritus, vulvar enlargement, comedones, prostatic hyperplasia, stranguria, and urinary obstruction in males	Clinical signs, abdominal palpation, elevations of one or more levels of circulating sex hormones, ultrasonography, pancytopenia may be present
Hyperestrogenism	Unmated females not stimulated to ovulate may result in prolonged estrus	Swollen vulva, alopecia, bone marrow suppression, anemia	Clinical signs, history, CBC
Hypersensitivity	Atopic dermatitis, food allergy	Pruritus	Rule out more common causes of pruritus, intradermal allergy testing, food trial

(continued on next page)

Table 10
(continued)

Disease/Condition	Causes	Clinical Signs/Properties	Diagnosis	Comments
Neoplasia				
Mast cell tumors		Small, round, slightly raised, dermal mass, Occasional yellow crusty surface or pruritic	Fine-needle aspirate, histopathology	Usually benign Can occur anywhere but common head, neck, shoulders, or trunk
Apocrine scent tumors	Adenocarcinoma, adenoma	Located in areas of high concentration of scent glands; head, neck, prepuce, vulva, perineum	Fine-needle aspirate, histopathology	Can exhibit rapid growth and be locally aggressive and metastatic
Basal cell tumor		Discrete, solitary, often pedunculated or ulcerated	Fine-needle aspirate, histopathology	
Cutaneous lymphoma		Nodules, ulcerated masses, swelling, pruritus, alopecia, erythema, scaling; most commonly affects feet and extremities	Cytology, histopathology	
Sebaceous adenomas/ epitheliomas		Mass may be ulcerated, have necrotic centers	Fine-needle aspirate, histopathology	
Environmental				
Seasonal alopecia	Seasonal molting	Bilaterally symmetric alopecia of tail, inguinal region, and perineum during breeding season	Clinical signs, history, season, ruling out other etiologies	
Telogen defluxion	2–3 mo after stressful event	Thinning of coat	History, ruling out other causes	
Nutritional				
Biotin deficiency	Raw eggs in diet	Bilaterally, symmetric alopecia	Dietary history, clinical signs	Compound in egg whites, avidin, binds dietary biotin

Data from Refs. [37,45–50]

  ○ For drier lesions, direct impressions can be attempted but acetate tape impressions may be preferred. Alternatively, a moistened swab can be used to collect a sample and contents rolled onto a slide.
2. Skin scrapings
   a. Very useful for detection of ectoparasites
   b. Given the thin skin of many exotic patients, some practitioners prefer to use scraping spatulas to perform skin scrapings
3. Bacterial culture and sensitivity
4. Fungal culture
5. Wood lamp
   a. Limited usefulness in small mammals given that *Trichophyton mentagrophytes* is the most common dermatophyte isolate in clinical cases
6. Trichogram
   a. Useful to evaluate hair structure
   b. Evaluation for broken or fractured hair ends that would help determine whether hair loss is traumatic. Evaluate for ectoparasites.
   c. Evaluation for evidence of dermatophytosis (fungal hyphae/ectothrix spores)
7. Acetate tape impression
   a. Useful for collection of surface-dwelling mites, such as *Cheyletiella* and *Myobia*
8. Skin biopsies for histopathology
9. Clinical pathology testing including complete blood count and biochemistry panel
10. Testing for adrenal disease in ferrets

Common Differential Diagnoses for Cutaneous Diseases

See **Table 6** for a review of common differential diagnoses for dermatologic diseases in rabbits, including *Cheyletiella parasitivorax* (**Fig. 9**). See **Table 7** for a review of common differential diagnoses for dermatologic diseases in guinea pigs, including *Gyropus ovalis* and noninflammatory flank alopecia (**Figs. 10** and **11**). See **Table 8** for a review of common differential diagnoses for dermatologic diseases in gerbils and hamsters, including demodicosis, (*Demodex aurati* and *Demodex criceti*, [**Fig. 12**]). See **Table 9** for a review of common differential diagnoses for dermatologic diseases in mice and rats, including *Myobia musculi* and *Polyplax spinulosa* (**Figs. 13** and **14**). See **Table 10** for a review of common differential diagnoses for dermatologic diseases

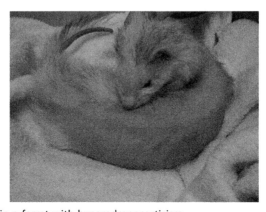

Fig. 15. Alopecia in a ferret with hyperadrenocorticism.

Table 11
Differential diagnoses for cutaneous diseases in chinchillas

Disease/Condition	Causes	Clinical Signs/Properties	Diagnosis
Bacterial			
Abscesses[a]	Bite wounds, dental disease; *Staphylococcus* and *Streptococcus* are common isolates	Soft fluctuant swelling	Fine-needle aspirate, culture/sensitivity, imaging
Moist dermatitis[a]	Staphylococcal infection caused by excessive salivation from dental disease	Moist erythematous dermatitis, ventral chin and neck	Clinical signs, culture/sensitivity
Fungal			
Dermatophytosis[a]	*Trichophyton mentagrophytes* most common, *Microsporum canis* and *Microsporum gypseum* less common	Alopecia; scaling; crusting and erythema around eyes, nose, mouth, legs, and feet	Trichogram, fungal culture
Husbandry-related			
Dietary deficiencies of fatty acids, zinc, and panthothenic acid[a]	Unbalanced diet	Patchy alopecia, scaly skin	History, clinical signs, and response to supplementation
Yellow ears, yellow fat[a]	Diet deficient in choline, methionine, or vitamin E; impaired metabolism of plant pigments leads to concentration of yellow-orange pigment in skin and fat	Yellowish discoloration of skin worse on the ventral abdomen and perineal, painful swellings on ventral abdomen	Clinical signs and history
Cotton fur syndrome[a]	High protein diet (crude protein >28%)	Wavy, weak hair that appears like cotton	Dietary analysis for protein levels and clinical signs
Fur chewing[a]	Barbering, may be related to overcrowding or other stressor	Traumatic alopecia	Trichogram
Matted fur[a]	Lack of dust baths, high relative humidity	Matted fur	Clinical signs and history
Miscellaneous			
Fur-slip[a]	Rough handling, frightened, trauma, fighting causes rapid shedding of patch of fur; natural defense mechanism	Well-circumscribed alopecia	History, clinical signs, and ruling out other differentials, especially dermatophytosis

[a] Meredith A. Dermatology of mammals. In: Patterson S, editor. Skin diseases of exotic pets. Ames (IA): Blackwell; 2006. p. 175–312.

in ferrets, including alopecia (**Fig. 15**). See **Table 11** for a review of common differential diagnoses for dermatologic diseases in chinchillas.

SUMMARY

Skin disease is an extremely common presenting complaint to the exotic animal practitioner. These cases may be challenging because dermatologic diseases are often multifactorial and many have underlying husbandry or environmental deficiencies that must be identified. A thorough diagnostic evaluation is critical for successful management of exotic animal cutaneous disease.

REFERENCES

1. White SD, Bourdeau P, Bruet V, et al. Reptiles with dermatological lesions: a retrospective study of 301 cases at two university veterinary teaching hospitals (1992-2008). Vet Dermatol 2011;22(2):150–61.
2. Hoppmann E, Barron HW. Dermatology in reptiles. J Exot Pet Med 2007;16(4): 210–24.
3. Goodman G. Dermatology of reptiles. In: Patterson S, editor. Skin diseases of exotic pets. Blackwell: Ames (IA); 2006. p. 73–118.
4. Johnston MS. Scales and sheds: the ins and outs of reptile skin disease. In: Proceedings North American Veterinary Dermatology Forum. Denver (CO): 2008. p. 62–6.
5. Mitchell M, Colombini S. Reptiles. In: Foster A, Foil C, editors. BSAVA manual of small animal dermatology. Gloucester (England): BSAVA; 2003. p. 269–75.
6. Gentz EJ. Medicine and surgery of amphibians. ILAR J 2007;48(3):255–9.
7. Wright KM. Pathology of amphibia. In: Wright KM, Whitaker BR, editors. Amphibian medicine and captive husbandry. Malabar (FL): Krieger; 2001. p. 401–85.
8. Pessier AP. Cytologic diagnosis of disease in amphibians. Vet Clin North Am Exot Anim Pract 2007;10:187–206.
9. Campbell CR, Voyles J, Cook DL, et al. Frog skin epithelium: electrolyte transport and chytridiomycosis. Int J Biochem Cell Biol 2012;44:431–4.
10. Clayton LA, Gore SR. Amphibian emergency medicine. Vet Clin North Am Exot Anim Pract 2007;10:587–620.
11. Wright KM. Anatomy for the clinician. In: Wright KM, Whitaker BR, editors. Amphibian medicine and captive husbandry. Malabar (FL): Krieger; 2001. p. 15–30.
12. Wright KM. Applied physiology. In: Wright KM, Whitaker BR, editors. Amphibian medicine and captive husbandry. Malabar (FL): Krieger; 2001. p. 31–4.
13. Wright KM. Clinical techniques. In: Wright KM, Whitaker BR, editors. Amphibian medicine and captive husbandry. Malabar (FL): Krieger; 2001. p. 89–110.
14. Conlon JM, Mechkarska M, King JD. Host-defense peptides in skin secretions of African clawed frogs (Xenopodinae, Pipidae). Gen Comp Endocrinol 2012;176: 513–8.
15. McKenzie VJ, Bowers RM, Fierer N, et al. Co-habiting amphibian species harbor unique skin bacterial communities in wild populations. ISME J 2012;6:588–96.
16. Prates I, Antoniazzi MM, Sciani JM, et al. Skin glands, poison and mimicry in dendrobatid and leptodactylid amphibians. J Morphol 2012;273:279–90.
17. Raspotnig G, Norton RA, Heethoff M. Oribatid mites and skin alkaloids in poison frogs. Biol Lett 2011;7(4):555–6.

18. Bennett TD. Frogs and toads. In: Meredith A, Johnson-Delaney C, editors. BSAVA manual of exotic pets. Gloucester (United Kingdom): British Small Animal Veterinary Association; 2010. p. 316–30.

19. de la Navarre BJ. Common procedures in reptiles and amphibians. Vet Clin North Am Exot Anim Pract 2006;9:237–67.

20. Wright KM. Restraint techniques and euthanasia. In: Wright KM, Whitaker BR, editors. Amphibian medicine and captive husbandry. Malabar (FL): Krieger; 2001. p. 111–22.

21. Pessier AP. An overview of amphibian skin disease. Semin Avian Exot Pet 2002; 11(3):162–74.

22. Klaphake E. Bacterial and parasitic diseases of amphibians. Vet Clin North Am Exot Anim Pract 2009;12:597–608.

23. McCampbell S. Clinical microbiology of amphibians for the exotic practice. In: Wright KM, Whitaker BR, editors. Amphibian medicine and captive husbandry. Malabar (FL): Krieger; 2001. p. 123–8.

24. Taylor S. Mycoses. In: Wright KM, Whitaker BR, editors. Amphibian medicine and captive husbandry. Malabar (FL): Krieger; 2001. p. 188–92.

25. Wright KM. Bacterial diseases. In: Wright KM, Whitaker BR, editors. Amphibian medicine and captive husbandry. Malabar (FL): Krieger; 2001. p. 160–79.

26. Johnson AJ, Wellehan JF. Amphibian virology. Vet Clin North Am Exot Anim Pract 2005;8:53–65.

27. Pessier AP, Mendelson JR III. Quarantine. In: Proceedings from Workshop on Infectious Diseases in Amphibian Survival Assurance Colonies and Reintroduction Programs. San Diego (CA): 2009. p. 69–101.

28. Pessier AP, Mendelson JR III. Diagnostic testing. In: Proceedings from Workshop on Infectious Diseases in Amphibian Survival Assurance Colonies and Reintroduction Programs. San Diego (CA): 2009. p. 102–58.

29. Searle CM, Gervasi SS, Hua J, et al. Differential host susceptibility to *Batrachochytrium dendrobatidis*, an emerging amphibian pathogen. Conserv Biol 2011; 25(5):965–74.

30. Palmeiro BS. Skin to fins: diving into pet fish dermatology. In: Proceedings North American Veterinary Dermatology Forum. Denver (CO): 2008. p. 55–9.

31. Wildgoose WH. Skin diseases. In: Wildgoose WH, editor. BSAVA manual of ornamental fish. 2nd edition. Gloucester (England): BSAVA; 2001. p. 269–75.

32. Forbes NA. Birds. In: Foster A, Foil C, editors. BSAVA manual of small animal dermatology. Gloucester (England): BSAVA; 2003. p. 256–67.

33. Fraser M. Dermatology of birds. In: Patterson S, editor. Skin diseases of exotic pets. Ames (IA): Blackwell; 2006. p. 3–14.

34. Nett CS, Tully T. Anatomy, clinical presentation and diagnostic approach to the feather picking pet bird. Comp Cont Educ Pract 2003;25(3):206–19.

35. Nett CS, Hodgin EC, Foil CS, et al. A modified biopsy technique to improve histopathological evaluation of avian skin. Vet Dermatol 2003;14:147–51.

36. Columbini S, Foil C, Hosgood G, et al. Intradermal skin testing in Hispaniolan parrots (Amazonia ventralis). Vet Dermatol 2000;11:271–6.

37. Meredith A. Dermatology of mammals. In: Patterson S, editor. Skin diseases of exotic pets. Ames (IA): Blackwell; 2006. p. 175–312.

38. Williams D. Reptiles. In: Foster A, Foil C, editors. BSAVA manual of small animal dermatology. Gloucester (England): BSAVA; 2003. p. 281–7.

39. Wright KM. Trauma. In: Wright KM, Whitaker BR, editors. Amphibian medicine and captive husbandry. Malabar (FL): Krieger; 2001. p. 233–8.

40. Johnson-Delaney C. Guinea pigs, chinchillas, degus and duprasi. In: Meredith A, Johnson-Delaney C, editors. BSAVA manual of exotic pets. Gloucester (United Kingdom): British Small Animal Veterinary Association; 2010. p. 28–62.
41. O'Rourke DP. Disease problems of guinea pigs. In: Quesenberry KE, Carpenter JW, editors. Ferrets, rabbits, and rodents: clinical medicine and surgery. 2nd edition. St Louis (MO): Saunders; 2003. p. 245–54.
42. Donnelly TM. Disease problems of small rodents. In: Quesenberry KE, Carpenter JW, editors. Ferrets, rabbits, and rodents: clinical medicine and surgery. 2nd edition. St Louis (MO): Saunders; 2003. p. 299–315.
43. Sayers I, Smith SA. Mice, rats, hamsters, and gerbils. In: Meredith A, Johnson-Delaney C, editors. BSAVA manual of exotic pets. Gloucester (United Kingdom): British Small Animal Veterinary Association; 2010. p. 1–27.
44. Garner M. Cytologic diagnosis of diseases of rabbits, guinea pigs, and rodents. Vet Clin North Am Exot Anim Pract 2007;10:25–49.
45. Antinoff N, Hahn K. Ferret oncology: disease, diagnostics, and therapeutics. Vet Clin North Am Exot Anim Pract 2004;7:579–625.
46. Orcutt C. Dermatologic diseases. In: Quesenberry KE, Carpenter JW, editors. Ferrets, rabbits, and rodents: clinical medicine and surgery. 2nd edition. St Louis (MO): Saunders; 2003. p. 107–14.
47. Pollock C. Emergency medicine of the ferret. Vet Clin North Am Exot Anim Pract 2004;10:463–500.
48. Quesenberry KE, Rosenthal KE. Endocrine diseases. In: Quesenberry KE, Carpenter JW, editors. Ferrets, rabbits, and rodents: clinical medicine and surgery. 2nd edition. St Louis (MO): Saunders; 2003. p. 79–90.
49. Schoemaker NJ. Ferrets, skunks, and otters. In: Meredith A, Johnson-Delaney C, editors. BSAVA manual of exotic pets. Gloucester (United Kingdom): British Small Animal Veterinary Association; 2010. p. 127–38.
50. Williams BH. Neoplasia. In: Quesenberry KE, Carpenter JW, editors. Ferrets, rabbits, and rodents: clinical medicine and surgery. 2nd edition. St Louis (MO): Saunders; 2003. p. 91–106.

Cutaneous Neoplasia in Ferrets, Rabbits, and Guinea Pigs

Sari Kanfer, DVM[a],*,

Drury R. Reavill, DVM, Diplomate, ABVP-Avian Practice, Diplomate, ACVP[b]

KEYWORDS

- Cutaneous neoplasia • Skin tumors • Ferrets • Rabbits • Guinea pigs

KEY POINTS

- Ferrets, rabbits, and guinea pigs develop several different types of cutaneous neoplasms, similar to other domesticated mammals.
- The most common skin tumors in ferrets, in order of frequency, are mast cell tumors, sebaceous epitheliomas, cutaneous hemangiomas, preputial gland tumors, and lymphoma.
- The most common skin tumors in rabbits, in order of frequency, are basal cell tumors, spindle cell sarcomas, collagenous hamartomas, squamous papillomas, and mammary gland adenocarcinomas.
- The most common skin tumors in guinea pigs, in order of frequency, are trichofolliculomas, lipomas, trichoepitheliomas, and mammary gland adenocarcinomas.
- The most frequently diagnosed skin tumors in the three species were benign.
- Rabbits had the highest percentage of malignant skin tumors.
- Knowledge of the frequency of cutaneous tumor types, and the behavior and treatment of these tumors, assists veterinarians when discussing prognosis and treatment options with owners.

INTRODUCTION

Small mammals remain popular as companion pets, being found in about 10% of US households. Many households on average may have one to two ferrets, rabbits, or guinea pigs.[1] Owners bond closely with their pets, and exotic pet medicine has advanced to the stage where clinicians can offer advanced veterinary care, including oncology, to owners that are interested in a high level of care for their beloved pet. Neoplasia involving the skin is grossly visible to owners, therefore they may be

Disclosures: The authors have nothing to disclose.
[a] Exotic Animal Care Center, 2121 East Foothill Boulevard, Pasadena, CA 91107, USA;
[b] Zoo/Exotic Pathology Service, 2825 KOVR Drive, West Sacramento, CA 95605, USA
* Corresponding author.
E-mail address: bunnyvet@yahoo.com

more likely to notice the disease and pursue treatment, such as surgical removal. This may be curative in many cases, but in others, additional treatment can be recommended based on tumor type. Histopathology also allows clinicians to give owners a prognosis. Familiarity with the incidence and pathogenicity of cutaneous neoplasias in these pets allows clinicians to help owners make more educated decisions regarding treatment. Surgical excision with good margins is generally curative for cutaneous neoplasms, but complete margins can be challenging in a small animal weighing only 1 kg. A 2-cm margin may be difficult to obtain, therefore tumor regrowth may occur. When excision is incomplete, or tumors recur, radiation therapy is a valuable treatment modality that exotic pets tolerate well. Radiation may be palliative, consisting of a few fractions, or definitive. For definitive radiation, daily anesthesia may be too stressful for exotic pets; a reduced schedule of three fractions a week for 4 weeks may be considered (Jarred Lyons, DVM, Dipl-ACVR [Radiation Oncology], Los Angeles, CA, personal communication, 2012).

Data on cutaneous neoplasia in ferrets, rabbits, and guinea pigs were collected from the database at Zoo/Exotic Pathology Service (ZEPS). Between 1998 and 2012, 763 ferret cases, 672 rabbit cases, and 133 guinea pig cases of cutaneous neoplasia were examined. Data were evaluated for gender and age predilection, and frequency of occurrence of the different tumor types. Tumors that may invade the skin, such as mammary gland neoplasias, were included in this study. This article lists all of the skin tumors in table format and discusses the most common tumors in more depth. The frequency, gross appearance and behavior of the tumors, cellular morphology, gender and age predilections, level of malignancy, and treatment recommendations are also discussed.

FERRETS

The frequency of the common cutaneous neoplasms reported in ferrets is described in **Table 1**. Out of 763 reported cases, a third were mast cell tumors, and another third were sebaceous epitheliomas, both benign tumors with an excellent prognosis. Sebaceous epitheliomas are also referred to as basal cell tumors with sebaceous and squamous differentiation. Another study, from 1987 to 1992, reported 58% basal cell tumors with sebaceous and squamous differentiation and 16% mast cell tumors, with 11% fibromas, 4% cutaneous hemangiomas, and a small number of other neoplasias.[2] Many ferrets may have multiple cutaneous tumors of differing types at the same time, and other concurrent noncutaneous neoplasia. Vaccine-induced fibrosarcomas were uncommon; only one case was seen in this study.

Mast Cell Tumors

Cutaneous mast cell tumors appear as small, flat or slightly raised, alopecic plaques that are variably pruritic and erythematous. They commonly look like a small darkly pigmented area of skin, or a small raised nodule that periodically bleeds then forms a scab (**Fig. 1**). They can be located anywhere on the head, torso, or limbs. On exfoliative cytology the commonly used metachromatic stains, such as toluidine blue or Giemsa, reveal few cytoplasmic granules. Histologically, mast cell tumors are composed of well-differentiated mast cells with a small number of scattered eosinophils within the dermis. The mast cells have a small number of faintly staining metachromatic cytoplasmic granules. A total of 66% of the ferrets that had mast cell tumors in this study were male, and the average age was 4.5 years. Mast cell tumors are benign; they do not spread locally or metastasize in ferrets.[2,3] Surgical excision is curative, but often is

Table 1
Cutaneous neoplasia in the ferret, 1998–2012

	Frequency (%)	No. Male	No. Female	Age Range (y)	Average Age (y)	Locations
Mast cell tumor	33	165	83	1–8	4.4	Face, ear, tail, limb, flank
Sebaceous epithelioma (basal cell tumor with sebaceous and squamous differentiation)	30	112	105	1–10	5.2	Face, ear, tail, limb, flank
Cutaneous hemangioma	8.5	34	27	2–8	4.7	Face, neck, ear, limb/feet
Preputial gland tumors, malignant	4	33	—	2–8	5.1	Prepuce
Lymphoma	2.5	7	12	3–8	5.8	Lymph nodes, inguinal, anal, periocular
Leiomyosarcoma	1.7	8	4	1–6	3.1	Not reported
Squamous cell carcinoma	1.7	6	6	3–7	4.5	Foot, lip, gingival
Spindle cell sarcoma	1.6	6	6	2–7	5.1	Foot, neck
Apocrine gland cystadenoma	1.4	4	5	2–5	3.5	Tail
Mammary gland adenoma	1.3	5	4	M 6–7 F 2.5–6	6.1 4.5	Mammary gland
Fibroma	1.1	7	2	3–6	4.5	Tail
Fibrosarcoma	1.1	6	3	M 2–6 F 6–9	4.3 7.5	Site not reported One vaccine induced
Leiomyoma	1.1	7	2	2–5	3.9	Head
Epitheliotrophic lymphoma	1	6	2	M 4–7 F 5–9	4.6 7	—
Squamous cell carcinoma in situ	1	3	4	3–8	5.7	Lip

Courtesy of Drury Reavill, DVM, West Sacramento, CA.

performed for comfort or cosmetic purposes because these tumors remain small and cause very few clinical signs.

Sebaceous Epitheliomas/Basal Cell Tumors with Sebaceous and Squamous Differentiation

These benign cutaneous tumors frequently appear as discrete, firm, nodular, wart-like or plaquelike masses, up to 1 cm in diameter (**Fig. 2**). They are frequently ulcerated and some may present pedunculated.[2] They can be found anywhere on the head, torso, or limbs, but have a predilection for the head and neck (**Fig. 3**). Sebaceous epitheliomas arise from pluripotential basaloid epithelial cells of sebaceous glands. In this study, the tumors were seen in nearly equal numbers

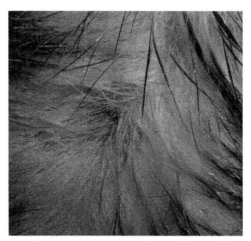

Fig. 1. Cutaneous mast cell tumor in a ferret. (*Courtesy of* Peter G. Fisher, DVM, Virginia Beach, VA.)

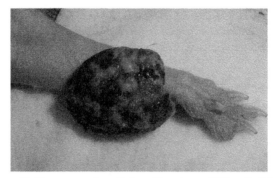

Fig. 2. Sebaceous epithelioma on a ferret's leg. (*Courtesy of* Peter G. Fisher, DVM, Virginia Beach, VA.)

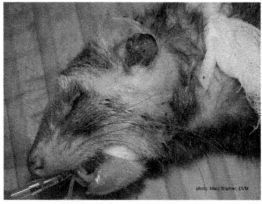

Fig. 3. Sebaceous epithelioma arising from a ferret's ear. (*Courtesy of* Marc Kramer, DVM, Miami, FL.)

of males and female ferrets, but in another study, 70% of the cases were female.[2] Found in ferrets of any age, these benign and slow-growing sebaceous epitheliomas do not metastasize but may be locally aggressive. Surgical excision is curative.

Cutaneous Hemangiomas

These appear as a small black mass, or a round red area of skin.[2] They may be found anywhere on the skin, but there is a slight predilection for the head, face, and feet. These masses are composed of blood-filled cavernous spaces lined by well-differentiated endothelial cells that readily hemorrhage when traumatized. They are seen in equal numbers of male and female ferrets, with an average age of 4.7 years. Because of benign behavior and lack of local growth, excision is curative. Ferrets rarely develop hemangiosarcomas (**Fig. 4**), but they appear similar to hemangiomas and, as typical for malignancies, are locally aggressive and may recur after apparently complete surgical removal.

Preputial Gland Tumors

The malignant tumors arising from the apocrine glands of the prepuce include carcinomas, adenocarcinomas, and cystadenocarcinomas. Small numbers of benign preputial adenomas were seen in other studies.[4,5] Malignant preputial tumors often start as a very small skin or subcutaneous nodule near the preputial orifice (**Fig. 5**A). Local growth is aggressive and fast, and there is a moderate potential for metastasis, especially to local tissues and lymph nodes (see **Fig. 5**B, C). Histologically, these tumors have an apocrine appearance of the cells with prominent apical protrusions. No age predilection was seen. These tumors are malignant, so early, wide, and deep surgical excision is necessary for complete remission. In many cases, a penile amputation and urethrostomy must be performed to obtain clean margins and prevent recurrence.[6,7] One case of preputial adenocarcinoma that recurred postsurgery was reportedly treated with radiation therapy.[8] The tumor regressed completely but returned in 4 months; a second course of radiation obtained an additional 2-month remission.

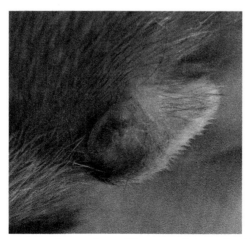

Fig. 4. Hemangiosarcoma on ferret pinna. (*Courtesy of* Peter G. Fisher, DVM, Virginia Beach, VA.)

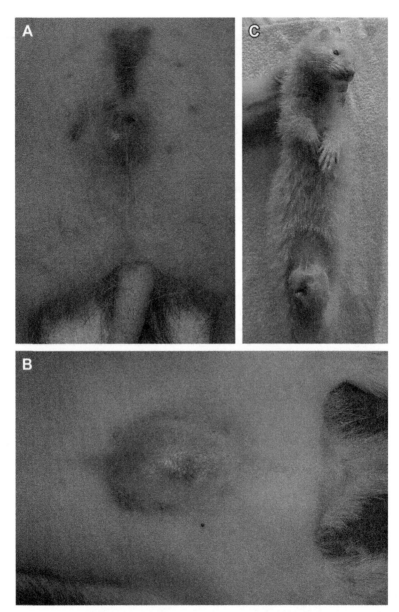

Fig. 5. (*A–C*) Preputial adenocarcinomas are locally aggressive tumors. (*Courtesy of* Peter G. Fisher, DVM, Virginia Beach, VA.)

Cutaneous Lymphoma (Nonepitheliotrophic)

Cutaneous lymphoma in ferrets indicates systemic disease. Lymphoma is a common malignant neoplasia in ferrets, and may be found in the lymph nodes, mediastinum, liver, spleen, or intestinal tract. In the present study, cutaneous lymphoma was found in a higher number of female ferrets, with an average age of 5.8 years for both genders. Palliative treatment with steroids may slow the course of disease. Injectable chemotherapy often helps, and several different protocols are listed in the literature.[9,10]

Epitheliotropic Lymphoma

Found in 1% of the submissions, epitheliotropic malignant lymphoma appears as diffuse generalized alopecia, erythema, erosions, crusts, and ulcerated plaques. All cases involved the feet. It is a neoplasm of T lymphocytes with a strong predilection for the epithelium, although this was not confirmed by immunohisto-chemistry in any of the cases diagnosed in the present study. In our study, 75% of the affected ferrets were male, with an average age of 4.6 years. Females tended to be affected later in life, with an average age of 7 years. Long-term prognosis is guarded, and ferrets may only live a few months after diagnosis. Treatment is frustrating because this neoplasia is relatively nonresponsive to corticosteroids. Supportive care, such as antibiotics and medicated shampoos, may keep pets comfortable. Treatment with isotretinoin has been beneficial in some cases.[11]

Leiomyosarcomas

These tumors may appear as raised pink skin nodules. They may be discrete or locally invasive, and are occasionally ulcerated. They can be found anywhere on the body but have a predilection for the head, neck, and limbs. Leiomyosarcomas arise from arrector pili smooth muscle of the follicle. They are twice as common in males as female ferrets, and can occur at any age. Leiomyosarcomas are considered malignant and can have a high mitotic index, but after surgical excision local recurrence and metastasis did not occur in two studies.[12,13] A case report from 2011 discussed a 2.5-year-old female spayed ferret with piloleiomyosarcoma that started on the tail and despite amputation, recurred on the torso several times over the next 3 years.[14] Because of the potential for recurrence, complete surgical excision is warranted, followed by monitoring for regrowth.

Mammary Tumors

Mammary gland tumors often present as a small nodule in the mammary tissue. They may get large and become ulcerated. Malignant adenocarcinomas and benign adenomas and fibroadenomas have all been described. In male ferrets, 70% of their mammary tumors were benign adenomas with 30% malignant adenocarcinomas. In female ferrets only benign tumors were reported in this study. Adenomas were most commonly seen in older males, 6 to 7 years, and younger females, 2 to 6 years of age. Adenomas are benign and surgical excision is curative. Adenocarcinomas have the potential for recurrence, especially if surgical margins are insufficient.

Numerous other cutaneous tumors were reported at less than 1% and were not listed in **Table 1**, including lipoma (0.9%); undifferentiated carcinoma (0.7%); hemangiosarcoma (0.6%); apocrine gland carcinoma (0.5%); basosquamous carcinoma (0.4%); round cell sarcoma (0.4%); undifferentiated sarcoma (0.4%); sebaceous gland adenoma (0.4%); squamous papilloma (0.4%); histiocytic malignant lymphoma (0.2%); histiocytic sarcoma (0.2%); mammary gland adenocarcinoma (0.2%); neurofibrosarcoma (0.2%); and perivulvar carcinoma (0.2%).

One of each of the following cutaneous tumors were seen: amelanotic malignant melanoma, anal gland adenocarcinoma, basal cell carcinoma, ceruminous gland adenocarcinoma and adenoma, collagen nevus, cystic adenocarcinoma, fibrolipoma, mammary fibroadenoma, meibomian gland carcinoma, melanocytoma, neurofibroma, extraskeletal osteoma, extraskeletal osteosarcoma, pilomatricoma, preputial adenoma, and sebaceous carcinoma.

RABBITS

The most common cutaneous neoplasms found in rabbits are listed in **Table 2**. Out of 672 cases, basal cell tumors (trichoblastomas) were the most frequently diagnosed at 20%, with spindle cell sarcomas at 9.5%, collagen nevi/hamartomas at 8.4%, squamous papillomas at 6.4%, and mammary carcinomas at 6%. Recently, most basal cell tumors have been reclassified as trichoblastomas based on the World Health Organization classification system.[15,16] A retrospective study of 184 cases of cutaneous neoplasia from the University of Pennsylvania during 1990 to 2006 reported some differences to our data.[17] They reported trichoblastomas as the most common tumors at 31.5%, followed by collagenous hamartomas (14.7%), Shope fibromas (10%), then lipomas (5.4%). Of the mesenchymal tumors they reported myxosarcomas (5%) and neurofibrosarcomas (4.3%) and did not list spindle cell sarcomas as a separate category. In our data spindle cell sarcomas (unclassified mesenchymal tumors) were at 9.5%; neurofibrosarcomas at 1.2%; and myxosarcomas at 1.2%.

Basal Cell Tumors/Trichoblastomas

These tumors are often pigmented, solitary, well-circumscribed intradermal masses. They may become very large and ulcerated. They can be found anywhere on the body but are more likely found on the head and neck and the forelegs. Trichoblastomas are derived from the primitive hair germ of embryonic follicular development. The tumors evaluated by ZEPS seemed to conform to the biologic behavior and histopathologic patterns of trichoblastomas as described in other species (**Fig. 6**). There was no sex predilection, and tumors were seen from 2 to 11 years of age, with an average of 6 years. These tumors are benign, and prognosis is excellent with complete surgical excision.

Spindle Cell Sarcomas

These mesenchymal tumors are formed by a neoplastic spindle cell population. In some cases, the cell of origin can be determined by hematoxylin and eosin examination (eg, fibrosarcomas, myxosarcomas, neurofibrosarcomas, and the muscle tumors). For others, the origin of the neoplastic cell population would require further evaluation (immunohistochemistry and electron microscopy) that was seldom explored in these clinical cases. This broad category of tumor type can be found anywhere on the body and most have a similar behavior. In the present study and other reports, these tumors tend to occur more frequently in the axillary, elbow, and shoulder area (**Fig. 7**).[18] They are firm subcutaneous masses that feel partially attached to deeper layers probably because of their growth pattern of fascicles of cells extending into the surrounding soft tissues (**Fig. 8**). They are malignant and grow very fast, becoming quite large. There is no age or gender predilection noted. The ideal treatment is early detection and wide, complete surgical excision followed by definitive radiation treatment. If untreated, rabbits may live comfortably for up to a year with a spindle cell sarcoma and palliative care; only when the tumor is very large does the rabbit seem to become systemically affected.

Collagenous Hamartomas/Collagen Nevi

These are benign, tumorlike lesions that are poorly characterized in rabbits. They are usually solitary dome- or gumdrop-shaped firm nodules in the skin, and they occur most frequently on the body and proximal limbs. Histologically, the skin masses are characterized by focal excess of dermal collagen and lack a discrete growth (**Fig. 9**). Based on our case submissions, 91% were male rabbits with an average

Table 2
Cutaneous neoplasia in the rabbit, 1998–2012

	Frequency (%)	No. Male	No. Female	Age Range (y)	Average Age (y)	Locations
Trichoblastoma (basal cell tumor, basal cell epithelioma)	20	69	64	2–11	6	Face, neck, axilla, shoulder, elbow, toe, dewlap
Spindle cell sarcoma (unclassified mesenchymal tumors)	9	36	24	2–11	7	Leg, shoulder, elbow, axilla, thorax, abdomen, face, neck
Collagenous hamartoma (collagen nevi)	8.4	51	5	0.8–11	5.8	Elbow, shoulder, mammary
Squamous papilloma	6	28	12	1–10	5	Ears, eyelid, conjunctiva, oral, toe, nose
Mammary gland adenocarcinoma	5.6	—	36	2–10	5.8	Mammary gland, axilla
Soft tissue sarcoma	5.6	21	17	1–10	6.4	Face, stifle, hock, flank, toe
Mammary gland adenoma	4.1	1	26	3–11	5.7	Mammary gland
Lipoma, often with steatitis, some infiltrative	4	18	8	2–15	5.6	Shoulder, stifle
Fibrosarcoma	3.4	17	6	4–10	6.3	Limb, oral, ear
Mammary gland carcinoma	3.2	—	23	1–12	6.2	Mammary gland
Basal cell carcinoma	2.7	7	10	2–11	6.6	Ear, axilla, toe, limb
Carcinoma (origin not determined)	2.7	4	14	1–10	6.1	Axilla, lip, submandibular, nasal canthus
Malignant melanoma	2.5	13	4	M 2–10 F 7–8	M 6.7 F 7.3	Eyelid, ear, toe
Squamous cell carcinoma	2.5	12	5	M 2–11 F 5–7.5	6 5.9	Ear, periocular, limb, genitals
Lymphoma	1.9	6	6	3–9	6	Cheek

Courtesy of Drury Reavill, DVM, West Sacramento, CA.

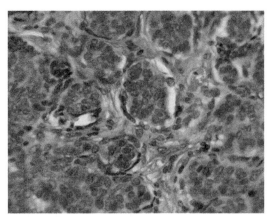

Fig. 6. Trichoblastoma demonstrating the serpiginous cords of basaloid trichoblasts forming small islands of cells (hematoxylin and eosin, original magnification ×40 [Obective]). (*Courtesy of* D. Reavill, DVM, West Sacramento, CA.)

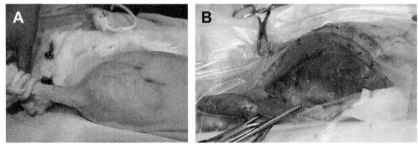

Fig. 7. (*A, B*) Preoperative and intraoperative views of large axillary mass in a 6-year-old rabbit. Histopathology diagnosed a poorly differentiated, high-grade spindle cell sarcoma, possibly anaplastic fibrosarcoma. This rabbit received a revised definitive course of radiation. The plan of 12 fractions of 4 Gy over 4 weeks was discontinued after eight fractions because of anorexia and gastrointestinal stasis.

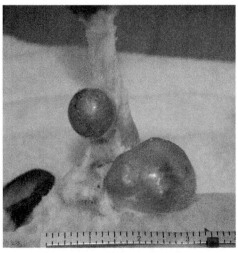

Fig. 8. Spindle cell tumor of left axilla and foreleg. This malignant tumor infiltrated the thoracic musculature.

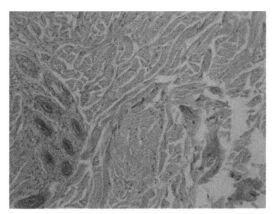

Fig. 9. Collagenous hamartoma is characterized by a nodule of haphazardly arranged collagen within the dermis (hematoxylin and eosin, original magnification ×4 [Obective]). (*Courtesy of* D. Reavill, DVM, West Sacramento, CA.)

age of 6 years. A report in the literature found these tumors occurred only in male rabbits, and they speculated that there may be possible hormonal influences.[17] In many cases, multiple nodules may develop, but complete surgical removal seems curative.

Squamous Papillomas

Benign warty growths, sometimes small, sometimes bigger with multiple projections, these tumors have a predilection for the head and mucosa (**Fig. 10**). It is probable that most, if not all of these masses are caused by the rabbit (Shope) papilloma virus, transmitted by insects or by direct contact through skin trauma.[17,19] Wild rabbits (*Sylvilagus*) are the natural reservoir. Squamous papillomas are characterized by multiple irregular papillary projections of hyperplastic stratified squamous epithelium. These papillary projections generally support thick dense overlying keratin (**Fig. 11**). In the present study, 70% of the cases were male, but there was no age predilection. These lesions are considered benign, and some may regress on their own after a few months. Surgical excision is mainly for cosmetic or diagnostic purposes.

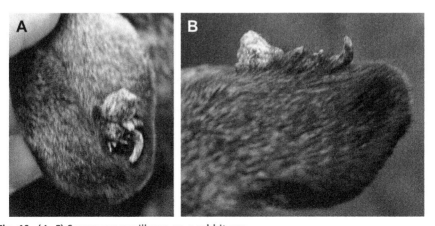

Fig. 10. (*A, B*) Squamous papilloma on a rabbit ear.

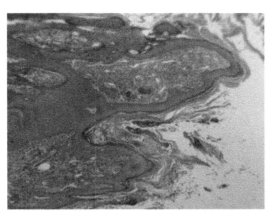

Fig. 11. Cutaneous papilloma is characterized by papillary fronds of hyperplastic epithelium supported on fibrovascular cores (hematoxylin and eosin, original magnification ×4 [Obective]). (*Courtesy of* D. Reavill, DVM, West Sacramento, CA.)

Mammary Tumors

Collectively, mammary tumors represented 14% of all cutaneous tumors in this study. Mammary tumors in rabbits start as a small nodule in one or more mammary glands, but can grow into a large mass before being discovered. If not removed, these tumors continue to grow and may become ulcerated. Mammary tumors are more commonly seen in female rabbits that are not spayed or have been spayed later in life. It is likely that the mammary tissue is stimulated by estrogens and progesterone, similar to what is seen in older unspayed canines and felines.[20–22] Among the female rabbits, 70% of the mammary tumors were malignant, including adenocarcinomas, carcinomas, and malignant mixed mammary tumors. In this study, mammary neoplasia was reported in one male rabbit and was identified as a benign papillary adenoma. The average age for affected female rabbits was 6 years; the single affected male rabbit was 4 years. Benign mammary gland tumors do not recur after complete surgical excision. Malignant mammary tumors may be more aggressive and eventually metastasize to other organs, such as the lungs and lymph nodes. If a single small nodule is present, a lumpectomy with complete margins can be performed, and if intact, an ovariohysterectomy should be performed. Spaying may not decrease the likelihood of future mammary tumor development, but treats or prevents the very common rabbit uterine diseases, such as adenocarcinoma and cystic endometrial hyperplasia. Because of prolonged sensitization of the mammary tissue with hormones, additional tumors may form in other mammary glands years after spaying, especially if the rabbit was spayed later in life. If multiple mammary glands are affected, a chain mastectomy may be necessary. If the mammary gland tumor cannot be completely excised, radiation can be effective to help stop or slow regrowth.[23] In cats and dogs when mammary gland tumors are nonresectable or have spread systemically, adjunctive treatments include chemotherapy with doxorubicin, a cyclooygenase-2 inhibitor, such as piroxicam or meloxicam, or the antiestrogen medication, tamoxifen.[24,25] No studies have yet been published regarding efficacy of these adjunctive treatments in rabbits.

Malignant Melanomas

Melanomas constituted 2.7% of cutaneous neoplasms submitted to ZEPS in this study. The initial appearance may be a small black freckle that remains the same for years then suddenly starts to grow (**Figs. 12** and **13**). They are usually found on

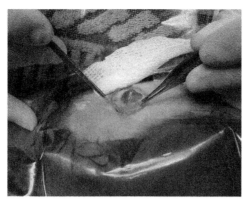

Fig. 12. Malignant melanoma on the lateral torso of a rabbit. (*Courtesy of* Peter G. Fisher, DVM, Virginia Beach, VA.)

the ear or eyelid, but have also been found on the toe and genital area. In the present study 76% of the rabbits with malignant melanoma were male, and tumors were seen as early as 2 years of age in male rabbits. Most of the male rabbits and all of the female rabbits developed melanomas later in life, averaging 7 years of age. Malignant melanomas tend to be locally invasive, with concurrent lymphatic invasion.[17] Complete excision when these tumors are small is ideal, because they may grow quickly. With tumors that are located on the face, good margins are difficult to attain, therefore regrowth may occur. Radiation postsurgery should be considered to attain better tumor control and longer remission time. If the tumor returns or is nonresectable, palliative radiation is helpful. A melanoma vaccine has been developed for use in dogs, but because it is of xenogenic origin it is considered safe in other species, such as rabbits.[26]

Cutaneous tumors reported in rabbits at less than 2% frequency were not listed in **Table 2** and include fibrolipoma (1.6%); fibroma (1.6%); basosquamous carcinoma (1.2%); myxosarcoma (1.2%); neurofibrosarcoma (1.2%); extraskeletal osteosarcoma

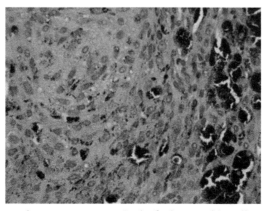

Fig. 13. Cutaneous melanomas are comprised of pleomorphic cells supporting variable amounts of cytoplasmic pigments (hematoxylin and eosin, original magnification ×40 [Obective]). (*Courtesy of* D. Reavill, DVM, West Sacramento, CA.)

(0.9%); melanocytoma (0.7%); spindle cell tumor (Shope fibromatosis) (0.7%); squamous cell carcinoma in situ (0.6%); apocrine gland adenoma (0.4%); epitheliotrophic lymphoma (0.4%); giant cell tumor of soft tissue (0.4%); malignant mixed mammary tumor (0.4%); myxoma (0.4%); trichoepithelioma (0.4%); adenoma (0.3%); hemangioma (0.3%); hemangiosarcoma (0.3%); keratoma (0.3%); leiomyosarcoma (0.3%); meibomian gland adenoma (0.3%); sebaceous carcinoma (0.3%); sebaceous cell epithelioma (0.3%); and trichoblastoma (0.3%).

One of each of the following cutaneous tumors were reported in the 14-year span of this study: carcinoma with squamous differentiation; cutaneous adenocarcinoma; neurofibroma; hemangiopericytoma; histiocytic sarcoma; keratoacanthoma; liposarcoma; mast cell tumor; mucoid fibrosarcoma; mucoid sarcoma; mucosal papilloma (conjunctiva); extraskeletal osteoma; and papillary adenocarcinoma.

GUINEA PIGS

The common cutaneous neoplasms reported in guinea pigs are described in **Table 3**. Out of 133 reported cases, most of these tumors are benign. Trichofolliculomas are the most commonly seen tumors, accounting for more than one-third of the reported

Table 3
Cutaneous neoplasia in the guinea pig, 1998–2012

	Frequency (%)	No. Male	No. Female	Age Range (y)	Average Age (y)	Locations
Trichofolliculoma	33	24	21	1–7	3.6	Dorsal and caudal hip
Lipoma, often with fibrosis and steatitis	25.5	15	19	1–6	3	Nipple, thorax
Trichoepithelioma	3.7	1	4	1–4	2.75	Not reported
Mammary gland adenocarcinoma	3.7	1	4	1–4.5	2.8	Mammary gland
Sebaceous adenoma	3	4	0	3–6	4	Not reported
Soft tissue sarcoma	3	3	1	2–4.5	3.4	Not reported
Fibrosarcoma	2.2	3	0	2–6	4	Not reported
Fibrolipoma	2.2	1	2	3–4	3.5	Not reported
Mammary gland adenoma/cystadenoma	2.2	1	2	3–4	3.75	Mammary gland
Carcinoma (origin not determined)	2.2	1	2	3–6	4.6	Not reported
Squamous cell carcinoma	2.2	2	1	2–6	4.5	Toe
Malignant melanoma	2.2	1	2	4–6.5	5.2	Not reported
Liposarcoma	1.5	2	0	4	4	Leg
Cutaneous hemangiosarcoma	1.5	2	0	1.5–4	2.75	Not reported
Epitheliotropic lymphoma	1.5	2	0	6	6	Not reported

Courtesy of Drury Reavill, DVM, West Sacramento, CA; and *Data from* Zoo/Exotic Pathology.

cutaneous tumors in this study. A total of 25.5% of the submissions were lipomas. Trichoepitheliomas and mammary gland adenocarcinomas were next at 3.7% each. A study from 1975 reported 21% trichoepitheliomas, 14% lipomas, and 14% mammary gland adenocarcinomas, and smaller numbers of seven other tumor types.[27]

Trichofolliculomas

These tumors frequently occur on the dorsal and caudal hip area and can become quite large, up to 4 cm in diameter or larger. Many of these tumors rupture and exude a white or gray thick sebaceous discharge, which can be confused with pus. Sometimes there is also associated chronic hemorrhage (**Fig. 14**). These benign hair follicle tumors are characterized by abortive follicular adnexal structures in walls of cysts lined by stratified squamous epithelium (**Fig. 15**). The core of the cyst is filled with clusters of irregular keratin debris (**Fig. 16**). There is no gender predilection noted, and they can occur at any age. Even though they are benign, these tumors continue to grow and may rupture; therefore, surgical removal is recommended. Complete surgical excision is curative.

Lipomas

A total of 25% of the cutaneous masses submitted were lipomas. They appear as soft to firm fatty masses in the skin or subcutaneous tissue. They may appear as a single mass or multiple nodules. Lipomas can occur anywhere, but have been most commonly reported in the inguinal lymph node area. Masses in these areas need to be differentiated from lymphoma or mammary gland tumors. Lipomas are benign connective tissue tumors composed of histologically normal adipose tissue (**Fig. 17**). They have been identified in equal numbers in male and female guinea pigs, and the average age is 3 years. Because they are benign, surgical removal may be recommended for cosmetic reasons or if the lipoma continues to grow, affecting ambulation and causing discomfort. Needle aspirate, biopsy, or excision may be indicated to differentiate a benign lipoma from a potentially malignant neoplasm. Liposarcomas have been diagnosed infrequently in guinea pigs; two cases were seen in the present study.

Trichoepitheliomas

These hair follicle tumors are not as common as trichofolliculomas, but are similar in being benign. Trichoepitheliomas differentiate toward all three segments of the hair

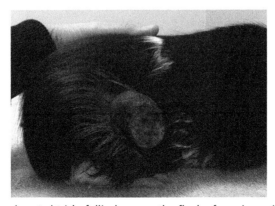

Fig. 14. Bleeding, ulcerated trichofolliculoma on the flank of a guinea pig.

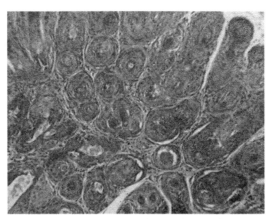

Fig. 15. A trichofolliculoma is formed by well-differentiated follicles that radiate out from a cystic core typically filled with keratin and hair fragments. The central area is to the top right border (hematoxylin and eosin, original magnification ×4 [Obective]). (*Courtesy of* D. Reavill, DVM, West Sacramento, CA.)

follicle (infundibulum, isthmus, and inferior segments). They are discrete masses comprised of mixtures of cystic structures and budding epithelial islands. In the present study they were seen primarily in female guinea pigs, with an average age of 2.75 years. Complete surgical removal is recommended because if the cysts rupture, the keratin elicits significant inflammation.

Mammary Gland Tumors

Mammary gland tumors constituted 6% of all cutaneous neoplasms in this study. Mammary tumors often start as a small nodule in the glandular tissue, but will continue to grow larger and can become ulcerated. They can affect one mammary gland or both

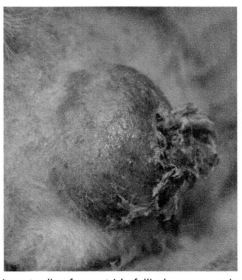

Fig. 16. Keratin debris protruding from a trichofolliculoma on a guinea pig's rump.

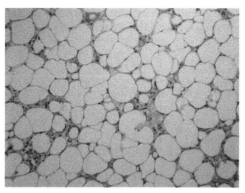

Fig. 17. A lipoma is lobules of mature lipocytes (hematoxylin and eosin, original magnification ×40 [Obective]). (*Courtesy of* D. Reavill, DVM, West Sacramento, CA.)

(**Fig. 18**). Similar to what is seen in other species, these tumors may develop under the influence of estrogen and progesterone.[28] In the present study, 66% of female guinea pig mammary tumors were malignant adenocarcinomas, and 33% were benign adenomas and cystadenomas. Females had a higher incidence of mammary tumors than male guinea pigs in this study, and we found one male with a malignant mammary tumor and one with a benign tumor. Another study from 2010[28] on 10 mammary gland tumors presents similar results: eight females and two males had mammary tumors. Five of the females had malignant tumors, and both of the males had malignant tumors. In contrast to the previous data, a review study found a higher total number of male guinea pigs (21) with mammary gland tumors than females (14). A total of 52% of the male guinea pigs had malignant mammary tumors, whereas only 36% of the females had a malignant tumor.[29] Mammary gland tumors are most frequently seen in animals 3 years and older. Surgical excision is ideal but clean margins may be difficult to obtain if the mass is large. Guinea pigs with malignant mammary tumors have a high incidence of disease recurrence after surgery; in one report three of the

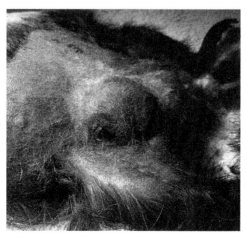

Fig. 18. Mammary gland tumor on a female guinea pig. (*Courtesy of* Peter G. Fisher, DVM, Virginia Beach, VA.)

four guinea pigs with follow-up data had tumor regrowth and died 2 to 5 months post-surgery.[28] Radiation treatment may be used, but guinea pigs do not tolerate chemotherapy very well. Nonsteroidal anti-inflammatory drugs may be used to palliate. Because of the guarded long-term prognosis with recurrent malignant mammary tumors, treatment is mainly palliative.

Other cutaneous tumors seen infrequently in guinea pigs, at one case each in the past 14 years, were not listed in **Table 3** and include apocrine gland adenoma, basal cell carcinoma, hemangioma, malignant lymphoma, myxosarcoma, neurofibrosarcoma, papillary cystadenocarcinoma, sebaceous gland epithelioma, schwannoma, spindle cell sarcoma, squamous papilloma, and tubulopapillary carcinoma.

SUMMARY

Similar to other domesticated mammals, ferrets, rabbits, and guinea pigs develop many common types of cutaneous neoplasms. In the present study we found that in all three species, the cutaneous masses found in the highest numbers were benign tumors. Rabbits had the highest percentage of malignancies; 46% of all cutaneous neoplasms in rabbits were malignant. In guinea pigs 26% of their skin masses were malignant, and ferrets had 19% malignancies.

Mammary gland tumors were seen at a frequency of 14% in rabbits, 6% in guinea pigs, and only 1.5% in ferrets in this study. In rabbits, mammary tumors were more common in female rabbits, and more likely to be malignant. In guinea pigs, our data showed a higher number of mammary tumors in females, 66% of which were malignant. Another study demonstrates a higher frequency of mammary tumors in male guinea pigs, with 52% of those being malignant. We saw small numbers of mammary tumors in ferrets, equally split among males and females. No female ferrets in our study were diagnosed with a malignant mammary tumor, but 30% of the male ferrets were.

Even though there are differences in tumor types and frequencies for ferrets, rabbits, and guinea pigs, the diagnostics do not differ from how veterinarians address cutaneous neoplasia in the more common domesticated species, such as dogs and cats. After a skin lesion is identified, an aspirate or biopsy should be performed to try and identify the tumor type. Malignant tumors require wide and deep surgical excision, although patient size may limit the ability to obtain adequate margins in these small animals. There is less evidence-based information on exotic mammal species than on dogs and cats in the literature regarding adjunctive treatments, such as chemotherapy and radiation, but more and more exotic pet veterinarians are extrapolating dosages and trying advanced modalities. Reports of successful chemotherapy have been cited in the ferret literature, but herbivorous rabbits and guinea pigs seem more sensitive to the toxic effects associated with chemotherapeutics. More is learned with every case treated. Although the patients may be smaller, they are no less deserving of high-quality medicine, and many owners care for them just as deeply as other pets.

REFERENCES

1. American Veterinary Medical Association. US Pet Ownership and Demographic Sourcebook. Schaumberg (IL): AVMA; 2012. p. 47–8.
2. Parker GA, Picut CA. Histopathologic features and post-surgical sequelae of 57 cutaneous neoplasms in ferrets (*Mustela putorius furo.*). Vet Pathol 1993;30(6): 499–504.

3. Stauber E, Robinette J, Basaraba R, et al. Mast cell tumors in three ferrets. J Am Vet Med Assoc 1990;196(5):766–7.
4. Li X, Fox JG, Padrid PA. Neoplastic diseases in ferrets: 574 cases (1968-1997). J Am Vet Med Assoc 1998;212(9):1402–6.
5. Williams BH. Pathology of the domestic ferret (*Mustela putorius furo*). In: Pathology of non-traditional pets, 2004 CL Davis ACVP Symposium.
6. Lightfoot T, Rubinstein J, Aiken S, et al. Soft tissue surgery in ferrets. In: Quesenberry KE, Carpenter JW, editors. Ferrets, rabbits and rodents: clinical medicine and surgery. 3rd edition. St. Louis (MO): Saunders Elsevier; 2012. p. 153–5.
7. Pinches MD, Liebenberg G, Stidworthy MF. What is your diagnosis? Preputial mass in a ferret. Vet Clin Pathol 2008;37(4):443–6.
8. Miller TA, Denman DL, Lewis GC Jr. Recurrent adenocarcinoma in a ferret. J Am Vet Med Assoc 1985;187(8):839–41.
9. Antinoff NA, Hahn K. Ferret oncology: diseases, diagnostics, and therapeutics. Vet Clin North Am Exot Anim Pract 2004;7:579–625.
10. Antinoff N, Williams BH. Neoplasia in ferrets. In: Quesenberry KE, Carpenter JW, editors. Ferrets, rabbits and rodents: clinical medicine and surgery. 3rd edition. St. Louis (MO): Saunders Elsevier; 2012. p. 103–22.
11. Orcutt C, Tater K. Dermatologic diseases in ferrets. In: Quesenberry KE, Carpenter JW, editors. Ferrets, rabbits and rodents: clinical medicine and surgery. 3rd edition. St. Louis (MO): Saunders Elsevier; 2012. p. 127–30.
12. Mikaelian I, Garner MM. Solitary dermal leiomyosarcomas in 12 ferrets. J Vet Diagn Invest 2002;14:262.
13. Rickman BH, Craig LE, Goldschmidt MH. Piloleiomyosarcoma in seven ferrets. Vet Pathol 2001;38(6):710–1.
14. Mialot M, Prata D, Girard-Luc A, et al. Multiple progressive piloleiomyomas in a ferret (*Mustela putorius furo*): a case report. Vet Dermatol 2011;22(1):100–3.
15. Goldschmidt MH, Dunstan RW, Stannard AA, et al. Histological classification of epithelial and melanocytic tumors of the skin of domestic animals. 2nd series. Washington, DC: World Health Organization, Armed Forces Institute of Pathology; 1998.
16. Bohn AA, Wills T, Caplazi P. Basal cell tumor or cutaneous basilar epithelial neoplasm? Rethinking the cytologic diagnosis of basal cell tumors. Vet Clin Pathol 2006;35(4):449–53.
17. von Bomhard W, Goldschmidt MH, Shofer FS, et al. Cutaneous neoplasms in pet rabbits: a retrospective study. Vet Pathol 2007;44:579.
18. Clippinger TL, Bennett RA, Alleman R, et al. Removal of a thymoma via median sternotomy in a rabbit with recurrent appendicular neurofibrosarcoma. J Am Vet Med Assoc 1998;213(8):1140–3.
19. Hess L, Tater K. Dermatologic diseases in rabbits. In: Quesenberry KE, Carpenter JW, editors. Ferrets, rabbits and rodents: clinical medicine and surgery. 3rd edition. St. Louis (MO): Saunders Elsevier; 2012. p. 240.
20. Mulligan RM. Mammary cancer in the dog: a study of 120 cases. Am J Vet Res 1975;36(9):1391–6.
21. Overley B, Shofer FS, Goldschmidt MH, et al. Association between ovariohysterectomy and feline mammary carcinoma. J Vet Intern Med 2005;19(4):560–3.
22. Bergman PJ. Mammary gland tumors: what you need to know. ABVP 2008.
23. Mauldin EA, Goldschmidt MH. A retrospective study of cutaneous neoplasms in domestic rabbits (1990-2001). Vet Dermatol 2002;13(4):214.

24. Borrego JF, Cartagena JC, Engel J. Treatment of feline mammary tumors using chemotherapy, surgery and a COX-2 inhibitor drug (meloxicam): a retrospective study of 23 cases (2002-2007). Vet Comp Oncol 2009;7(4):213–21.

25. Tonetti DA, Jordan VC. The estrogen receptor: a logical target for the prevention of breast cancer with antiestrogens. J Mammary Gland Biol Neoplasia 1999;4(4): 401–13.

26. Phillips JC, Lembcke LM, Noltenius CE, et al. Evaluation of tyrosinase expression in canine and equine melanocytic tumors. Am J Vet Res 2012;73(2):272–8.

27. Kitchen DN, Carlton WW, Bickford AA. A report of fourteen spontaneous tumors of the guinea pig. Lab Anim Sci 1975;25(1):92–102.

28. Suarez-Bonnet A, Martin de las Mulas J, Millan MY, et al. Morphological and immunohistochemical characterization of spontaneous mammary gland tumors in the guinea pig (Cavia porcellus). Vet Pathol 2010;47(2):298–305.

29. Gibbons PM, Garner MM. Mammary gland tumors in guinea pigs (Cavia porcellus). In: Proceedings for the annual AEMV conference. Milwaukee (WI): 2009. p. 83.

Erythema Multiforme in a Ferret (*Mustela putorius furo*)

Peter G. Fisher, DVM, ABVP- ECP

KEYWORDS

- Ferret • Erythema multiforme • Hypersensitivity • Immune disease
- Dermatopathology • Adrenal disease • Hyperadrenocorticism

KEY POINTS

- Erythema multiforme is an uncommon skin disease that most dermatopathologists think is a host-specific hypersensitivity reaction induced by various antigens that alter keratinocytes, making them targets of an aberrant immune response.
- In veterinary medicine, erythema multiforme has been more commonly reported in dogs than in cats, and is typically associated with drug administration (eg, ampicillin, cephalexin, trimethoprim-sulfonamide, griseofulvin, acepromazine, enrofloxacin, and lincomycin), although many cases remain idiopathic.
- The onset of clinical signs is typically acute with erythematous macules and papules developing rapidly and often becoming annular or serpiginous as they coalesce in partially symmetric patterns.
- On skin biopsy histology, individual cell necrosis of keratinocytes, or apoptosis, and lymphocyte satellitosis are the most characteristic histologic lesions of erythema multiforme.
- Adrenal disease should be considered as a primary underlying cause of erythema multiforme in the ferret.

INTRODUCTION

Erythema multiforme (EM) is an uncommon skin disease that most dermatopathologists think is a host-specific hypersensitivity reaction induced by various antigens that alter keratinocytes, making them targets of an aberrant immune response. Reported in humans and various animal species, including the dog, cat, and horse,[1] it is currently thought that the process of cell death occurring in EM results from an initiation of a death program through cell-mediated or unknown factors.[2] It has been documented that the cell-mediated response in EM has a Th1 cytokine pattern.[3,4] The T cell–mediated response is directed at keratinocytes that may express antigens

Disclosures: The author has nothing to disclose.
Pet Care Veterinary Hospital, Inc., 5201-A, Virginia Beach Boulevard, Virginia Beach, VA 23462, USA
E-mail address: pfisher@petcarevb.com

in a novel way because of drug administration, infection, or neoplasia resulting in apoptosis (single-cell necrosis) of keratinocytes.[3] The more severe the clinical presentation of EM, the more likely it is to be associated with an adverse drug reaction.[3,5]

Among animals, EM has been more commonly reported in dogs than in cats, but in both species the disease is:

- Most commonly associated with drug administration; ampicillin, cephalexin, trimethoprim-sulfonamide, griseofulvin, acepromazine, enrofloxacin, and lincomycin all have been reported as initiating factors.

Other less common initiators include:

- Neoplasia[2]
- Bacterial infection[6]
- Fungal infection[7]
- Viral infection[8]
- Idiopathic[6]
- Insecticidal dips[9]
- Food hypersensitivities[10]

Breed or sex predilection has not been noted for any of the forms of EM.[2]

Lesions of EM usually develop after 7 to 18 days of exposure to the causative agent,[6,11] although lesions may develop as soon as day 1 after exposure if the animal has been previously exposed.[5,6] The ferret reported here developed lesions 12 weeks after having undergone surgery for gastric trichobezoars and partial resection of a grossly enlarged right adrenal gland, during which time it was exposed to various drugs including dexmedetomidine, burtorphanol, isoflurane, famotidine, cefazolin, and meloxicam. Polydioxanone suture (PDS) was used during surgery. Because of the length of time between drug exposure and onset of clinical signs, it is unlikely that drug administration was responsible for the EM in this ferret.

CLINICAL HISTORY AND PHYSICAL EXAMINATION FINDINGS

A 5-year-old neutered male with a body weight of 1.2 kg initially presented with a sudden onset of scabbing and erythema of the ventral inguinal area. The skin of the dorsum was not affected and there were no dermal signs typical of ferret hyperadrenocorticism. On initial presentation the body temperature was normal and the ferret was bright and alert. Pruritus was not reported, and external parasites were not seen on physical examination or multiple skin scrapings. On gross examination, several papules were seen with varying degrees of scale and scabbing. Dermal tape preparation cytology showed cornified epithelial cells and occasional cocci bacteria. Because of the close resemblance of the ferret's gross dermal lesions to those of epidermal collarettes commonly associated with superficial pyoderma typical of the canine, the ferret was placed on cefadroxil (Cefadrops, Fort Dodge Animal Health, Fort Dodge, IA) at 10 mg/kg every 12 hours with instructions to reevaluate clinical signs in 1 week.

CLINICAL COURSE

A medical progress examination 1 week later revealed a worsening of the dermatitis. The dermatitis, manifested as erythematous papules and scabs, had progressed to involve the inguinal (**Fig. 1**A) and axillary regions (see **Fig. 1**B) and ventromedial aspect of the limbs. In addition, all four feet showed foot pad thickening with hyperkeratosis as well as dermal inflammation between the pads (**Fig. 2**A). The ear pinna were

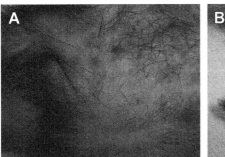
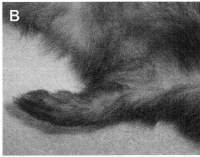

Fig. 1. One week after initial presentation for a dermatitis of unknown origin, this 5-year-old ferret presented with a worsening of clinical signs seen here as erythematous macules and papules in the inguinal area (*A*) and the axillary area (*B*). The dermatitis had worsened in spite of antibacterial therapy. This image is of the inguinal area.

inflamed and showed evidence of hyperkeratosis (see **Fig. 2**B). Because of the uncommon presentation the ferret was sedated with dexmedetomidine and anesthetized with isoflurane and multiple surgical skin biopsies were taken and submitted to a pathologist knowledgeable in dermatopathology (Tammy Johnson, DVM, DACVP). After biopsy, the ferret was placed on the antiinflammatory drug prednisolone (Lloyd Inc, Shenandoah, IA) 1.25 mg/kg every 12 hours, and an antibiotic, enrofloxacin (Wedgwood compounding pharmacy, Swedesboro, NJ) 10 mg//kg every 12 hours pending results of histopathology.

Skin biopsy histopathology was consistent with a severe manifestation of EM. On review of medical records and on questioning the owner there was no known history of recent drug or chemical exposure as a potential underlying cause. Tissue samples were submitted to 2 other pathologists, both familiar with ferret tissues: Robert Schmidt, DVM, PhD, DACVP, Zoo/Exotic Pathology Service, and Bruce Williams, DVM, DACVP, Armed Forces Institute of Pathology, for a second opinion. Both pathologist agreed, particularly Dr Williams, that dermatohistopathology was consistent with EM.

On medical progress examination 10 days after biopsy the dermatitis showed a partial response to prednisolone and enrofloxacin therapy (**Figs. 3** and **4**). A decrease in

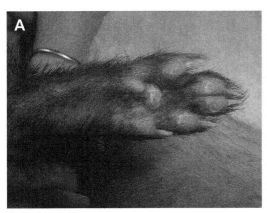
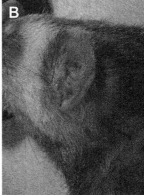

Fig. 2. Hyperkeratosis and erythema of the foot pads (*A*) and ear pinna (*B*) were other manifestations of the dermatitis seen in this 5-year-old ferret.

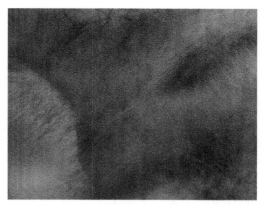

Fig. 3. The skin lesions had shown signs of significant improvement after 10 days of gluco-corticoid therapy.

the degree of erythema and scabbing of the dermis along the ventrum was noted and the severity of foot and ear lesions was diminished. The prednisolone was continued at 1.25 mg/kg every 12 hours for 4 more weeks. During this time the owner decreased the dose (without consulting a veterinarian) to once daily because of associated weight gain and difficulty ambulating. Azathioprine (Mylan Pharmaceuticals, Morgantown, WV) at 1 mg every 24 hours was added to the immunosuppressive therapy protocol. Six weeks after instituting azathioprine therapy there was no clinical improvement in the dermatologic lesions and the drug was stopped. Throughout the therapy with

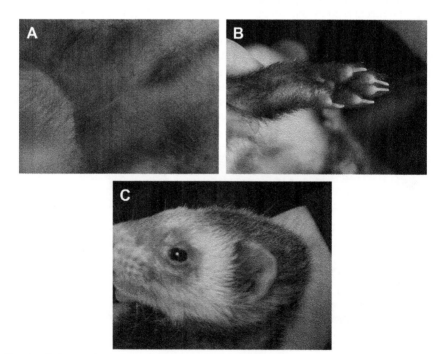

Fig. 4. All dermatologic lesions including the skin (*A*), foot pads (*B*), and the ear pinna (*C*) had significantly improved 1 week after instituting glucocorticoid therapy.

concurrent prednisolone and azathioprine the dermal lesions waxed and waned but never completely resolved.

Ten weeks into immunosuppressive therapy the ferret became pruritic and clinical signs worsened again (**Fig. 5**) in spite of prednisolone therapy. Because a partial right adrenalectomy had been performed 12 weeks before onset of clinical signs, an adrenal panel was submitted to the Clinical Endocrinology Service at the University of Tennessee. Pending results of the adrenal panel, oral cyclosporine (Atopica, Novartis Animal Health, Greensboro, NC) therapy was initiated at 2. 5 mg every 12 hours and prednisolone therapy was maintained at 1.25 mg/kg every 12 hours.

Results of the ferret adrenal panel were consistent with hyperadrenocorticism. Medical treatment options, including the use of melatonin and leuprolide acetate for depot suspension, were discussed with the owner. The owner opted to treat the ferret with a melatonin implant (Ferretonin 5.4 mg melatonin per implant, Melatek LLC, Fort Collins, CO) because her spouse was in the military and they had recently received orders to relocate and were afraid they would not be able to follow up on future leuprolide therapy. At the time of case presentation, use of deslorelin acetate implants for medical treatment of ferret adrenal disease had not been published.

Because of adverse signs associated with the prednisolone, and because long-term concurrent use of cyclosporine with glucocorticoids may predispose to the development of potentially severe opportunistic infections,[12] attempts were made to wean off the prednisolone. However, skin lesions worsened in spite of the added cyclosporine therapy, and the concurrent use of prednisolone was continued. Cyclosporine blood levels were not run because of financial constraints and lack of information on therapeutic cyclosporine blood levels at the time of case presentation. Two additional months of concurrent prednisolone and cyclosporine therapy did not improve the appearance of skin lesions (**Fig. 6**) and the owner elected euthanasia. The owner did not give permission for a necropsy.

LABORATORY FINDINGS AND DIAGNOSIS

A normal complete blood count and serum chemistry analysis had been assessed 12 weeks before case presentation and were not repeated. On initial examination

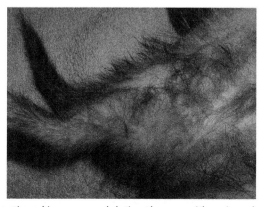

Fig. 5. In spite of continued immunomodulating therapy with various drugs including prednisolone, azathioprine, and cyclosporine, the dermal lesions never resolved completely and waxed and waned in severity. The dermatitis was worsening again after 10 weeks of immunosuppressive therapy.

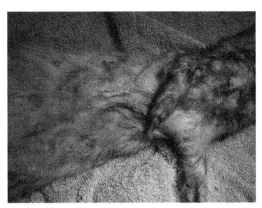

Fig. 6. Clinical appearance of the EM major at the time of euthanasia. The dermatitis had worsened to include urticarial plaques and ulcerations.

multiple skin scraping were performed but failed to identify ectoparasites. Skin cytology revealed bacterial cocci in low numbers and keratinized epithelial cells in moderate numbers.

Skin biopsy histopathology showed severe multifocal to confluent and moderate to severe epidermal keratinocyte necrosis and bulla formation, severe superficial/interface dermatitis, and mild to moderate hyperkeratosis and parakeratosis of the skin. The pathologist commented that histopathology was consistent with a severe manifestation of EM, especially if the case history supported an association with recent drug or chemical administration or other problem known to be associated with EM. An autoimmune disease, particularly pemphigus vulgaris, or early epitheliotropic lymphoma would be other primary differentials. No bacterial organisms were identified in examined tissue sections. Opinions from 2 other pathologists supported the diagnosis of EM.

Because of a suspicion of recurring adrenal disease and failure of the patient to respond to immunosuppressive drug therapy, an adrenal panel was submitted to the Clinical Endocrinology Service at the University of Tennessee 10 weeks after initial presentation. Results of the ferret adrenal panel were consistent with hyperadrenocorticism (**Table 1**).

DISCUSSION

The onset of clinical signs associated with EM is typically acute because erythematous macules and papules develop rapidly and often become annular or serpiginous

Table 1		
Results of adrenal hormone panel from the Clinical Endocrinology Service, University of Tennessee		
Test	**Result**	**Normal Range**
Estradiol	406.0 pmol/L	30–180 pmol/L
17-Hydroxyprogesterone	1.73 nmol/L	0–0.8 nmol/L
Androstenedione	86.2 nmol/L	0–15 nmol/L

as they coalesce in partially symmetric patterns.[2,3] The gross dermal lesions most commonly associated with EM include:

- Erythematous macules and papules: rapid development
- Urticarial plaques[2]
- Crusting commonly occurs as the lesions spread peripherally and form arciform patterns
- Epidermal collarettes
- Annular target lesions with central clearing
- Ulcers (less commonly) may eventuate from the urticarial and plaquelike lesions[2]
- Some lesions, especially in cats, become bullous, with detachment and necrosis of the epidermis[6]

More recent nomenclature categorizes EM clinically based on severity of lesions. In EM minor, characteristic lesions involve only 1 mucosal surface and affect less than 10% of the body surface. EM major has clinically similar lesions with more than 1 mucosal surfaced affected, 10% to 50% of the body surface affected, and less than 10% epithelial detachment.[3,13] According to this definition, the ferret in this case report fits a diagnosis of EM major.

Because of the pleomorphic nature of EM, clinical differential diagnoses are varied and include:

- Superficial pyoderma
- Bacterial folliculitis
- Epitheliotropic lymphoma
- Early-stage bullous immune-mediated skin diseases (pemphigus vulgaris, bullous pemphigoid, and systemic lupus erythematosus)

Definitive diagnosis of EM is based on history; physical examination; laboratory testing including skin scrapings, tape prep cytology, and dermatophyte culture to rule out other causes of skin disorder; and skin biopsy. Skin biopsy histologic findings associated with EM include:

- Maculopapular lesions are characterized histologically by hydropic interface dermatitis with prominent single-cell apoptosis of keratinocytes at all levels of the epidermis[12] and lymphocytic migration into the affected epidermis (many times surrounding the necrotic keratinocytes, a term known as satellitosis) (**Figs. 7–9**). Individual cell necrosis of keratinocytes, or apoptosis, and lymphocyte satellitosis are the most characteristic histologic lesions of EM.[3]
- Eosinophils, solitary or grouped, may be present at all levels of the epidermis.
- Urticarial lesions are characterized by hydropic interface dermatitis and striking dermal edema.[12]
- Vesiculobullous lesions are characterized by segmental full-thickness coagulation necrosis of epithelium. A superficial perivascular to interstitial accumulation of predominantly lymphohistiocytic cells is typical, and subepidermal cleft and vesicle formation may occur owing to separation of the necrotic epithelium from the underlying connective tissue at the basement membrane zone (**Fig. 10**).[12]
- Progression of keratinocyte necrosis usually leads to ulceration.
- Secondary neutrophilic infiltration and crusting are observed. Some affected animals have full-thickness necrosis of the epidermis, a typical finding with toxic epidermal necrolysis, which tends to manifest clinically as a more severe dermatopathy than EM.[6]

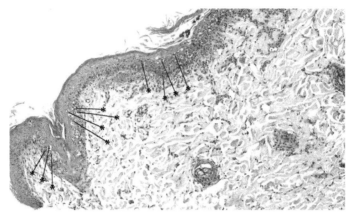

Fig. 7. All the individually apoptotic keratinocytes, located throughout the full thickness of the epidermis and not just located at basal epidermis as typically occurs with lupoid diseases. These keratinocytes are darkly eosinophilic (*pink to red*), rounded, and retracted from the surrounding cells, as shown by clear halolike areas, with dark-staining condensed nuclei. These apoptotic cells are surrounded by characteristic small dark cells (lymphocytes), called lymphocyte satellitosis.

The progression of EM varies from case to case, from mild to severe forms. A thorough search for underlying infectious disease or neoplasia is warranted if there is no history of drug administration before onset of clinical signs. Prognosis is good to guarded depending on whether or not an underlying cause can be identified.

Options for treatment of EM include:

- Whenever possible identify and correct any underlying cause.
- Appropriate symptomatic and supportive care in the form of fluids, antibiotics, parenteral nutrition, and soothing topical medications is instituted as needed.
- The use of immunosuppressive drugs, especially glucocorticoids, in the treatment of EM continues to be controversial; however, successful management of EM with high doses of glucocorticoids has been reported in the dog.[11]

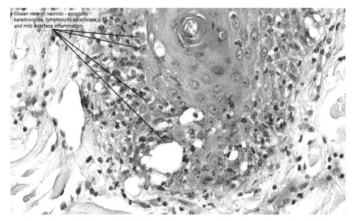

Fig. 8. Loss of epidermal-dermal BM junction caused by lymphocytic inflammation. BM, Basement Membrane.

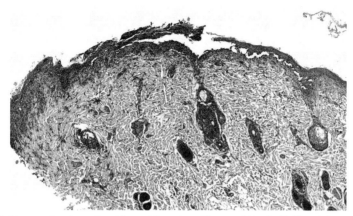

Fig. 9. Clefting at the dermal-epidermal junction. The resulting bullalike clefts are a useful artifact to recognize because they only occur at sites of severe interface inflammation and basement membrane damage, a lesion typical of immune-mediated skin disease.

- Immunomodulating drugs such as prednisolone,[12] azathioprine,[12] cyclosporine,[14] and human immunoglobulin[6] have all been used to treat EM with varying success in both dogs and cats.

The author is aware of 1 of case of EM being diagnosed in the ferret (Jennifer Graham, DVM, Associate Professor of Zoological Companion Animal Medicine, Tufts Cummings School of Veterinary Medicine, North Grafton, MA, personal communication, 2012). This ferret was also concurrently diagnosed with adrenal disease and, when treated with a gonadotropin-releasing hormone analogue, leuprolide acetate (30 day depot Lupron, Tap Pharmaceuticals, Lake Forrest, IL), the dermatologic lesions associated with EM resolved. This case was lost to long-term follow-up so it is unknown whether clinical EM ever recurred. As a result of this communication and the information gained in this case study, the author thinks that underlying adrenal disease should be considered as a primary underlying cause of EM in the ferret, and

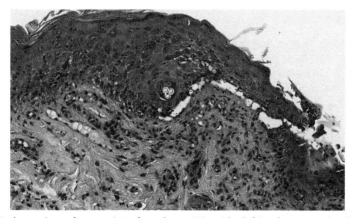

Fig. 10. A closer view of severe interface dermatitis with clefting between the dermis and epidermis. The small blue cells at this junction are lymphocytes. Note severe bubbling or vacuolation along the basal epidermis.

pursuit of a definitive diagnosis of adrenal disease via hormonal or ultrasonographic analysis should be the goal in any suspect case. In retrospect, the author would have more aggressively treated the hyperadrenocorticism with a gonadotropin-releasing hormone analogue, leuprolide acetate (Lupron), or, now that it is approved for the use in the United States, deslorelin acetate (Suprelorin F, Virbac Animal Health, Fort Worth, TX), because more definitive work has substantiated the ability of these drugs to suppress the hormones associated with adrenal disease compared with the melatonin implant. In addition, it would have been ideal to run cyclosporine blood levels in spite of therapeutic levels for the ferret being unknown at the time of case presentation. Cyclosporine is thought to be a safe and effective immunosuppressive therapy for many immune-mediated skin diseases,[14] including EM. The failure to respond to cyclosporine is difficult to judge because therapeutic blood levels of this drug were not assayed. More recently measurements of serum cyclosporine in the ferret have been published.[15]

SUMMARY

This is the first known published report of EM in the ferret. EM is typically a disease of multifactorial cause and, in this case, could have been a manifestation of underlying adrenal disease because no other history of recent drug or chemical exposure could be confirmed. Identification of an underlying cause and addressing this problem is always the primary goal in treatment of this disease. The prognosis for animals with EM is unpredictable, depending on the distribution and severity of clinical signs, identification of an underlying cause, and response to immunosuppressive therapy. In this ferret, prednisolone therapy improved clinical signs associated with disease but the patient never experienced a complete resolution of dermal lesions. Failure to appropriately treat a potential underlying cause (adrenal disease) and poor owner compliance with immunosuppressive therapy may also have contributed to the failure of this case to improve.

ACKNOWLEDGMENTS

The author thanks Tammy Johnson, DVM, Diplomate, American College of Veterinary Pathologists, for her help in preparing the histopathology images for this article.

REFERENCES

1. Marshall C. Erythema multiforme in two horses. J S Afr Vet Assoc 1991;62(3): 133–6.
2. Gross TL, Irhke PJ, Walder E. Necrotizing diseases of the epidermis. Erythema Multiforme. In: Gross TL, Irhke PJ, Walder E, editors. Veterinary dermatopathology. Philadelphia: Saunders; 1992. p. 41–6.
3. Outerbridge CA. Cutaneous manifestations of internal diseases. In: Morris DO, Kennis RA, editors. Clinical dermatology. VCNA, Small Animal Practice. Philadelphia: Elsevier; 2013. p. 135–52.
4. Caproni M, Torchia D, Schincaglia E, et al. Expression of cytokines and chemokine receptors in the cutaneous lesions of erythema multiforme and Stevens-Johnson syndrome/toxic epidermal necrolysis. Br J Dermatol 2006;155:722–8.
5. Hinn AC, Olivry T, Luther PB, et al. Erythema multiforme, Stevens-Johnson syndrome, and toxic epidermal necrolysis in the dog: clinical classification, drug exposure, and histopathological correlations. Vet Allergy Clin Immunol 1998;6: 13–20.

6. Byrne KP, Giger U. Use of human immunoglobulin for treatment of severe erythema multiforme in a cat. J Am Vet Med Assoc 2002;220(2):197–201.
7. Contreras-Barrera ME, Moreno-Coutino G, Torres-Guerrero DE, et al. Erythema multiforme secondary to cutaneous *Trichophyton mentagrophytes* infection. Rev Iberoam Micol 2009;26(2):149–51.
8. Favrot C, Olivry T, Dunston SM, et al. Parvovirus infection of keratinocytes as a cause of canine erythema multiforme. Vet Pathol 2000;37(6):647–9.
9. Rosenbaum MR, Kerlin RL. Erythema multiforme major and disseminated intravascular coagulation in a dog following application of D-limonene-based insecticidal dip. J Am Vet Med Assoc 1995;207(10):1315–9.
10. Itoh T, Nibe K, Kojimoto A, et al. Erythema multiforme possibly triggered by food substances in a dog. J Vet Med Sci 2006;68(8):869–71.
11. Scott DW, Miller WH. Erythema mulitforme in dogs and cats literature review and case material from Cornell University College of Veterinary Medicine (1988–1996). Vet Dermatol 1999;10:297–309.
12. Scott DW, Miller WH, Griffen CE. Immune-mediated disorders. In: Scott DW, Miller WH, Griffen CE, editors. Small animal dermatology. 6th edition. Philadelphia: Saunders; 2001. p. 667–779.
13. Gross TL, Irhke PJ, Walder E, et al. Skin diseases of the dog and cat. Clinical and histopathologic diagnosis. 2nd edition. Ames (IA): Blackwell Science; 2005.
14. Palmeiro BS. Cyclosproine in veterinary dermatology. In: Morris DO, Kennis RA, editors. Clinical dermatology. VCNA, Small Animal Practice. Philadelphia: Elsevier; 2013. p. 153–71.
15. Malka S, Hawkins MG, Zabolotzky SM, et al. Immune-mediated pure red cell aplasia in a domestic ferret. J Am Vet Med Assoc 2010;237(6):695–700.

Ectoparasites in Small Exotic Mammals

Michael Fehr, PhD, DVM, Dip ECZM (small mammals)*,
Saskia Koestlinger, DVM

KEYWORDS

- Dermatologic diseases • Arachnida • Insects • Pruritus • Dermatitis • Mites • Lice
- Ectoparasites

KEY POINTS

- Ectoparasites can cause significant clinical signs in small exotic mammals as a result of associated skin puncturing, epidermal lesions, or dermal surface scavenging, with or without the ingestion of blood, lymph, sebaceous secretions, and skin debris.
- Pruritic dermatoses resulting from a cell-mediated hypersensitivity to parasite antigen include erythema, excoriations, crusts, hyperkeratosis, alopecia, secondary bacterial dermatitis, and, in guinea pigs, seizure-like behavior.
- Diagnosis is mainly based on direct and microscopic visualization of ectoparasites, microscopy of trichograms, tape preparations, and skin scrapings.
- For prevention of reinfestation, treatment of all in-house pets, dogs, cats, and so forth, cleaning of cages and environment, and, if necessary, professional disinfection of the living quarters is advised.
- Lack of licensed antiparasiticides for use in exotic species in most countries requires off-label use of adequate pharmaceuticals.
- Therapeutic options are based on the topical application of appropriate acaricidal drops, sprays, or spot-on products, oral or parenteral parasiticides, or bathing or powdering.
- In certain species drug contraindications have to be considered, based on reported adverse reactions.

INTRODUCTION

Dermatologic diseases often disrupt the skin barrier, thus endangering the patient's quality of life, especially when severe pruritus occurs.[1,2] Ectoparasites inhabiting the fur and/or skin live on the outer surface or burrow into cutaneous layers of the affected host. Intense host irritation is caused by piercing, sucking, and chewing lymph, blood,

Disclosures: The author has nothing to disclose.
Clinic for Exotic Pets, Reptiles and Birds, University of Veterinary Medicine Hannover, Buenteweg 9, D-30559 Hannover, Germany
* Corresponding author.
E-mail address: Michael.Fehr@tiho-hannover.de

or skin debris. The digging of tunnels and burrowing in the skin associated with some ectoparasites leads to self-trauma and potential secondary bacterial dermatitis. Saliva components of ectoparasites can also induce allergic reactions with severe skin inflammation. Transmission can occur directly by contact with an infested animal of the same species, other household pets, or wild animals, or indirectly through infested food or a contaminated environment (eg, bedding material). Transmission may also be airborne in origin or via fomites such as the clothing or shoes of people. In cases of ectoparasitic skin disease in small exotic mammals, mites, lice, fleas, ticks, fly strikes, or helminths all have to be considered.[3]

A few characteristics of common ectoparasites in small mammals are worthy of mention. Insects belong to the hexapoda: adults are characterized by 3 pairs of legs with a well-developed body structure comprising a segmented head, thorax, and abdomen. On the other hand, adult arachnida are characterized by 4 pairs of legs; the head and thorax are fused to form the cephalothorax, with different parts of the body merging into each other.[4]

MITES

Various species of mites with various morphologic differences can be found in small exotic mammals. The typical life cycle of 4 developmental stages consists of egg deposition, hatchling larva with 3 pairs of legs, 1 or more nymph stages with 4 pair of legs, and adults. Living and feeding habits of mites vary; adults may live on the skin surface, in dermal tunnels, or in the environment, and only feed on the host.[4]

Burrowing Mites

Demodectidae
Demodex spp (D aurati, D caviae, D cunicoli, D criceti, D merioni, D ratti, D ratticola) Clinical demodicosis in exotic mammals, with the exception of hamsters, is rare. Infection in other species such as ferrets, gerbils, guinea pigs, rabbits, and brown rats is most often associated with concurrent immunosuppression resulting from such factors as overcrowding, poor nutrition and husbandry, or concurrent disease.[3,5–13] Case studies have associated demodectic mite infections in ferrets with repeated glucocorticoid-containing ointment application for recurrent ear-mite infections[14] or in ferrets with concurrent adrenal disease or lymphoma.[15]

Owen and Young[16] reported a high infestation incidence of Demodex criceti and Demodex aurati mites in hamsters, even without clinical signs, in Great Britain. Infected small mammals will be presented with a history of local alopecia and pruritus,[14] which can be localized around the eyes, mouth, and tail.[15] Skin lesions may be detected in areas of heavy mite burdens. Hamsters may be presented with alopecia, beginning on the lumbosacral area and extending up the back, sometimes with scaling, focal ulceration, and a dry, scabby dermatitis resulting from secondary bacterial infection.[16–19] Lesions can also occur on face, thorax, abdomen, or limbs (**Figs. 1–3**). Demodex ratti is common on the eye lid, ear canal and back, Demodex norvegicus at the anal and genital region, and Demodex ratticola at the nose and mouth region. Sometimes lethargy, anorexia, and mild to severe pruritus can be observed.[20]

Deep skin scraping on direct potassium hydroxide (KOH) preparation for microscopic detection of mites and/or skin biopsies is mandatory for definitive diagnosis.[20] Microscopy may reveal large bodied Demodex mites similar to Demodex canis, nymphs, larvae, and/or ova. D criceti has a shorter length (80–110 µm) than D aurati (150–200 µm). D criceti has a short blunt abdomen and is a resident of the epidermis,

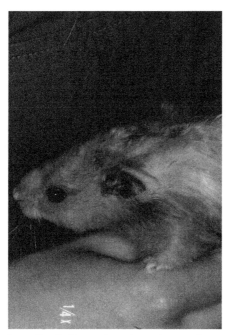

Fig. 1. Teddy hamster demodicosis. Focal alopecia on face and nose. (*Courtesy of* Michael Fehr, PhD, Hannover, Germany.)

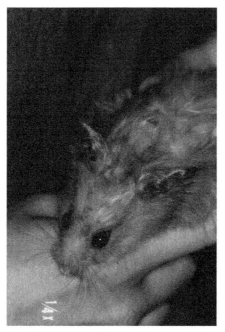

Fig. 2. Teddy hamster *Demodex aurati* with skin-scraping wound on the neck. (*Courtesy of* Michael Fehr, PhD, Hannover, Germany.)

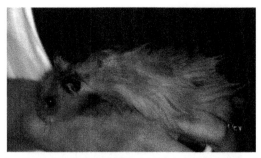

Fig. 3. Teddy hamster *Demodex aurati*, whole body view. (*Courtesy of* Michael Fehr, PhD, Hannover, Germany.)

inhabiting the keratin and pits of the epidermal surface. *D aurati* is cigar-shaped and lives in hair follicles (**Fig. 4**).[21]

Sarcoptidae

Sarcoptes scabiei, Notoedres cati Skin mange caused by *Sarcoptes* spp can be responsible for high losses in affected rabbitries or ferret shelters. Mite exposure results from contact with infected conspecifics, infected carrier species such as dogs, or bedding/fomites. Occasionally sarcoptic mange may be encountered in the ferret; it is somewhat more common in feral ferrets in Europe but also has been reported in domestic ferrets in Australia and the United States. Zoonotic potential exists with this mite.

Clinically, some ferrets will display intense itching accompanied by a scabby yellow and red rash. This rash may appear on the face and ears (**Figs. 5** and **6**). If it is confined to the feet and toes it is called footrot. In these cases paws become swollen and inflamed (**Fig. 7**); in severe cases skin is crusty, and nails may become deformed or even slough.

Rabbits with *Notoedres cati* infections develop cutaneous lesions characterized by hypotrichosis, erythema, and thick brown to gray crusting lesions. *Notoedres* infestation in hamsters occurs after direct contact. In the female hamster clinical signs most commonly are associated with the ears; in male hamsters signs may extend from the nose to the tail, with a scabby dermatitis and severe pruritus.[22]

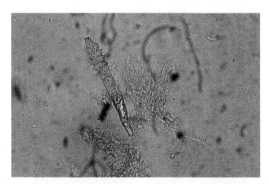

Fig. 4. Microscopic view of teddy hamster *Demodex aurati*, which is cigar-shaped with 4 pairs of stout legs (original magnification ×100). (*Courtesy of* Michael Fehr, PhD, Hannover, Germany.)

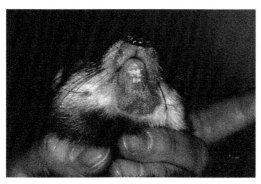

Fig. 5. Ferret *Sarcoptes* sp infestation of the mouth region with alopecia and erythema. (*Courtesy of* Michael Fehr, PhD, Hannover, Germany.)

Diagnosis can be difficult, and multiple skin scrapings may be necessary to reveal the disease. *Sarcoptes* spp have a round body, short legs, and a larger pretarsus than other mites, with bell-shaped suckers on pedicles (**Fig. 8**).[22,23] *Notoedres* spp are considerably smaller than *Sarcoptes* spp, the dorsal striations of *Notoedres cati* have a thumbprint-like appearance owing to a concentric ring formation. The anal opening is dorsal, instead of terminal as in *Sarcoptes* spp.[22,23]

Sarcoptidae: *Trixacarus caviae* In guinea pigs *Trixacarus caviae* is the most important mange ectoparasite found in Australia,[24,25] Austria,[26] Denmark,[27–29] Germany,[30] the United States[31,32] and even in wild guinea pigs in Peru.[33] Asymptomatic carriers exist, and individuals or groups of guinea pigs kept for longer times in isolation suddenly can develop clinical signs, often after stressful situations such as hypovitaminosis C, pregnancy, or suboptimal husbandry. Because *Trixacarus* spp burrow and tunnel into the skin, they often elicit a cell-mediated immune response resulting in a severe pruritus with subsequent erythema, crusts, hyperkeratosis, alopecia, and secondary bacterial dermatitis (**Figs. 9–13**). Scratching-induced self-trauma lesions on the head and neck may be the first clinical signs. Affected animals often lose body weight, and in severe cases intense pruritus has been associated with seizure-like behavior.[34] Deep, bloody skin scrapings are necessary for the confirmation of diagnosis (mix the material collected with 10% KOH solution on a slide, warm up under a Bunsen burner, and

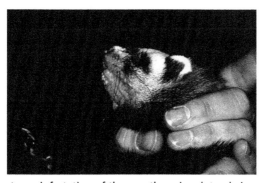

Fig. 6. Ferret *Sarcoptes* sp infestation of the mouth region; lateral view of alopecia and erythema. (*Courtesy of* Michael Fehr, PhD, Hannover, Germany.)

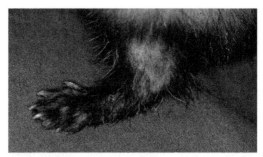

Fig. 7. Ferret *Sarcoptes* sp infestation with alopecia, erythema, and footrot. (*Courtesy of* Michael Fehr, PhD, Hannover, Germany.)

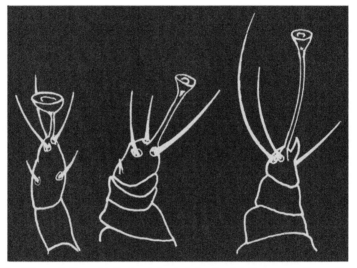

Fig. 8. Mite differentiation aid. Pretarsi short stalks, leg I + II stronger than others = *Chorioptes* spp; pretarsi long on leg I + II, anus dorsal = *Notoedres* spp; short stubby legs, long stalks, anus terminal = *Sarcoptes* spp. (*Courtesy of* Michael Fehr, PhD, Hannover, Germany.)

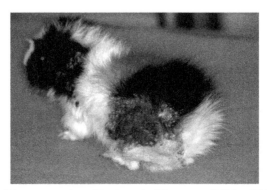

Fig. 9. Guinea pig *Trixacarus caviae* with alopecia. (*Courtesy of* Michael Fehr, PhD, Hannover, Germany.)

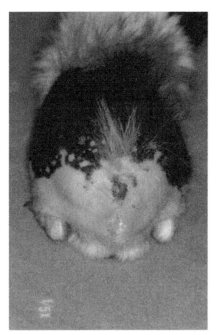

Fig. 10. Guinea pig lumbar region. (*Courtesy of* Michael Fehr, PhD, Hannover, Germany.)

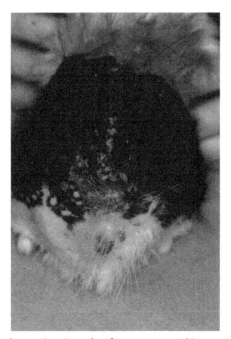

Fig. 11. Guinea pig lumbar region 2 weeks after treatment. (*Courtesy of* Michael Fehr, PhD, Hannover, Germany.)

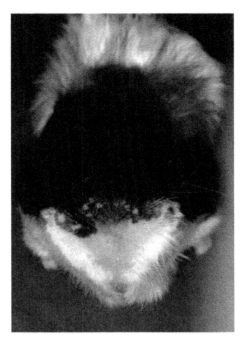

Fig. 12. Guinea pig lumbar region 4 weeks after treatment. (*Courtesy of* Michael Fehr, PhD, Hannover, Germany.)

apply to a coverslip) (**Figs. 14** and **15**). *T caviae* mites are smaller in size than *Sarcoptes scabiei*.[27,34]

Sucking Mites

Psoroptidae
Otodectes cynotis The ear-mite infestation with the psoroptidae, *Otodectes cynoti*, affects ferrets as well as other small animals. Frequently it can be detected in the external auditory meatus in young and elderly ferrets that have close contact with infected ferrets, cats, or dogs. Adult mites are about 0.3 mm in length and therefore too small to be seen with the naked eye. The mites often create an abundance of

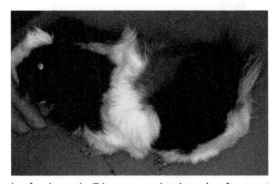

Fig. 13. Whole body of guinea pig *Trixacarus caviae* 4 weeks after treatment. (*Courtesy of* Michael Fehr, PhD, Hannover, Germany.)

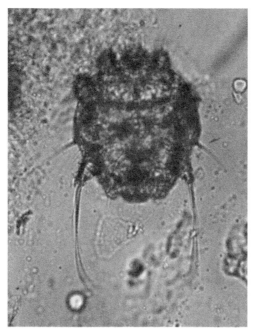

Fig. 14. Microscopic view of *Trixacarus caviae*—1 (original magnification ×400). (*Courtesy of* Michael Fehr, PhD, Hannover, Germany.)

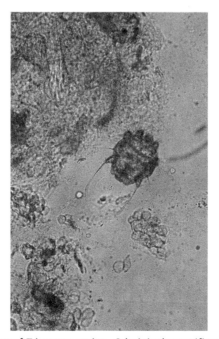

Fig. 15. Microscopic view of *Trixacarus caviae*—2 (original magnification ×200). (*Courtesy of* Michael Fehr, PhD, Hannover, Germany.)

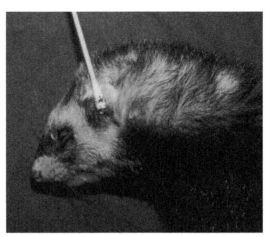

Fig. 16. Otodectic mange in ferret, with brownish waxy ear-canal exudate. (*Courtesy of* Michael Fehr, PhD, Hannover, Germany.)

dark, crumbly or black waxy debris in the ear canal of their host, although healthy ferrets normally have a dark-brown earwax as well (**Figs. 16** and **17**). Because mites feed on ear debris and their presence within the ear canal is irritating, infected ferrets may present with a history of rubbing and/or scratching of the ears with or without head shaking. In rare cases convulsions have been reported.[35,36] Mites may occasionally spread to other parts of the head, neck, and body. In severe cases the mites may

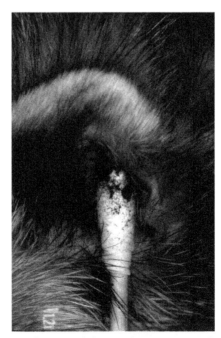

Fig. 17. Otodectic mange in ferret, with brownish waxy ear canal exudate (close-up view). (*Courtesy of* Michael Fehr, PhD, Hannover, Germany.)

destroy the eardrum, causing much deeper infections of middle or inner ear.[37] Ear-mite infection is found throughout the world. Transmission may occur through direct contact, especially of infested females to their kits. Diagnosis is easily made by collecting some of the ear debris and microscopic examination in KOH or liquid paraffin. *Otodectes* sp do not have jointed pretarsi, and the sucker-like pulvillus is cup-shaped, as opposed to trumpet-shaped *Psoroptes* spp infestation. In adult females the third and fourth legs end with a pair of whip-like setae (**Fig. 18**).

Psoroptes cuniculi, Chorioptes cuniculi Psoroptidae are nonburrowing mites, between 1 and 2 mm long, with long legs, especially the third and fourth, usually seen by direct microscopy. Direct detection of white-moving specks is possible.[3,38] Ear-mite infestation in rabbits, also called ear canker, can be mild (**Figs. 19–21**) to severe (**Fig. 22**), resulting in reddish-brown crusting lesions of the ear canal, pruritus, and head shaking. Infestation may also spread to ectopic regions causing alopecia, head tilt, or an aural hematoma.[3]

Caparinia tripilis, Caparinia erinacei *Caparinia* is the most common mite affecting the pet African hedgehog.[39–42] Similar to the Sarcoptidae, these mites burrow into the skin where they form clusters. Hedgehogs with mite infestation show alopecia, spine loss, asbestos-like powdery deposits around the eyes and nose, and encrusted skin lesions especially at the ears (**Figs. 23** and **24**). Pruritus may cause self-trauma resulting in a crusty, scabby dermatitis, with or without a secondary bacterial dermatitis, in rare cases even resulting in host fatality. Mixed mite infestations are also possible.[39] In the United States *Chorioptes* spp can be found in African hedgehogs, with spine loss, crusting, and flaking.[43]

Skin-scraping samples from severely affected areas and microscopic examination may confirm diagnosis (**Figs. 25–28**) Morphologically, pedicles of adult mites are short and unjointed. Tarsal caruncles are bell-shaped on all legs of males (**Fig. 29**), but are absent on legs III and IV of females.

Listrophoridae
Myocoptes musculinus, Myobia musculi, Radfordia ensifera, Notoedres muris Listrophoridae that infest fur-bearing animals have specialized mouth parts

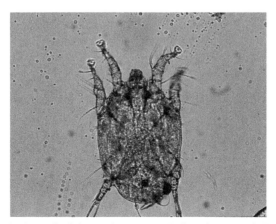

Fig. 18. Microscopic view of adult *Otodectes cynotis*, female, ventral view, third + fourth leg ending with a pair of whip-like setae (original magnification ×100). (*Courtesy of Michael Fehr, PhD, Hannover, Germany.*)

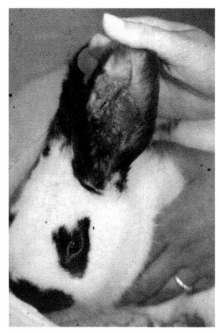

Fig. 19. Rabbit *Psoroptes cuniculi* infestation. (*Courtesy of* Michael Fehr, PhD, Hannover, Germany.)

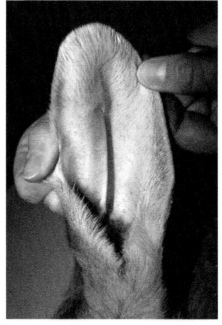

Fig. 20. Rabbit *Psoroptes* spp infestation of left ear canal. (*Courtesy of* Michael Fehr, PhD, Hannover, Germany.)

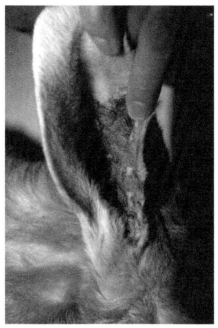

Fig. 21. Rabbit *Psoroptes* spp infestation of right ear canal. (*Courtesy of* Michael Fehr, PhD, Hannover, Germany.)

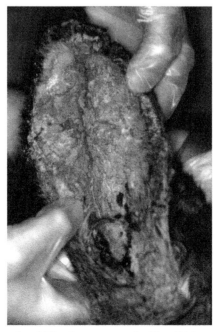

Fig. 22. Heavy ear mange in rabbit; pinnae covered with a thick crust. (*Courtesy of* Michael Fehr, PhD, Hannover, Germany.)

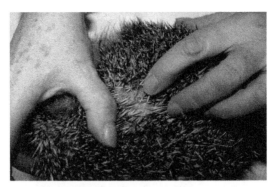

Fig. 23. European hedgehog with yellow-white powdery deposits between the spikes. (*Courtesy of* Michael Fehr, PhD, Hannover, Germany.)

and legs modified for grasping hairs. Fur mites are found to occur more often in mice than in rats, with *Myocoptes* and *Radfordia* being most commonly reported.[3,44] Fur-mite infestation is characterized by alopecia, excoriations, dermatitis, and a dull hair coat. Skin lesions can be detected in all areas of the body, but especially the ears and head (*Myobia musculi*) or along the back (*Myocoptes musculinus*). In chronic cases dermal ulceration may develop (**Figs. 30–32**).

Diagnosis is made by detection of mites on skin scrapes or tape strippings, and examination of collected specimens by microscopy. The first pair of legs is modified to allow the mite to attach itself to the hair of its host.

Surface Mites: Fur Mites

Cheyletiella parasitivorax

Cheyletiella parasitivorax is a mobile fur mite feeding on the skin, creating gray-white flaky, sometimes oily skin scaling with a powdery appearance.[45] When mites can be seen moving under the scales, it is known as "walking dandruff." Distribution of alopecia and scales typically shows a symmetric V-pattern on shoulder and dorsum. The mite is zoonotic and can cause an itching dermatitis even in dogs, cats, and humans.[46] The mite is yellowish, ovoid, about 0.5 mm long to 0.15 mm wide. Eggs are fixed to the

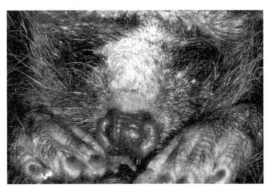

Fig. 24. European hedgehog with yellow-white deposits around eyes and nose. (*Courtesy of* Michael Fehr, PhD, Hannover, Germany.)

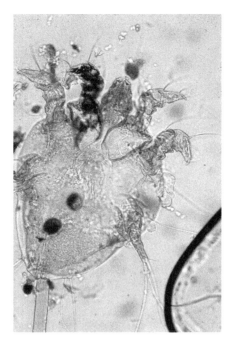

Fig. 25. Microscopic view of hedgehog *Caparinia triplis*—1 (original magnification ×400). (*Courtesy of* Michael Fehr, PhD, Hannover, Germany.)

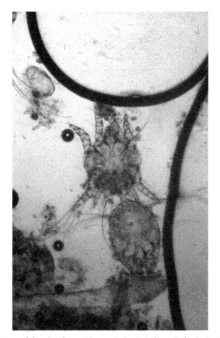

Fig. 26. Microscopic view of hedgehog *Caparinia triplis*—2 (original magnification ×100). (*Courtesy of* Michael Fehr, PhD, Hannover, Germany.)

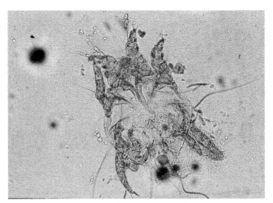

Fig. 27. Microscopic view of *Caparinia triplis*—3 (original magnification ×100). (*Courtesy of* Michael Fehr, PhD, Hannover, Germany.)

hair shaft a few millimeters above the skin layer. For detection, dandruff is combed out onto dark paper and the mite movements and microscopy scrapings observed.[3]

Leporacarus gibbus

Leporacarus gibbus is another rabbit fur mite. Affected animals show a scaly alopecia, and sometimes self-mutilating behavior deriving from a hypersensitivity reaction is recognized.[46] The mite is ovoid, brownish, 0.6 mm long, and up to 0.2 mm broad. The female mite fixes the eggs to hair shafts. This mite is not zoonotic.[4]

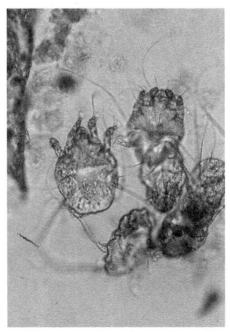

Fig. 28. Microscopic view of *Caparinia triplis*—4 (original magnification ×100). (*Courtesy of* Michael Fehr, PhD, Hannover, Germany.)

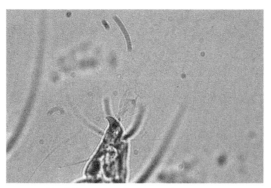

Fig. 29. Microscopic view of bell-like caruncles on male *Caparinia triplis* (original magnification ×600). (*Courtesy of* Michael Fehr, PhD, Hannover, Germany.)

Chirodiscoides caviae

The so-called guinea pig fur mite *Chirodiscoides caviae* can be found clinging to the hair shaft in animals immunosuppressed or with poor condition. Rough hair coat, erythema, alopecia, and scratching-induced dermatitis,[47] as well as concurrent infestation with lice (*Gyropus ovalis*, *Gliricola porcelli*) are common clinical findings (**Figs. 33–41**).[48]

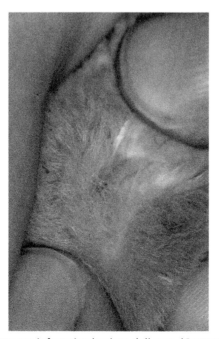

Fig. 30. Mouse *Myocoptes* spp infestation leads to dull coat. (*Courtesy of* Michael Fehr, PhD, Hannover, Germany.)

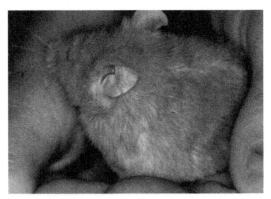

Fig. 31. Mouse *Myocoptes* infestation with alopecia excoriation near the ear. (*Courtesy of* Michael Fehr, PhD, Hannover, Germany.)

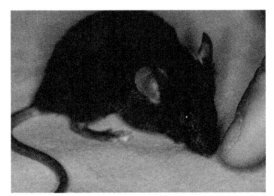

Fig. 32. Mouse *Myocoptes* spp infestation. (*Courtesy of* Michael Fehr, PhD, Hannover, Germany.)

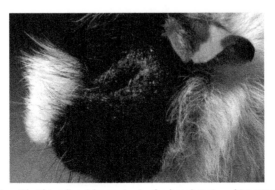

Fig. 33. Guinea pig with *Chirodiscoides caviae* in the head region. (*Courtesy of* Michael Fehr, PhD, Hannover, Germany.)

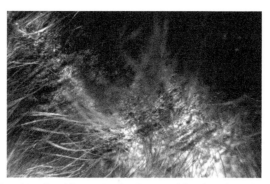

Fig. 34. Guinea pig *Chirodiscoides caviae* leads to scabby skin, hyperkeratosis, and crusts. (*Courtesy of* Michael Fehr, PhD, Hannover, Germany.)

Ornithonyssus bacoti, Ornithonyssus sylvarium, Dermanyssus gallinae

Avian mites can feed on mammals (including men) if the usual bird host is unavailable. One case reports a *Dermanyssus gallinae* infestation in birds with transmission to degus kept together in the same household.[49] The tropical rat mite, *Ornithonyssus bacoti* can affect humans as well as degus, gerbils, hamsters, pygmy African hedgehogs, mice, and rats.[50–56]

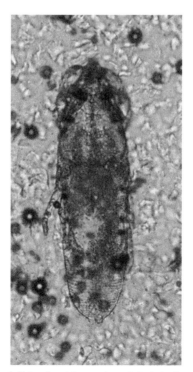

Fig. 35. Microscopic view of *Chirodiscoides caviae*—1 (original magnification ×400). (*Courtesy of* Michael Fehr, PhD, Hannover, Germany.)

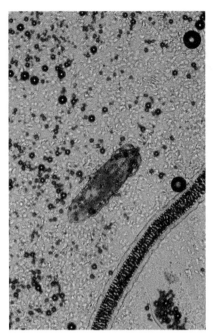

Fig. 36. Microscopic view of *Chirodiscoides caviae*—2 (original magnification ×200). (*Courtesy of* Michael Fehr, PhD, Hannover, Germany.)

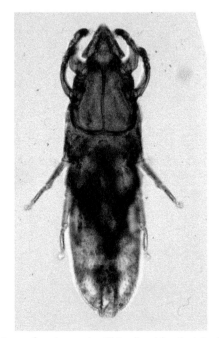

Fig. 37. Microscopic view of guinea pig *Chirodiscoides* (original magnification ×400). (*Courtesy of* Michael Fehr, PhD, Hannover, Germany.)

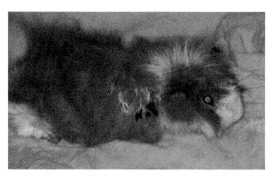

Fig. 38. Guinea pig *Gliricola porcelli* infestation. (*Courtesy of* Michael Fehr, PhD, Hannover, Germany.)

Humans, particularly children in close body contact with their pet rodents, may present with cutaneous lesions such as red papules partly with a central vesicle, predominantly displayed. Hamsters, mice, and rats mostly show nonspecific signs such as increased restlessness, unusual grooming behavior, itching, and shaggy coat (**Figs. 42** and **43**).[57]

The rat mites can be detected on the skin, in the bedding, or in cage wedges. Because of the mite's size (0.7–1.1 mm long), detection of adult parasites is possible by macroscopic examination of host and environment. Diagnosis by naked eye or

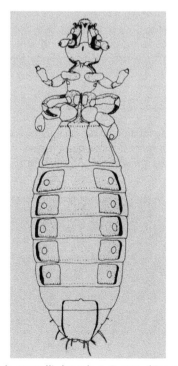

Fig. 39. Drawing of *Gliricola porcelli*, length 1–2 mm. (*Courtesy of* Michael Fehr, PhD, Hannover, Germany.)

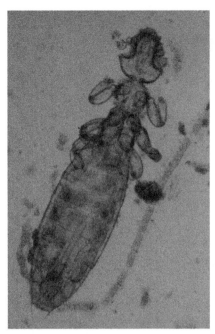

Fig. 40. Microscopic view of lice egg cemented to hair in a guinea pig (original magnification ×400). (*Courtesy of* Michael Fehr, PhD, Hannover, Germany.)

microscopy may show black-colored or (after a heavy blood meal) red-colored mites, with a typical dorsal shield tapering posteriorly and a hairy dorsum. On microscopy *O bacoti* is a hairy mite with a narrow dorsal shield tapering posteriorly (**Figs. 44** and **45**).[47]

Other Mites

Acarus furis

Acarus furis is a nonparasitic mite frequently contaminating animal food and bedding. In cases of optimal environmental conditions these mites can multiply to vast numbers. Jacklin[58] reported a case of nonpruritic dermatitis with alopecia, scaling,

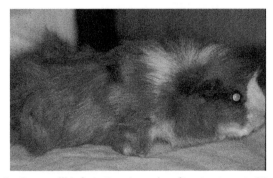

Fig. 41. Guinea pig *G porcelli* infestation 4 weeks after treatment. (*Courtesy of* Michael Fehr, PhD, Hannover, Germany.)

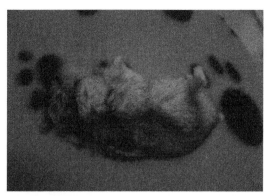

Fig. 42. Dwarf Russian hamster (*Phodophus sungorus*) *Ornithonyssus bacoti* infestation. (*Courtesy of* Michael Fehr, PhD, Hannover, Germany.)

and skin thickening affecting the tail of 3 gerbils. Numerous oval-shaped, 0.3-mm long mites were detected.

Atricholaelaps chinchillae
In addition to mites associated with skin disease, the mite *Atricholaelaps chinchillae* has been reported to occur on the skin of wild chinchillas in Peru.[59]

LICE

According to their feeding manner, lice belong to either the suborder Anoplura (sucking lice), which are characterized by a head that is narrower than the abdomen and thorax, or Mallophaga (chewing lice), which have a head that is as wide as their thorax. Because the females glue the eggs to the hairs, diagnosis is easier by confirming these nits with a magnifying glass. With a strip of adhesive tape, hairs can be detached in the region of crust formation and examined under a microscope.[4]

Polyplax Serrata (Mice, Rat), Polyplax spinulosa (Rat)
Polyplax serrata and *Polyplax spinulosa* are the most common blood-sucking lice in mice and rats.[3] Young, underfed hosts are more often diseased. Severe anemia,

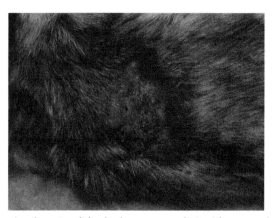

Fig. 43. Dwarf Russian hamster (*Phodophus sungorus*) *Ornithonyssus bacoti* infestation, showing scratch wound. (*Courtesy of* Michael Fehr, PhD, Hannover, Germany.)

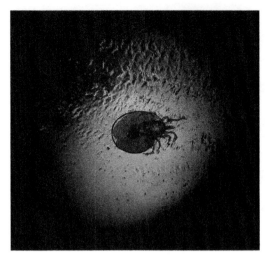

Fig. 44. Microscopic view of *Ornithonyssus bacoti* infestation—1 (original magnification ×100). (*Courtesy of* Michael Fehr, PhD, Hannover, Germany.)

alopecia, and pruritus can be detected. Constant scratching, particularly behind the ears, is often noted. Lice are 0.6 to 1.5 mm long and yellow-brown in color (**Figs. 46–49**). The head is eyeless with prominent 5-segmented antennae. Eggs are glued to the hairs (**Figs. 50** and **51**).[46,60]

Gyropus ovalis, Gliricola porcelli
In guinea pigs, lice infestations with the debris-feeding lice *Gliricola porcelli* or *Gyropus ovalis* are common. Adults of both species are up to 1.5 mm long (*Gyropus* slightly smaller), yellow-gray in color, and often attached to the hair shafts.[61]

Haemodipsus ventricosus
The rabbit louse, *Haemodipsus ventricosus*, is infrequently found on dwarf rabbits. Adult mites measure between 1.5 and 2.0 mm, have a head with short antennae,

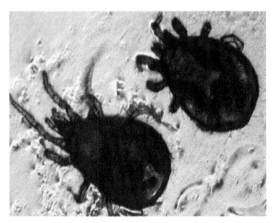

Fig. 45. Microscopic view of *Ornithonyssus bacoti* infestation—2 (original magnification ×200). (*Courtesy of* Michael Fehr, PhD, Hannover, Germany.)

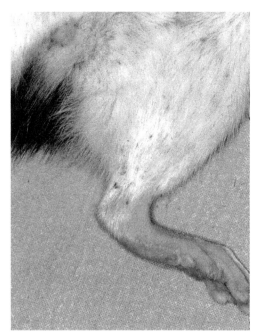

Fig. 46. Rat *Polyplax* spp infestation on the leg. (*Courtesy of* Michael Fehr, PhD, Hannover, Germany.)

and 3 pairs of strong legs with hook-like claws. Eggs are glued to the hairs. This sucking louse can also function as a vector of diseases (eg, tularemia) in animals and humans.[4]

TICKS
Ixodes ricinus, Ixodes hexagonus, Ripicephalus sanguineus, Haemaphysalis erninacei, Haemaphysalis leporisplalustris, Dermacentor variabilis

Ticks may be diagnosed in ferrets, hedgehogs, and rabbits housed outdoors, or in hunting ferrets (**Figs. 52–54**). *Ixodes ricinus* is the most common tick species found

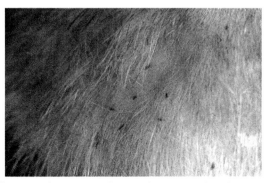

Fig. 47. Rat *Polyplax* spp infestation: red stage. (*Courtesy of* Michael Fehr, PhD, Hannover, Germany.)

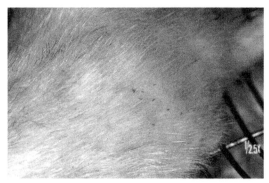

Fig. 48. Rat *Polyplax* spp infestation: yellow-brown nymphal stage (dorsal body). (*Courtesy of* Michael Fehr, PhD, Hannover, Germany.)

in central Europe, but *Ripicephalus* sp, *Haemaphysalis* sp, and others are also common.[62–64] In the northeastern United States rabbits are commonly parasitized by *Ixodes scapularis*, *Ixodes dentatus*, *Haemaphysalis leporisplalustris*, or *Dermacentor variabilis*.[65] In hedgehogs mostly *I ricinus* infestations are diagnosed, and rarely *Ixodes hexagonus*.

There are also no clinical cases of Lyme disease in rabbits, but the isolation of antibodies to antigens of *Borrelia burgdorferi* were reported in Chinese rabbits[66] and in cottontail rabbits captured in New York.[65] No cases of Lyme disease in ferrets or hedgehogs have been reported.[35]

Because all ticks mentioned may also be found on cats and dogs, as well as other vertebrate hosts, they may serve as a biological vector for *Borrelia* sp or other tick-borne diseases, and may also play a role in human zoonosis. These mammalian hosts and related lagomorphs should therefore be monitored closely.[65]

FLEAS
Ctenocephalides spp, Ceratophyllus sciorum, Pulex irritans, Nosopsylla spp, Spilopsyllus cuniculi, Xenopsylla spp

Flea infestation in chinchillas, ferrets, hedgehogs, mice, and rats by direct transmission, or indirectly via a flea-infested environment, can be detected. Captive chinchillas, mice, rats, rabbits and so forth that are housed with infested dogs or cats may also become infested with *Ctenocephalides* spp. If exposed to wild rats or

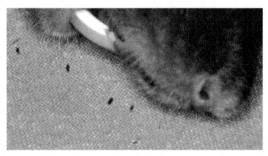

Fig. 49. Rat *Polyplax* lice, 0.6–1.5 mm in length. (*Courtesy of* Michael Fehr, PhD, Hannover, Germany.)

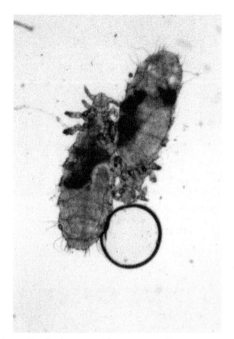

Fig. 50. Microscopic view of *Polyplax* sp, with segmented antennae and distinct ventral sternal plate (original magnification ×100). (*Courtesy of* Michael Fehr, PhD, Hannover, Germany.)

mice, *Nosopsylla* spp or *Xenopsylla* spp can be detected in pet rodents. Wild rabbits infested with the rabbit flea *Spilopsyllus cuniculi* may serve as an important vector in the transmission of myxomatosis.[67]

Flea infestation may be asymptomatic but can also cause clinical signs, with affected animals showing dull hair coats, pruritus, flea-bite hypersensitivities, and secondary bacterial dermatitis. In severe cases anemia and death can occur. Identification of fleas or flea excrement confirms the diagnosis. Diagnosis is easy because fleas can directly be detected on hairless regions such as ears, or by evidence of flea excrement when the fur is grossly examined (**Figs. 55–57**).

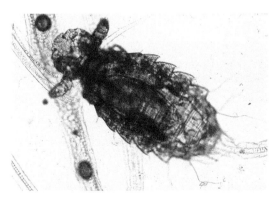

Fig. 51. Microscopic view of *Polyplax* spp infestation (original magnification ×150). (*Courtesy of* Michael Fehr, PhD, Hannover, Germany.)

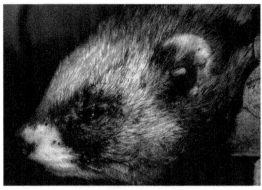

Fig. 52. Adult *Ixodes ricinus* infestation on a ferret. Gray fed females, unfed adults, and larvae. (*Courtesy of* Michael Fehr, PhD, Hannover, Germany.)

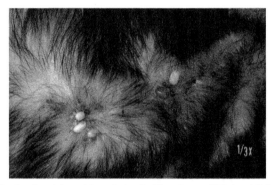

Fig. 53. Ferret ticks *Ixodes ricinus* (dorsal view). (*Courtesy of* Michael Fehr, PhD, Hannover, Germany.)

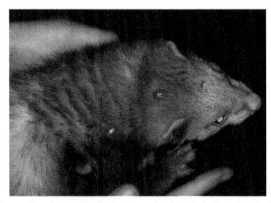

Fig. 54. Ferret ticks *Ixodes ricinus* on the body region, with fed and unfed adults and larvae. (*Courtesy of* Michael Fehr, PhD, Hannover, Germany.)

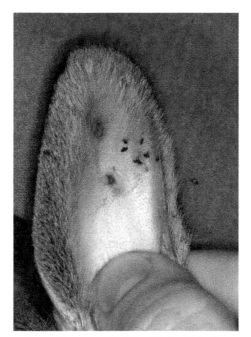

Fig. 55. Rabbit with ear fleas. (*Courtesy of* Michael Fehr, PhD, Hannover, Germany.)

Archeopsylla erinacei, Ceratophyllus gallinae, Ctenocephalides felis

Nearly every wild living hedgehog is infested with ticks and fleas.

Archeopsylla erinacei, Ceratophyllus gallinae, and *Ctenocephalides felis* flea infestations were detected in 76 hedgehogs in Germany.[63] Macroscopic detection of ectoparasites between the spines is diagnostic (**Figs. 58** and **59**).

HELMINTHS
Hypodema spp, Cuterebra spp, Dracunculus insignis

Cuterebriasis can occur if ferrets, rabbits, and so forth are housed outdoors in times of warm weather. The hatched larvae of cuterebra flies can crawl into the fur, then enter the subcutis through body openings. The resultant swelling has a typical breathing hole visible at the skin surface. Larvae of 1 to 3 cm length can be visualized within

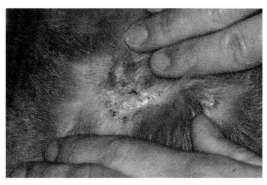

Fig. 56. Rabbit flea excreta, neck region. (*Courtesy of* Michael Fehr, PhD, Hannover, Germany.)

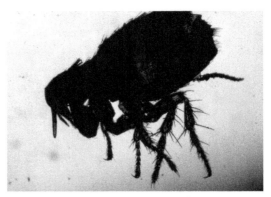

Fig. 57. Microscopic view of rabbit flea (original magnification ×10). (*Courtesy of* Michael Fehr, PhD, Hannover, Germany.)

the lesion. Extraction of larvae without damage, followed by debridement of necrotic tissue, can be done after incising the skin through the breathing hole. Fly control, wound care, and (possibly) antibiotics are required.[3]

THERAPY

The treatment of ectoparasites in small mammals is challenging, because many products are not licensed for the use in exotic companion mammals, and as a result care should be taken to prescribe appropriate safe products (see **Tables 1–9** in the Appendix). Treatment options in small exotic mammals with ectoparasites correspond to options in dogs and cats with the same disease. Topical solutions and, if possible, sprays should be applied to the back of the neck so that the animal cannot reach the treatment region, thus avoiding licking of the agent. Shampooing can be very stressful to these small animals, resulting in panic reactions, broken legs, or even cardiac arrest. If large enough, ectoparasites can be removed by physically combing them out or with the help of forceps. The environment must be thoroughly cleaned, with vacuuming of carpets and the application of acaricides recommended. Potential sources of contamination such as bedding and towels must be removed, and if necessary washed at temperatures higher than 60°C/140°F.[4] All household pets should be treated to avoid recontamination. In cases of *O bacoti* infestations, the help of an exterminator is advised.[46]

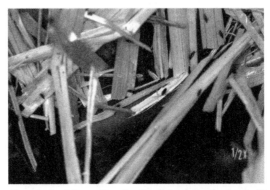

Fig. 58. Hedgehog fleas in bedding after death of host (hedgehog). (*Courtesy of* Michael Fehr, PhD, Hannover, Germany.)

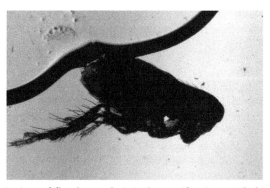

Fig. 59. Microscopic view of flea larvae (original magnification ×10). (*Courtesy of* Michael Fehr, PhD, Hannover, Germany.)

DRUG CONTRAINDICATIONS

Evidence-based studies of acaricide drug interactions in small mammals are sparse; contraindications for drug use therefore are mainly based on clinical reports. In certain species drug contraindications have to be considered, based on reported adverse product reactions. Dichlorvos-impregnated flea collars should not be used in ferrets.[35] Ivermectin should not be applied on pregnant ferrets, owing to the increased rate of congenital defects.[72] Because of reports of adverse reactions, including deaths, associated with the use of fipronil (Frontline) in rabbits, it is not recommended for use in this species, especially young, debilitated, and underweight rabbits.[119–121,130,131] Adverse reactions to fipronil have also been reported in sick hedgehogs.[120,132] The use of flea collars in rabbits should be avoided because of chemical skin burning. Pyrethrin-based flea powders should also be cautioned because of reported adverse side effects including seizures, tremors, and limb paralysis.[4]

SUMMARY

Small exotic mammals can be infested with a variety of skin parasites (mites, lice, fleas, ticks, helminths) that inhabit the fur and/or skin. Parasite-associated skin puncturing, epidermal lesions, or dermal surface scavenging, with or without the ingestion of blood, lymph, sebaceous secretions, and skin debris, often leads to pruritic dermatoses. In some cases a cell-mediated hypersensitivity to parasite antigen may induce dermal erythema, excoriations, crusts, hyperkeratosis, alopecia, and secondary bacterial dermatitis. In guinea pigs intense pruritus has been associated with seizure-like behavior. Diagnosis is mainly based on direct and microscopic visualization of ectoparasites, microscopic examination of trichograms, tape preparations, and deep skin scrapings. At present, a lack of licensed antiparasiticides for use in exotic species in most countries requires off-label use of many of the effective pharmaceuticals recommended for treatment. For prevention of reinfestation the treatment of all housed pets, cleaning of cages and the environment, and, if necessary, professional disinfection of the living quarters is advised.

REFERENCES

1. Barron HW. Dermatologic disease in exotic pets: an introduction. J Exotic Pet Med 2007;16(4):209.

2. Hill PB, Eden CA, Huntley S, et al. Survey of the prevalence, diagnosis and treatment of dermatological conditions in small animals in general practice. Vet Rec 2006;158(16):533–9.
3. Hoppmann E, Barron HW. Ferret and rabbit dermatology. J Exotic Pet Med 2007;16(4):225–55.
4. Van Praag E, Maurer A, Saarony T. Skin diseases of rabbits. Switzerland: MediRabbit.com; 2010.
5. Reynold SL, Gainer JH. Dermatitis of Mongolian gerbils (Meriones unguiculatus) caused by Demodex sp'. Scientific sessions of the 19th Annual Meeting of Am Assoc Lab Anim Sci, Las Vegas, Nevada, 1968, No. 150.
6. Schwarzbrott SS, Wagner JE, Frisk CS. Demodicosis in the Mongolian gerbil (*Meriones unguiculatus*): a case report. Lab Anim Sci 1974;24(4):666–8.
7. Walberg JA, Stark DM, Desch C, et al. Demodicosis in laboratory rats (*Rattus norvegicus*). Lab Anim Sci 1981;31:60–2.
8. Häfeli W. Demodicosis in guinea pigs. Kleintierpraxis 1989;34:337–8.
9. Bukva V. Demodex species parasitizing the brown rat. Folia Parasitol (Praha) 1995;42:149–60.
10. Zwart P, Treiber A. Gerbil. In: Gabrisch K, Zwart P, editors. Heimtierkrankheiten. Hannover (Germany): Schlütersche; 2008. p. 163–82.
11. Harvey RG. *Demodex cuniculi* in dwarf rabbits (*Oryctolagus cuniculus*). J Small Anim Pract 1990;31:204–7.
12. Schönfelder J, Henneveld K, Schönfelder A, et al. Concurrent infestation of *Demodex caviae* and *Chirodiscoides caviae* in a guinea pig. Tierarztl Prax 2010; 91(1):28–30.
13. Charlesworth EN, Clegern RW. Tropical rat mite dermatitis. Arch Dermatol 1977; 113:937–8.
14. Noli C, van der Horst HH, Willemse T. Demodicosis in ferrets (*Mustela putorius furo*). Vet Q 1996;18(1):28–31.
15. Beaufrere H, Neta M, Smith DA, et al. Demodectic mange associated with lymphoma in a ferret. J Exotic Pet Med 2009;18(1):57–61.
16. Owen D, Young C. The occurrence of *Demodex aurati* and *Demodex criceti* in the Syrian hamster (*Mesocricetus auratus*) in United Kingdom. Vet Rec 1973; 92:282–4.
17. Nutting WB. *Demodex aurati* sp. nov. and *D. criceti*, ectoparasites of the golden hamster (*Mesocricetus auratus*). Parasitology 1961;51:515–22.
18. Estes PC, Richter CB, Franklin JA. Demodectis mange in the golden hamster. Lab Anim Sci 1971;21:825–8.
19. Hasegawa T. A case report of the management of demodicosis in the golden hamster. J Vet Med Sci 1995;57(2):337–8.
20. Karaer Z, Kurtdede A, Ural K, et al. Demodicosis in a golden (Syrian) hamster (*Mesocricetus auratus*). Ankara Üniv Vet Fak Derg 2009;56:227–9.
21. Sarashina T, Sato K. Demodicosis in the golden hamster. Nippon Juigaku Zasshi 1986;48:619–22.
22. Beco L, Petite A, Olivry T. Comparison of subcutaneous ivermectin and oral moxidectin for the treatment of notoedric acariasis in hamsters. Vet Rec 2001; 149(11):324–7.
23. Rosen LB. Dermatologic manifestations of zoonotic diseases in exotic animals. J Exotic Pet Med 2011;20(1):9–13.
24. Collins GH, Rothwell TLW. Trixacarus caviae in guinea pigs. Austr Vet J 1982;58: 120–2.

25. Shipstone M. *Trixacarus caviae* infestation in guinea pig: failure to respond to ivermectine administration. Austr Vet Pract 1997;27:143–6.

26. Hinaidy K, Loupal G. Occurrence of mange in guinea pigs caused by Trixacarus caviae in Austria. Tieraerztl Prax 1988;16:93–6.

27. Hansen KA, deTengnagel LF. Mange mite infestation of guinea pigs caused by *Trixacaraus* (*Caviacoptes*) *caviae*: diagnosis and therapy. Europ J Comp Anim Pract 1992;2(2):21–2.

28. Hirsjavi P, Phyala L. Ivermectin treatment of a colony of guinea pigs infested with fur mite (*Chirodiscoides caviae*). Lab Anim 1995;29:200–3.

29. Honda M, Namikawa K, Hirata H, et al. An outbreak of *Trixacarus caviae* infestation of guinea pigs at an animal petting facility and an evaluation of the safety and suitable dose of seleamectin treatment. J Parasitol 2011;97(4):731–4.

30. Schossier N, Fehr M. The management of sarcoptes mange in guinea pigs with Amitraz and Ivermectin. Kleintierpraxis 1989;34(11):569–72.

31. Kummel BA, Estes SA, Arlian LG. *Trixacarus caviae* infestation of guinea pigs. J Am Vet Med Assoc 1980;177:903–8.

32. Zajac A, Williams JF, Williams CSF. Mange caused by *Trixacarus caviae* in guinea pigs. J Am Vet Med Assoc 1980;177:898–900.

33. Dittmar de la Cruz K, Ribbeck R, Daugschies A. Presence and distribution of ectoparasites in guinea pigs (*Cavia* spp.) in Peru, South America. Berl Munch Tierarztl Wochenschr 2003;116(3):102–7.

34. Esher D, Bdolah-Abram T. Comparison of efficacy, safety, and convenience of selamectin versus ivermectin for treatment of *Trixacarus caviae* mange in pet guinea pigs (*Cavia procellus*). J Am Vet Med Assoc 2012;241(8):1056–8.

35. Paterson S. Skin diseases in exotic pets. Oxford (United Kingdom): Blackwell; 2006. p. 223–4.

36. Moormann-Roest H. Ferrets. In: Gabrisch K, Zwart P, editors. Krankheiten der Heimtiere. Hannover (Germany): Schlüetersche; 2008. p. 263–306.

37. Kelleher SA. Skin diseases of the ferret. Vet Clin North Am Exot Anim Pract 2001; 4(2):565–72.

38. Hutchinson MJ, Jacobs DE, Bell GD, et al. Evaluation of imidacloprid for the treatment and prevention of cat flea (*Ctenocephalides felis felis*) infestations on rabbits. Vet Rec 2001;148(22):695–6.

39. Heath AC, Rush-Munro RM, Rutherford DM. The hedgehog: a new host record for *Notoedres muris* (Acari, Sarcoptidae). N Z Entomol 1971;5:100–3.

40. Ivey E, Carpenter JW. African hedgehogs. In: Quesenberry KE, Carpenter JW, editors. Ferrets, rabbits, and rodents. 3rd edition. St Louis (MO): Elsevier; 2012. p. 411–27.

41. Kim DH, Oh DS, Ahn KS, et al. An outbreak of *Caparinia tripilis* in a colony of African Pygmy hedgehogs (*Atelerix albiventris*) from Korea. Korean J Parasitol 2012;50(2):151–6.

42. Hoefer HL. Hedgehogs. Vet Clin North Am Small Anim Pract 1994;24(1):113–20.

43. Larson RS, Carpenter JW. Husbandry and medical management of African hedgehogs. Vet Med 1999;94:877–90.

44. Bornstein S. Mange in domesticated rats. Vet Rec 1997;140(1):28–9.

45. Mellgren M, Bergvall K. Treatment of rabbit cheyletiellosis with selamectin or ivermectin: a retrospective study. Acta Vet Scand 2008;50:1.

46. Beck W. Case report: pediculosis by *Polyplax*-lice (Anoplura: Hoplopleuridae) in mouse and rat—biology of *Polyplax* sp., pathogenesis, clinical features, diagnosis and treatment. Kleintierpraxis 1999;44:461–7.

47. Beck W. Mass infestation by tropical rat mite, *Ornithonyssus bacoti* (Acari: Macronyssidae), in gerbil—experiences to the treatment with selamectin (Stronghold^R). Kleintierpraxis 2002;47:607–13.

48. White SD, Bourdeau PJ, Meredith A. Dermatologic problems in guinea pigs. Compend Contin Educ Pract Vet 2003;25(9):690–700.

49. Sassenburg L. Degu. In: Gabrisch K, Zwart P, editors. Diseases of exotic pets. Hannover (Germany): Schluetersche; 2008. p. 215–38.

50. Keefe TJ, Scanlon JE, Wetherald LD. *Ornithonyssus bacoti* (Hirst) infestation in mouse and hamster colonies. Lab Anim Care 1964;14:366–9.

51. Beck W. Common ectoparasitic diseases and dematophytosis in small mammals, birds and reptiles. Prakt Tierarzt 2003;10:752–62.

52. Beck W, Fölster-Holst R. Tropical rat mites (*Ornithonyssus bacoti*)—serious ectoparasites. J Dtsch Dermatol Ges 2009;7(8):67–70.

53. Hill WA, Randolph MM, Boyd KL, et al. Use of permethrin eradicated the tropical rat mite (Ornithonyssus bacoti) from a colony of mutagenized and transgenic mice. Contemp Top Lab Anim Sci 2005;44(5):31–4.

54. Creel NB, Crowe MA, Mullen GR. Pet hamsters as a source of rate mite dermatitis. Cutis 2003;71:457–61.

55. Lucky AW, Savers C, Arcus JD, et al. Avian mite bites acquired from a new source—pet gerbils: report of 2 cases and review of the literature. Arch Dermatol 2001;137(2):167–70.

56. Leonatti SR. *Ornithonyssus bacoti* mite infestation in an African pygmy hedgehog. Exotic DVM 2007;9:3–4.

57. Baumstark J, Beck W, Hofmann H. Outbreak of tropical rat mite (*Ornithonyssus bacoti*) dermatitis in a house for disabled persons. Dermatology 2007;215:66–8.

58. Jacklin MR. Demodicosis sassociated with acarus farris in gerbils. J Small Anim Pract 1977;38(9):410–1.

59. Strandtmann RW. *Atricholaelps traubi* and *A. chinchillulae*, from calloscirurus and the chinchilla respectively. Proc Entomol Soc Wash 1948;50:187–92.

60. Levine JF, Lage AL. House mouse mites infesting laboratory rodents. Lab Anim Sci 1984;34(4):393–4.

61. Kim SH, Jun HK, Yoo MJ, et al. Use of a formulation containing imidacloprid and moxidectin in the treatment of lice infestation in guinea pigs. Vet Dermatol 2008; 19:187–8.

62. Loewenstein M, Prosl H, Loupal G. Parasitoses of the hedgehog and their control. Wien Tierärzl Wschr 1991;78:127–35.

63. Visser M, Rehbein S, Wiedemann C. Species of flea (siphonaptera) infesting pets and hedgehogs in Germany. J Vet Med B Infect Dis Vet Public Health 2001;48(3):197–202.

64. Staley EC, Staley EE, Behr MJ. Use of permethrin as a miticide in the African hedgehog (Atelerix albiventris). Vet Hum Toxicol 1994;36:138.

65. Magnarelli LA, Norris SJ, Fikrig E. Serum antibodies to whole-cell and recombinant antigens of *Borrelia burgdorferi* in cottontail rabbits. J Wildl Dis 2012;48(1): 12–20.

66. Zhan L, Chu CY, Zuo SQ, et al. *Anaplasma phagocytophilum* and *Borrelia burgdorferi* in rabbits from southeastern China. Vet Parasitol 2009;162(3–4):354–6.

67. Sobey WR, Conolly D. Myxomatosis: the introduction of the European rabbit flea *Spilopsyllus cuniculi* (Dale) into wild rabbit populations in Australia. J Hyg (Lond) 1971;69(3):331–46.

68. Fox JG. Outbreak of tropical rat mite dermatitis in laboratory personnel. Arch Dermatol 1982;118:767–8.

69. Jacklin MR. Dermatosis associated with *Acarus farris* in gerbils. J Small Anim Pract 1977;38(9):410–1.
70. Castro F, Gonzalez A, et al. Contribution to the knowledge of the genus Hoplopleura Enderlein, 1904, (Anolpura, Holopleuridae): a new species parasitic on Octodontidae (Rodentiae). Rev Bras Entomol 1998;41:2–4.
71. Goff M, Ebb J Jr. A new species of *Paraguacarus* (Acari; Trombiculidae) from a degu (Mammalia: Rodentia) collected in Chile. J Vec Ecol 1989;14(1):93–4.
72. Orcutt C, Tater K. Dermatologic diseases. In: Quesenberry KE, Carpenter JW, editors. Ferrets, rabbits, and rodents. Clinical medicine and surgery. St Louis (MO): Elsevier; p. 122–31.
73. Patterson MM, Kirchain SM. Comparison of three treatments for control of ear mites in ferrets. Lab Anim Sci 1999;49:655–7.
74. Miller DS, Eagle RP, Zabel S, et al. Efficacy and safety of selamectin in the treatment of *Otodectes cynotis* infestation in domestic ferrets. Vet Rec 2006;159(22): 748–50.
75. Oglesbee BL. The 5-minute veterinary consult. Ferret and rabbit. Ames (IA): Blackwell; 2006. p. 157–8.
76. Wenzel U, Heine J, Mwengel H, et al. Efficacy of imidacloprid 10%/mioxidectin 1% (Advocate/Advantage Mulit) against fleas (*Cteneocephalides felis felis*) on ferrets (*Mustela putorius furo*). Parasitol Res 2008;103:231.
77. Fisher MA, Jacobs DE, Hutchinson MJ, et al. Efficacy of imidacloprid on ferrets experimentally infested with the cat flea *Cteneocephalides felis*. Comp Cintinun Educ Pract Vet Suppl 2001;23(4A):8–10.
78. Martin AL, Irizarry-Rovira AR, Bevier DE, et al. Histology of ferret skin: preweaning to adulthood. Vet Dermatol 2007;18:401–11.
79. Larsen KS, Siggurdsson H, Mencke N. Efficacy of imidacloprid, imidacloprid/permethrin and phoxim for flea control in the Mustelidae (ferrets, mink). Parasitol Res 2005;97(Suppl 1):107–12.
80. Molnar V, Pazar P, Rigo D, et al. Autochthonous *Dirofilaria immitis* infection in a ferret with aberrant larval migration in Europe. J Small Anim Pract 2010;51:393–6.
81. Fain A, Hovell GJ, Hyatt KH. A new sarcoptid mite producing mange in albino guinea-pigs. Acta Zool Pathol Antverp 1972;56:73–82.
82. McKellar QA, Midgley DM, Galbraith EA, et al. Clinical and pharmacological properties of ivermectin in rabbits and guinea pigs. Vet Rec 1992;130(4):71–3.
83. Esghar D, Bdolah-Abram T. Comparison of efficacy, safety, and convenience of selamectin versus ivermectin for treatment of Trixacarus caviae mange in pet guinea pigs (Cavia porcellus). J Am Vet Med Assoc 2012;241(8):1056–8.
84. Haefeli W. Demodicosis in guinea pigs. Kleintierpraxis 1989;34:337–8.
85. Schoenfelder J, Hennveld K, Schönfelder AJ, et al. Concurrent infestation of Demodex caviae and Chirodiscoides caviae in a guinea pig. Tieraerztl Prax 2010;38(K):28–30.
86. Beck W. Fur mites (*Chirodiscoides caviae*) in guinea pigs. Kleintiermedizin 2002;1:10–4.
87. Timm KI. Pruritus in Rabbits. Rodents and Ferrets. vet Clin North Am Small Anim Pract 1988;18(5):1077–91.
88. Letcher JD. Amitraz as a treatment for acariasis in African hedgehogs (*Atelerix albiventris*). J Zoo Wildl Med 1988;19:24–9.
89. Hoefer HL. Hedgehogs. Vet Clin North An Small Anim Pract 1984;24(1):113–20.
90. Arbona R, Lipman NS, Riedel ER, et al. Treatment and eradication of murine fur mites: toxicologic evaluations of ivermectin-compounded feed. J Am Assoc Lab Anim Sci 2010;49:564–70.

91. Baumanns V, Havenaar R, Rooymanns TP. The effectiveness of Ivomec and Neguvon in the control of murine mites. Lab Anim 1988;11:243–5.

92. Wing SR, Courtney CH, Young M. Effect of ivermectin on murine mites. J Am Vet Med Assoc 1985;187:1191–2.

93. Cole JS, Sabol-Jones M, Karolewski B, et al. Ornithonyssus bacoti infestation and elimination from a mouse colony. Cotemp Top Lab Anim Sci 2005;44(5): 27–30.

94. West WL, Schofield JC, Bennet BT. Efficacy of the "micro-dot" technique for administering topical 1% ivermectin for the control of pinworms and fur mites in mice. Contemp Top Lab Anim Sci 1992;31:7–10.

95. Gönenc B, Sarimehmetoglu HO, Ica A, et al. Efficacy of selamectin against mites (*Myobia musculi, Myoptes musculinus* and *Ratfordia ensifera*) and nematodes (*Aspiculuris tetraptera* and *Syphacia abvelata*) in mice. Lab Anim 2006; 40:201–13.

96. Kondo S, Taylor A, Chun S. Elimination of an infestation of rat fur mites (*Ratfordia ensifera*) from a colony of Long Evans rats, using the micro-dot technique for topical administration of 1% ivermectin. Contemp Top Lab Anim Sci 1998;37: 58–61.

97. Brown C, Donelley TM. Disease problems of small rodents. In: Quesenberry KE, Carpenter JW, editors. Ferrets, rabbits, and rodents. 3rd edition. St Louis (MO): Elsevier; 2012. p. 354–72.

98. Cohen SR. Cheyletiella dermatitis: a mite infestation of rabbit, cat, dog, and man. Arch Dermatol 1980;116(4):435–7.

99. Ellis C, Mori M. Skin diseases of rodents and small exotic mammals. Vet Clin North Am Exot Anim Pract 2001;4(2):493–502.

100. Fisher M, Beck W, Hutchinson MJ. Efficacy and safety of selamectin (Stronghold^R/Revolution^{TM}) used off-label in exotic pets. Int J Appl Res Vet Med 2007;5(3):87–96.

101. Paterson S. Skin diseases and treatments of guinea pigs. In: Patterson S, editor. Skin Diseases of Exotic Pets. Oxford (UK): Blackwell Science; 2006. p. 232–50.

102. MacHole EJ. Mange in domesticated rats. Vet Rec 1996;138:312–3.

103. Sparrow S. Diseases of rodents. J Small Anim Pract 1980;21:1–16.

104. Meredith A. Dermatology of mammals. In: Paterson S, editor. Skin diseases of exotic pets. Ames (IA): Blackwell Publishing; 2006. p. 175–324.

105. Hoppmann E, Barron HW. Ferret and Rabbit Dermatology. J Exotic Pet Med 2007;16(4):225–37.

106. Kurtdede A, Karaer Z, Acar A, et al. Use of selamectin for the treatment of psoroptic and sarcoptic mite infestation in rabbits. Vet Dermatol 2007;18:18–22.

107. Mousa S, Gada N, Sokkar L, et al. Efficacy of a single injectable dose of ivermectin for psoroptic and sarcoptic mange in rabbits. Assiut Vet Med J 1986; 17(33):237–9.

108. Patel A, Robinson KJ. Dermatosis associated with *Listrophorus gibbus* in the rabbit. J Small Anim Pract 1993;34:409–11.

109. Curtis SK, Housley R. Brooks DL. Use of ivermectin for treatment of ear mite infestation in rabbits. J Am Vet Med Assoc 1990;196:1139–40.

110. Beck W, Möbius S, Hansen O, et al. Efficacy of a formulation containing imidacloprid and moxidectin (Advocate^R) against naturally acquired ear mange in rabbits. Kleintierpraxis 2006;51(5):256–62.

111. Prosl H, Kangout AG. Therapy of ear mange in rabbits with ivermectine. Berl Munch Tierarztl Wochenschr 1985;98:45–7.

112. Sang-Hun K, Hyung-Kyou J, Kun-Ho S, et al. Prevalence of fur mites in pet rabbits in South Korea. Vet Dermatol 2008;19(3):189–90.
113. Cutler SL. Ectopic *Psoroptes cuniculi* infestation in a pet rabbit. J Small Anim Pract 1998;39:86–7.
114. Farmaki R, Koutinas F, Papazahariadou G, et al. Effectiveness of a selamectin spot-on formulation in rabbits with sarcoptic mange. Vet Rec 2009;164(4):431–2.
115. McTier TL, Hair JA, Walstrom DJ, et al. Efficacy and safety of topical administration of selamectin for treatment of ear mite infestation in rabbits. J Am Vet Med Assoc 2003;223(3):322–4.
116. Wagner R, Wendlberger U. Field efficacy of moxidectin in dogs and rabbits naturally infested with *Sarcoptes* spp., *Demodex* spp. and *Psoroptes* spp. mites. Vet Parasitol 2000;93(2):149–58.
117. White SD, Bourdeau PJ, Meredith A. Dermatologic problems in rabbits. Sem Avian Exotic Pet Med 2002;11(3):141–50.
118. Wright FC, Riner JC. Comparative efficacy of injection routes and doses of ivermectin against *Psoroptes* in rabbits. Am J Vet Res 1985;46:752–4.
119. Cooper PE, Penaliggon J. Use of frontline spray on rabbits. Vet Rec 1997;140: 535–6.
120. Beck CW. Efficacy of fipronil (FRONTLINE[R]) against ectoparasites: application against lice, mites, and mallophages in diverse small mammals. Tierarztl Umsch 2000;55:244–50.
121. Johnston MS. Clinical toxicoses of domestic rabbits. Vet Clin North Am Exot Anim Pract 2008;11(2):315–26.
122. Timm KI. Pruritus in rabbits, rodents and ferrets. Vet Clin North Am Small Anim Pract 1988;18(5):1077–91.
123. Kennedy AH. Chinchilla diseases and ailments. Toronto: Fur Trade Journal of Canada; 1952. p. 259.
124. Birke LL, Molina PE, Baker DG, et al. Comparison of selamectin and imidacloprid plus permethrin in eliminating *Leporacarus gibus* infestation in laboratory rabbits (*Oryctolagus cuniculus*). J Am Assoc Lab Anim Sci 2009;48(6):757–62.
125. Cole JS, Sabol-Jones M, Karolewski B, et al. Ornithonyssus bacoti infestation and elimination from a mouse colony. Contemp Top Lab Anim Sci 2005;44(5): 27–30.
126. Hansen O, Mencke N, Pfister K, et al. Efficacy of a formulation containing Imidacloprid and Permethrin against naturally acquired ectoparasite infestations (*Ctencephalides felis*, *Cheyletiella parasitivorax*, and *Listrophorus gibbus*) in rabbits. Int J Appl Res Vet Med 2006;4(4):320–5.
127. Carpenter JW, Dryden MW, KuKanich B. Pharmacokinetics, efficacy, and adverse effects of selamectin following topical administration in flea-infested rabbits. Am J Vet Res 2012;73(4):562–6.
128. Pinter L. *Leporacarus gibus* and *Spilopsyllus cuniculi* infestation in a pet rabbit. J Small Anim Pract 1999;40(5):220–1.
129. Jenkins JR. Skin disorders of the rabbit. Vet Clin North Am Exot Anim Pract 2001;4(2):543–63.
130. Curtis SK. Diagnostic exercise: moist dermatitis on the hind quarters of a rabbit. Lab Anim Sci 1991;41(6):623–4.
131. Curtis SK, Housley R, Brooks DL. Use of ivermectin for treatment of ear mite infestation in rabbits. J Am Vet Med Assoc 1990;196(7):1139–40.
132. Hatch C, Doode DJ. Fleas on hedgehogs and dogs. Vet Rec 1986;119(7): 162–4.

APPENDIX

Table 1
Treatment of ectoparasites in chinchillas

Species	Ectoparasite	Clinical Signs	Treatment	Comments
Chinchilla *Chinchilla lanigera* (long-tailed chinchilla) *Chinchilla brevicaudata* (short-tailed chinchilla)	*Atricholaelaps chinchillae* booklouse *Liposcelis* sp	Affected animals lost weight, with fur developing a dull lusterless appearance. Pruritus and secondary self-trauma–induced dermatitis	No treatment recommendation	Described in free-ranging chinchillas in Peru
Chinchilla	*Ctenocephalides* spp infestations are possible in chinchillas housed with dogs and cats	Secondary anemia and flea-allergic dermatitis may develop	Pyrethrin or Carbaryl-based products for use in cats are recommended Selamectin 6–12 mg/kg (Beck, personal communication, 2013)	Flea dips are not safe. Affected and all in-contact animals should be treated
Chinchilla	*Cheyletiella* spp		Imidacloprid up to 40 mg topically	

Adapted from Refs.[3,35,59]

Table 2
Treatment of ectoparasites in gerbils

Species	Ectoparasite	Clinical Signs	Treatment	Comments
Gerbil *Meriones unguiculatus*	*Demodex merioni*	Pruritus, alopecia, dermatitis, pigmentation change	Ivermectin 0.2 mg/kg PO, SC Every 7 d for at least 3 wk or 1 wk post negative skin scrape Amitraz topical 100 ppm, 3–6 times at 2-wk intervals	Often an underlying disease, old age, immunosuppression have to be considered
Gerbil	*Ornithonyssus bacoti* *Ornithonyssus sylvarium*	Pruritus, excoriation head, ear, nose	Selamectin 15 mg spot-on 1 drop	Clean the environment, use acaricides
Gerbil *Meriones unguicukatus*	*Ctenocephalides* spp	Dull hair coat, patchy alopecia, skin erythema, severe pruritus	Fipronil spray or Carbaryl powder 5%	Treat all in-contact animals
Gerbil	*Acarus farris*	Scaling, alopecia, skin thickening on the tail Excoriation	Ivermectin 0.2 mg/kg PO, SC Fipronil spray	Decrease humidity, introduce new food

Abbreviations: PO, by mouth; SC, subcutaneously.
Adapted from Refs.[3,6,10,35,47,55,68,69]

Table 3
Treatment of ectoparasites in degus

Species	Ectoparasite	Clinical Signs	Treatment	Comments
Degu *Octodon degus*	Hoplopleura (Anolpura, Holopleuridae) Paraguacarus (Acari, Trombiculidae)	Not described	No treatment recommendation	Some new parasitic species on free-living degus are described: the genus Hoplopleura (Anolpura, Holopleuridae) and Paraguacarus (Acari, Trombiculidae)
Degu	*Dermanyssus gallinae*	Pruritus, anemia, secondary self-trauma–induced dermatitis	Ivermectin 0.2 mg/kg SC or spot-on	Affected birds in the same household have to be treated

Adapted from Refs.[49,70,71]

Table 4
Treatment of ectoparasites in ferrets and mink

Species	Ectoparasite	Clinical Signs	Treatment	Comments
Ferret *Mustela putorius furo*	*Otodectes cynotis*	Brown earwax, inflammation ulceration of ear canal. Pruritus, head shaking, convulsions, alopecia Secondary self-trauma–induced dermatitis	Ivermectin 0.2–0.4 mg/kg SC Repeated every 2 wk for 3 treatments Ivermectin 1% diluted in 1:10 propylene glycol topical Fipronil 2 drops per ear or 2–3 sprays per ferret of 2.5 g/L Imidacloprid 1 cat dose (40 mg) divided onto 2 or 3 spots on dorsum Permethrin/pyrethrins topical every 7 d, use products safe for kittens	Ectopic disease on the feet or tail tip. Topical treatment often is ineffective because of small ear canal All household pets must be treated at the same time
Ferret *Mustela putorius furo*	*Otodectes cynotis*	Alopecia of the face and tail	Ivermectin 50 μg/kg orally every 24 h, can be increased up to 300 μg/kg orally	Described in association with lymphoma in a ferret
Ferret *Mustela putorius furo*	*Otodectes cynotis*	Brown-black earwax, pruritus, head shaking, convulsions	Selamectin 15 mg BW 400–1300 g Selamectin 30 mg BW >1300 g Selamectin 45 mg In the dorsal interscapular area every 30 d	Don't use local therapeutics in case of ear drum perforation, Kits up to 400 g should not be treated
Ferret *Mustela putorius furo*	*Sarcoptes scabiei*	Pruritus, alopecia, lichenification, crusts, paw inflammation, "foot rot," nail deformation and slough	Ivermectin 0.2–0.4 mg/kg SC Repeated every 7–14 d for 3 doses Selamectin 15 mg BW 400–1300 g Selamectin 30 mg BW >1300 g	Clean environment and in-contact animals Prednisone as a symptomatic therapy to relieve pruritus can help at 0.25–1 mg/kg BW every 24 h PO

Animal	Ectoparasite	Clinical signs	Treatment	Notes
Ferret *Mustela putorius furo*	*Ixodes ricinus*	Anemia	Ivermectin 0.4 mg/kg BW SC Fipronil spray	Ferrets had a long-term treatment with triamcinolone. 3 final treatments with Amitraz 0.0375% every 5 d. *Demodex* sp were detected in 9 of 25 healthy ferrets in the facial, caudal abdominal, perianal skin
Ferret *Mustela putorius furo*	*Ctenocephalides* spp., *Ceratophyllus sciorum*, *Pulex irritans*	Intense pruritus, less commonly flea-bite hypersensitivities with papulocrustous dermatitis	Imidacloprid 10%/moxidectin 1% after 2 wk 100%, after 4 wk >90% preventive effectivity Imidacloprid 10% (40% for cats) 0.4 mL local on skin at the base of skull Selamectin 6 or 18 mg/kg BW monthly or Fipronil	
Ferret *Mustela putorius furo*	*Demodex* sp	Alopecia, mild yellow-brown seborrhea, cast formation	Amitraz 0.0125%–0.025% dippings 3 times at 7-d intervals	Ferrets had a long-term treatment with triamcinolone. 3 final treatments with Amitraz 0.0375% every 5 d. *Demodex* sp were detected in 9 of 25 healthy ferrets in the facial, caudal abdominal, perianal skin
Mink *Mustela vision*	*Ceratophyllus sciurorum*	Pruritus, anemia	Imidacloprid 10% solution, imidacloprid 10%/permethrin 50% solution, phoxim 0.05%–0.1%	90%–99% success rate

Abbreviation: BW, body weight.
Adapted from Refs. [14,15,35,36,47,51,72–80]

Table 5
Treatment of ectoparasites in guinea pigs

Species	Ectoparasite	Clinical Signs	Treatment	Comments
Guinea pig *Cavia porcellus*	*Trixacarus caviae, Sarcoptes scabiei*	Pruritus, (in severe cases convulsions) Erythema, crusts, hyperkeratosis Alopecia, secondary dermatitis, later lethargy, exitus letalis possible	Selamectin 15 mg/kg Ivermectin 0.4–0.5 mg/kg SC every 7–10 d for 2–3 times Fipronil spray (whole body) 2 times 10 d apart Amitraz 0.025% bath, 3 times 7 d apart	*Trixacarus caviae* Most common and most important ectoparasitic disease in guinea pig No drug detection in plasma after orally or topically administered Ivermectin Clean environment No fipronil in case of open skin wounds Selamectin better owner compliance, no need for repeated therapy, effective, but currently not approved for use in guinea pig
Guinea pig *Cavia porcellus*	*Demodex caviae*	Asymptomatic, alopecia, erythema, papules, crusts	Selamectin 15 mg/kg every 2 wk	Concurrent infestation of *Demodex caviae* and *Chirodiscoides caviae*
Guinea pig *Cavia porcellus*	*Chirodiscoides caviae*	Subclinical, severe cases alopecia, erythema	Selamectin 15 mg/kg once	
Guinea pig *Cavia porcellus*	Lice *Gyropus ovalis, Gliricola porcelli*	Usually unaffected, may be pruritic	Imidacloprid 10% + moxidectin 1% solution 0.05 mL once	

Adapted from Refs.[3,8,12,24,26,27,30–32,34,51,61,81–86]

Table 6
Treatment of ectoparasites in hamsters

Species	Ectoparasite	Clinical Signs	Treatment	Comments
Hamster *Mesocricetus auratus*	*Demodex criceti* *Demodex aurati*	Alopecia, scaling, focal ulceration, dry scabby dermatitis, pigmentation	Amitraz 0.013% topical bath	No drug detection in plasma after orally or topically administered ivermectin Clean environment No fipronil in case of open skin wounds
Hamster *Mesocricetus auratus*	*Ornithonyssus bacati*	Pruritus, erythema, papules, crusts	Fipronil spray indirectly applied by a soaked swab wiped over the whole body 2 times 10 d apart. Ivermectin 0.2 mg/kg BW subcutaneously 3 times 7 d apart	All in-housed pets, hamsters must be treated, the cages cleaned and the apartments professionally disinfected
Hamster	*Notoedres* spp	Pruritus, erythema, papules, yellow crusts	Ivermectin 0.4 mg/kg BW subcutaneously once for 8 wk Moxidectin 0.4 mg/kg PO once a week for 8 wk	Only 60%–70% success rate after 8 wk

Adapted from Refs.[3,17,18,20–22,35,51,54,82,87]

Table 7
Treatment of ectoparasites in hedgehogs

Species	Ectoparasite	Clinical Signs	Treatment	Comments
Hedgehog *Erinacaeus europaeus* *Atelerix albiventris*	*Notoedres muris* *Caparinia tripilis,* *Caparinia erinacei* *Demodex erinacei* *Chorioptes* spp *Ornithonyssus bacoti*	Pruritus, scales, white to brownish crusts, secondary, dry scabby dermatitis, quill and hair loss, deformation of ears	Ivermectin 0.2–0.4 mg/kg PO, SC Amitraz 0.3% topical bath weekly for 2–3 (5) wk Fipronil spray (one spray on the dorsum, repeated after 10 d) Selamectin 6 mg/kg Phoxim bath 1:1000 mL water once a week 2 times	Do not use fipronil in hedgehogs
Hedgehog *Erinacaeus europaeus*	*Archeopsylla ernicaei,* *Ceratophyllus gallinae,* *Ctenocephalides felis* *Ixodes hexagonus,* *Ixodes ricinus,* *Rhipicephalus sanguineus,* *Haemaphysalis erinaceii*	Anemia, pruritus	Selamectin 6 mg/kg Phoxim bath 1:1000 mL water once a week 2 times[51] Fipronil spray or pyrethrin	

Adapted from Refs.[35,39–41,43,51,56,88,89]

Table 8
Treatment of ectoparasites in mice and rats

Species	Ectoparasite	Clinical Signs	Treatment	Comments
Mouse (M) Mus musculus	Myocoptes musculinus M Myobia musculi M	Localized pruritus, alopecia, ulcerative dermatitis, lymphadenopathy, weight loss Self-induced trauma, dermatitis, anemia (in lice infestations) Severe pruritus	Ivermectin 0.2–0.4 mg/kg PO or SC every 7–14 d 2–3 treatments Ivermectin 32 mg/mL water PO 10 d, 2 times repeated after 7 d Ivermectin solution 1%, 1 drop (0.03 mL) 2 times 7–14 d apart on to the neck or behind the ear Selamectin 12 –2 4 mg/kg PO Moxidectin 0.5% solution local at 0.5 mg/kg repeated after 10 d Moxidectin 0.5% solution at 2.0/kg PO	In mice Myocoptes musculinus and Myobia musculi are most common Fur mite eradication in large colonies by medical feed is recommended
Mouse (M) Mus musculus Rat (R) Rattus norvegicus	Ratfordia affinis M Ratfordia ensifera R	Localized pruritus, alopecia, ulcerative dermatitis, lymphadenopathy, weight loss	Ivermectin solution 1%, 1 drop (0.03 mL) 2 times 7–14 d apart on to the neck or behind the ear Ivermectin 0.08% (sheep drench) at 4 mL (3.2 mg) per liter of drinking water, PO One week on, 1 wk off, 1 wk on Selamectin 12–24 mg/kg PO	In rats Ratfordia ensifera are most common
Mouse (M) Mus musculus Rat (R) Rattus norvegicus	Polyplax serrata M Polyplax spinulosa R	Severe pruritus, alopecia, dermatitis Anemia	Fipronil spray indirectly applied by a soaked swab wiped over the whole body 2 times 10 d apart	
	Notoedres muris M Liponyssus bacoti, Liponyssoides sanguineus M, R			
	Demodex ratti R[7,9] Ornithonyssus bacoti M, R			
	Archeopsylla Leptospylla segnis, Ctenophthalmus assimilis M, R			

Adapted from Refs.[3,35,46,51,52,60,90–105]

Table 9
Treatment of ectoparasites in rabbits

Species	Ectoparasite	Clinical Signs	Treatment	Comments
Rabbit *Oryctolagus cuniculus*	*Psoroptes cuniculi*	Pruritus, head shaking, mild to thick crust formation in the ear canal (eardrum perforation, otitis media, meningitis), ear drooping may spread to face, neck, abdomen	Imidacloprid 10 mg/kg + moxidectin 1 mg/kg solution local on the neck 3 times repeated after 4 wk Ivermectin 0.2–0.4 mg/kg SC every 7–14 d 2–3 times Ivermectin 0.4 mg/kg SC + fipronil spray 3 mL/kg, fipronil treatment every 2 mo later Selamectin 6–18 mg/kg spot on the neck Moxidectin 0.2 mg/kg PO once every 10 d for 2 times	Ivermectin does not kill *P cuniculi* eggs which hatch in 4 d, but sufficient concentration in skin (13 d) and ears (9 d) will destroy new generations Do not use fipronil; adverse reactions including deaths in young, debilitated, underweight rabbits are reported
Rabbit *Oryctolagus cuniculus*	*Notoedres cati, Sarcoptes scabiei*	Intense pruritus First lesions on nose, lips, then face, feet, alopecia, white-yellow crusts, dermatitis	Selamectin 6–18 mg/kg spot on the neck[45,106] Imidacloprid 10 mg/kg + moxidectin 1 mg/kg solution local on the neck 3 times repeated after 4 wk Ivermectin 0.2–0.4 mg/kg SC every 10–14 d for 3 treatments	
Rabbit *Oryctolagus cuniculus*	*Cheyletiella parasitvorax*	Mild to severe crust, scaly dry pruritic dermatitis, "powdery appearance," patchy alopecia, broken hairs	Selamectin 6–18 mg/kg spot on the neck Ivermectin 0.2–0.4 mg/kg SC every 7–14 d 2–3 treatments Doramectin 0.5 mg/kg SC repeated after 7–10 d Imidacloprid 14.8–22.2 mg/kg + permethrin 74.1–111.1 mg/kg solution	

Animal	Parasite	Clinical signs	Treatment
Rabbit *Oryctolagus cuniculus*	*Demodex cuniculi*	Alopecia, seborrhea sicca, pruritus	Amitraz 0.05% water solution weekly once for 6 occasions
Rabbit *Oryctolagus cuniculus*	*Ornithonyssus bacoti*	Intense pruritus Skin excoriations, dermatitis	Pyrethrin spray weekly 8 times, pyrethrin spray of all premises (floor, walls, adjacent hallways etc)
Rabbit *Oryctolagus cuniculus*	*Ctenocephalides* spp, *Nosopsyllus* spp, *Xenopsylla* spp	Mild to severe crust and scale formation Self-induced trauma, flea dermatitis, flea feces, anemia	Selamectin 20 mg/kg SC every 7 d
Rabbit *Oryctolagus cuniculus*	*Listrophorus gibbus*	Mild to severe crust and scale formation Self-induced trauma, dermatitis	Imidacloprid 16 mg + permethrin 50 mg spot-on solution per rabbit on the neck Imidacloprid 14.8–22.2 mg/kg + permethrin 74.1–111.1 mg/kg solution
Rabbit *Oryctolagus cuniculus*	*Cuterebra* spp	Multiple, subcutis swellings, skin perforation (breathing hole)	Enlarge breathing hole via incision, extract larva with forceps, debride necrotic tissue
Rabbit *Oryctolagus cuniculus*	*Ixodes* spp	Can be found especially on ears, eyes, nose, and perineum	Ivermectin 0.4 mg/kg SC

Adapted from Refs. [3,4,11,35,45,46,51,52,60,82,103,106–132]

Chrysosporium Anamorph *Nannizziopsis vriesii*

An Emerging Fungal Pathogen of Captive and Wild Reptiles

Mark A. Mitchell, DVM, MS, PhD, DECZM (Herpetology)[a],*,
Michael R. Walden, MS, DVM, PhD[b]

KEYWORDS

- *Chrysosporium* anamorph *Nannizziopsis vriesii* • Diagnostic testing • Fungus
- Pathogen • Reptile

KEY POINTS

- *Chrysosporium* anamorph *Nannizziopsis vriesii* is an obligate fungal pathogen of reptiles.
- *Chrysosporium* anamorph *N vriesii* is typically locally invasive, but can cause systemic disease.
- Diagnosing *Chrysosporium* anamorph *N vriesii* can be done using culture, histopathology, and polymerase chain reaction assays.
- Itraconazle and voriconazole are commonly used to treat affected reptiles.

When veterinary clinicians consider different pathogens in a differential diagnosis list for reptiles, fungi tend to be the group placed lowest on the list. The primary reason for this is because fungi are generally considered to be opportunistic pathogens in reptiles, rather than obligate pathogens such as viruses, parasites, and bacteria. One exception to this is *Chrysosporium* anamorph *Nannizziopsis vriesii* (CANV). This fungus was originally considered a ubiquitous organism found in the soil and associated with infections in invertebrates, but is now considered to be an obligate pathogen of reptiles.[1] Over the past 15 years, this fungus has been shown to be an emerging pathogen in captive reptiles, and has also recently been identified in wild reptiles.[2] Because of the emergence of this pathogen in both captive and wild reptiles, veterinarians need to familiarize themselves with the clinical presentation of affected animals, diagnostic

[a] Department of Veterinary Clinical Medicine, University of Illinois, College of Veterinary Medicine, 1008 West Hazelwood Drive, Urbana, IL 61802, USA; [b] USDA-FSIS, Cargill Meat Solutions, 2510 East Lake Shore Drive, Waco, TX 76705, USA
* Corresponding author.
E-mail address: mmitch@illinois.edu

Vet Clin Exot Anim 16 (2013) 659–668
http://dx.doi.org/10.1016/j.cvex.2013.05.013
1094-9194/13/$ – see front matter © 2013 Elsevier Inc. All rights reserved.

methods used to confirm the presence of CANV in affected animals, and the different treatment methods against this fungus.

To date, there has been little research to characterize the epidemiology of CANV in reptiles, with most the articles published on the subject being case reports. Although case reports are often viewed as having limited value regarding their contribution to characterizing the epidemiology of a disease, the author finds that the information provided in case reports serves as an important first step to outline many of the important factors (eg, range of hosts, sources of infection, clinical signs, diagnostics, therapeutics) required to develop an understanding of the relationship between animals and pathogens. This article reviews what is known about CANV in reptiles to develop an understanding of the epidemiology of this organism in reptiles.

THE PATHOGEN

CANV is an ascomycetous fungus. A hallmark of this genus is keratinolytic activity, which is a primary reason why this organism is a pathogen of invertebrates and lower vertebrates, such as reptiles. The outer layer of the stratum corneum of reptiles is composed of keratin, which serves as an appropriate substrate for the fungus. *Chrysosporium* spp have restricted growth at 37°C, which is also why this fungus has a predilection for lower vertebrates and invertebrates. Hospitalizing reptiles at increased temperatures (37–39°C) during treatment may help the patient eliminate the fungus; however, it is important to know whether the patient can tolerate these warmer temperatures. This genus is naturally resistant to cycloheximides, which are protein biosynthesis inhibitors in eukaryotes. The life cycle of this fungus involves the formation of clavate or pyriform single-celled or 2-celled aleurioconidia, and alternate and fission arthroconidia.

CANV has been suggested as an obligate fungal pathogen of reptiles based on preliminary epidemiologic studies with this organism. Pare and colleagues[3] evaluated the mycobiota of skin in different reptiles and found that the organism was rare compared with other organisms such as *Aspergillus* spp, *Paecilomyces* spp, and *Penicillium* spp. In total, 127 reptile (36 lizards; 91 snakes) sheds were evaluated and only 1 CANV was isolated, from an African rock python (*Python sebae*). However, in the same animals, 50 different genera of fungi were recovered from the skin sheds, suggesting that fungi are common skin inhabitants of reptiles. The investigators concluded that the rarity of CANV suggests that it is not an opportunistic fungal infection only taking advantage of injuries to the integument, but an obligate pathogen that infects reptiles after exposure. The study was based on the submission of shed skins through the mail, so it is possible that the recovery rate of CANV could have been affected by environmental temperature, shipping conditions, or competition with other microflora. For this reason, follow up studies to evaluate the prevalence of CANV on healthy skin samples are needed.

To confirm whether CANV is an obligate pathogen of reptiles requires the fulfillment of the Koch postulate, and this has been done in at least 1 species.[4] Pare and colleagues[4] were able to infect veiled chameleons (*Chamaeleo calyptratus*) through environmental exposure or direct application of the fungus to intact or abraded skin. The infection was similar to that described for clinical cases in which initial or early infections were in the stratum corneum and stratum germinativum and later infections led to necrosis and granuloma formation in the deeper tissues. CANV was also contagious by both direct contact and through fomite contact. Because many reptile owners maintain more than one animal in their collection, education regarding minimizing exposure to the pathogen through good hygiene practices is essential to minimizing the dissemination of the fungus through a collection.

Clinical Signs

Reptiles infected with CANV can present with a range of clinical signs, from focal skin lesions to systemic disease (rarely). In some cases, the clinical signs seem to be order specific or even genera specific. The most common clinical signs are associated with the integument. Crust formation, color change, and necrosis are commonly seen. As is common with fungal skin lesions, CANV infections of the integument tend to start as focal lesions that spread from a central point. However, by the time the animals present, the lesions can be variable and generalized. Because of the invasive nature of this fungus, it is common to see pyogranulomatous disease as it invades through the epidermis and dermis (**Fig. 1**). Once the fungus invades through the integument it can spread locally or systemically. Most reports suggest that the fungus is locally invasive; however, in one case, granulomas associated with this fungus were identified in the lung of a jewel chameleon (*Chamaeleo lateralis*),[1] and in another it was associated with a hepatic granuloma in a bearded dragon.[5] This article provides a more specific review based on the different orders of reptiles found to be infected with CANV.

LIZARDS

A review of the literature finds that at least 11 different species of lizards have been diagnosed with CANV (**Table 1**). In the author's experience, bearded dragons and chameleons tend to be the most common case presentations. Bearded dragons affected with CANV typically present with dermatitis characterized by crusts, ulcers, and pyogranulomatous disease. Both central inland bearded dragons (*Pogona vitticeps*) and coastal bearded dragons (*Pogona barbata*) have been reported to be infected with CANV.[5,6] Originally described as yellow fungus disease, the crusts found on bearded dragons tend to have a yellow coloration (**Fig. 2**). Lesions in bearded dragons are often multifocal and may include the head, oral cavity, limbs, ventrum, or dorsum (**Fig. 3**). Infections in bearded dragons tend to be aggressive and disseminate into the subcutaneous tissues, muscle, and bones.[5] As mentioned previously, there is at least one report of dissemination systemically into the liver of a bearded dragon.[5]

Chameleons are the other group of lizards that seem to be highly susceptible to CANV infections, and infections do not seem to be limited to a group from a single native origin (see **Table 1**). Affected chameleons often present with focal to multifocal necrotic (black) areas of skin surrounded by crusts (**Fig. 4**). The lesions may be found on both the body and limbs/tail.[1]

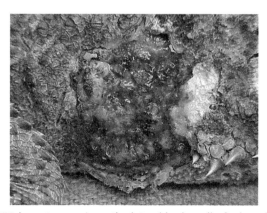

Fig. 1. Severe CANV dermatomycosis on the lateral body wall of a bearded dragon.

Table 1
Species of reptiles found to be infected with CANV

Common Name	Scientific Name
Lizards	
Amevia	*Amevia chaitzarni*[9]
Day geckos	*Phelsuma* spp[3]
Green iguanas	*Iguana iguana*[8]
Central inland bearded dragon	*Pogona vitticeps*[5]
Coastal bearded dragon	*Pogona barbata*[6]
Panther chameleon	*Furcifer pardalis*[1]
Jackson's chameleon	*Chamaeleo jacksoni*[1]
Jeweled chameleon	*C lateralis*[1]
Parson's chameleon	*Chamaeleo parsonii*[1]
Veiled chameleon	*C calyptratus*[4]
Girdled lizard	*Cordylus giganteus*[7]
Snakes	
Ball pythons	*Python regius*[3]
Garter snakes	*Thamnophis* sp[3]
Brown tree snake	*Boiga irregularis*[12]
Milk snake	*Lampropeltis triangulum*[3]
Corn snake	*Pantherophis guttatus*[3]
Tentacle snakes	*Erpeton tentaculatum*[10]
Eastern massasauga rattlesnakes[a]	*Sistrurus catenatus catenatus*[2]
Boa constrictor	*Boa constrictor*[11]
File snakes	*Achrochordus* sp[6]
Crocodilians	
Saltwater crocodiles	*Crocodylus porsus*[13]

[a] Chrysosporium sp.

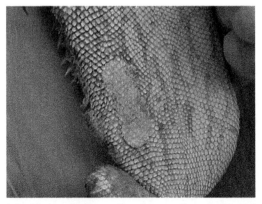

Fig. 2. CANV was originally described as yellow fungus disease of bearded dragons because of the yellow coloration associated with the crusts found on these animals.

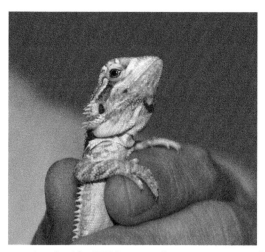

Fig. 3. The lesions associated with CANV on reptiles can occur anywhere on the body, although lesions on the head seem to be most common. Note the crust in the gular area and the lesions at the commissure of the mouth.

Other species of lizards that have been reported to develop CANV infections in captivity include day geckos (*Phelsuma* sp),[1] a wild-caught girdled lizard (*Cordylus giganteus*) after being held in captivity for 2 years,[7] green iguanas (*Iguana iguana*),[8] and an amevia (*Amevia chaitzarni*).[9] The lesions in these animals were similar to those described for bearded dragons and chameleons and included crusting and ulcerative dermatitis lesions on the head and body. In many of the cases, preliminary diagnostics were focused on bacterial dermatitis. It is important for clinicians to consider CANV dermatitis in lizards presenting to their practices, especially when antibacterial treatment is unrewarding.

SNAKES

A review of the literature finds that at least 9 different species of snakes have been diagnosed with CANV (see **Table 1**). Although the distribution of CANV lesions in snakes seems to be primarily associated with the head,[2,10,11] in at least some cases

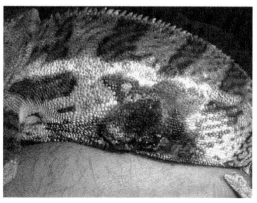

Fig. 4. A chameleon with dermatomycosis associated with CANV. Note the black (necrotic) central lesion and surrounding crust.

it can be found elsewhere on the body (eg, ventrum).[12] Lesions are similar to those described with necrotizing dermatitis (a generic disease syndrome in snakes) and may include erythema, plaque and crust formation, and the presence of vesicles. Because of the low specificity associated with these clinical signs, it is important to perform preliminary cytology to rule out potential fungal pathogens or submit fungal culture samples when screening potential pathogens for dermatitis in snakes. As mentioned earlier, site specificity for lesions in snakes seems to be the around the head. The location of the lesions on the head may provide insight into the source of exposure for these animals. For example, snakes actively burrowing may stir up the fungus from the substrate. Research to investigate sources of exposure in these animals is needed. Compared with the other groups of reptiles infected with CANV, there seems to be a higher mortality with this disease in snakes.

A *Chrysosporium* sp recently identified in protected eastern massasauga snakes (*Sistrurus catenatus catenatus*) is of special concern.[2] This case represents the first report of this genus of fungus infecting wild animals. Although not diagnosed as CANV, the clinical disease reported in the snakes was similar to that described for other reptiles, including ulcerative dermatitis, crust formation, and granulomas.

CROCODILIANS

There is a single report of CANV infection in captive saltwater crocodiles (*Crocodylus porosus*).[13] The lesions were associated with the skin and mortalities (n = 48) were recorded. Infections were recorded twice on the farm 3 years apart. High-density production facilities, such as those used for the crocodilian leather industry, may be highly susceptible to CANV infections. In these cases, any scarring to the leather from the infections could cause financial loss to the producer.

Diagnostic Testing

A thorough diagnostic work-up is recommended for reptiles presenting with suspected CANV infections. A complete blood count and plasma biochemistry panel can provide insight into the general physiologic status of the reptile. Anemia of chronic disease is a common finding. However, most of these cases tend to be regenerative in nature. Screening blood smears for the presence of active (3+ to 4+ on a 1–4+ scale) anisocytosis and poikilocytosis helps characterize the patient's response to the anemia. Affected reptiles also frequently present with inflammatory leukograms. Although the white blood cell counts are often not severely increased, affected animals tend to have a heterophilia, lymphocytosis, and monocytosis. Animals that are not eating or have generalized lesions tend to be dehydrated at presentation. Increased packed cell volume, total protein, albumin, sodium, and chloride levels are common in affected patients. Hyperglobulinemia and an inverse albumin/globulin ration are also commonly observed in affected reptiles.

Survey radiographs can be used to assess the extent of soft tissue involvement and characterize any bony involvement.[2] Osteomyelitis is common in reptiles infected with CANV, and radiographs can be used to assess the integrity of the bone when planning medical and surgical options for a case. Advanced imaging such as computed tomography can also be used to better characterize the extent of lesions (especially bony involvement) when used with iodinated radiocontrast solution.

Biopsy and screening of the sample are required to make a diagnosis. Full-thickness biopsy samples can be submitted for culture, histopathology, and/or polymerase chain reaction (PCR) testing. Parallel testing strategies using all three of these modalities should be considered the gold standard for diagnosing CANV in reptiles.

Culture remains the definitive method of diagnosing CANV. The methods used to culture often start with a Sabouraud dextrose agar or a potato dextrose agar. Incubation temperatures range from 25 to 35°C, with the higher temperatures being more commonly used for certain species (eg, bearded dragons).[5] It is important to discuss incubation temperature with the laboratory processing a sample, because CANV does not grow well at greater than 37°C and false-negative results could occur in cases in which incubation temperature is too high. Culture length may vary from 24 to 48 hours up to 5 to 7 days, with lower temperature requiring longer culture times. Colonies tend to be white and cottony in appearance. Secondary cultures are often done to further evaluate the morphology and morphometry of the fungus. Phytone yeast extract can be used for this purpose. When colonies are evaluated under light microscopy they tend to be pyriform to cylindrical, sessile, and have aleuroconidia on branched hyphae.

Histopathology can be used in combination with the other methods to guide the clinician and pathologist in pursuing a diagnosis of CANV. This fungus is aggressive and intralesional fungi can be seen with periodic acid-Schiff staining. Affected tissues tend to have a mixture of inflammatory cells, such as macrophages and heterophils, and the fungus (**Fig. 5**). Granuloma formation is common.

PCR assay can be used to detect CANV in cases in which culture is difficult or unrewarding. Previous studies have found it possible to confirm the presence of CANV by testing the internal transcribed spacer (ITS1-5.8S-ITS2) region of the fungus.[8] Of the three diagnostic methods mentioned, PCR is most likely the assay with the highest sensitivity. Culture tends to have lower sensitivities because of the potential for misclassification of cases as false-negatives. In contrast, the specificity of culture would be expected to be higher than PCR and thus culture would be less susceptible to false-positives. This tendency suggests that positive results obtained from culture should be considered highly likely to be positives, whereas negative results on PCR are more likely to be true-negatives. In addition, culture is needed to provide an isolate for antifungal sensitivity testing. As mentioned previously, using a parallel testing strategy that combines culture, histopathology, and PCR results provides the veterinary clinician with the most robust results. The author has found the University of Texas Fungus Laboratory (San Antonio, TX) to be an excellent resource for culture and PCR testing.

Therapy

There have been a variety of different treatment recommendations made for managing CANV in reptiles.[1,5,7,13] Treatment typically consists of both topical and systemic

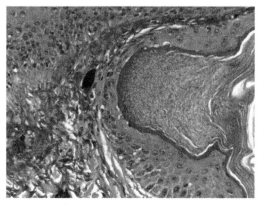

Fig. 5. CANV is an aggressive fungus. Note how the organism is invading through the stratum corneum (hematoxylin and eosin, 400×).

antifungals. Most treatment regimens use a systemic antifungal such as ketocona-zole, itraconazole, or voriconazole. The triazoles are important antifungal com-pounds because they selectively affect a compound unique to fungi, ergosterol. When using triazoles it is important to consider the side effects. The most common clinical signs associated with triazole toxicity are anorexia and depression. Affected animals tend to develop mild hepatitis as a result of the toxicity. Screening animals' liver functions before initiating treatment and during/after treatment is recommended (discussed later).

Of the triazoles, the author could only find a single reference to using ketoconazole for treating CANV infections in reptiles. The ketoconazole had been used to success-fully treat 2 green iguanas with confirmed CANV infections.[8] In the past, ketocona-zole was used as the drug of choice for treating fungal diseases in vertebrates; however, newer drugs with fewer side effects have since been developed (eg, itraco-nazole and voriconazole) to replace it. It is important to consider ketoconazole when performing antifungal sensitivity testing in cases in which resistance is found to other antifungals.

Most of the reports focused on treating CANV infections in reptiles used itracona-zole. Previous reports cite success treating CANV infections in chameleons with itra-conazole.[1] In bearded dragons, itraconazole has been used with mixed results. Bowman and colleagues[5] used 10 mg/kg itraconazole by mouth every 24 hours in 2 bearded dragons, with poor results, and 5 mg/kg by mouth every 48 hours in 1 animal with positive results. The author has likewise seen mixed results using these doses. Whether or not the drug dosing had an effect on the outcomes is unknown but, based on the postmortem examinations of the animals reported in the literature, it was not expected. The azoles are known for causing toxicity to vertebrates, especially at the level of the liver, so it is important to monitor animals closely. The best methods for monitoring animals are to closely observe their attitude and appetite, serially measure clinical chemistries, and collect liver biopsies to measure drug levels. Reptiles with hepatic disease secondary to drug toxicity are often depressed and anorexic. The clinical chemistries commonly used to assess liver disease include aspartate amino-transferase (AST), gamma glutyltransaminase (GGT), and bile acids. Although AST and GGT are not liver specific, they may be helpful in combination with other param-eters. Bile acid testing is the most useful chemistry for evaluating liver function, and should be performed if secondary liver disease is suspected. It is important to be sure that the assay being run measures the bile acids produced by the species being tested, because false-negatives may occur with this assay. Liver biopsies can be used to assess the liver for disease and concentrations of the drugs measured to determine whether the drug is accumulating to unsafe levels. To minimize the risk of side effects with itraconazole, lower doses at less frequent intervals are recommended. Pulse ther-apy is another potential consideration for reducing toxic side effects associated with itraconazole.

Voriconazole is a triazole that is being used more frequently by clinicians because it seems to have a lower incidence of side effects compared with other antifungals, such as itraconazole and ketoconazole. Voriconazole inhibits P450 dependent 14-alpha-sterol demethylase, leading to an increase in 14-alpha methylated sterols and a loss of ergosterol. In a wild-caught, captive girdled lizard (*Cordylus gigan-teus*), 10 mg/kg voriconazole by mouth was found to reach minimum inhibitory concentrations.[7] The study also showed how it was possible to create a patient-specific testing strategy to treat CANV. Additional studies in bearded dragons have likewise found the 10 mg/kg voriconazole by mouth every 24 hours achieved minimum inhibitory concentrations appropriate to treat CANV.[14] Bearded dragons treated with 10 mg/kg voriconazole were more likely to survive than dragons treated with 5 mg/kg itraconazole once daily.

The risk factors most commonly associated with CANV in reptiles are substandard husbandry, improper diet, and environmental stressors.[5] These same risk factors are associated with many of the disease processes reported with reptiles and show that striving to provide optimal diet and husbandry is essential to minimizing the introduction and dissemination of disease. However, it is important to determine more specific risk factors associated with this debilitating and potentially fatal pathogen. Substrate likely plays an important role, so it is important for future research to evaluate different substrates under different conditions (eg, temperature and humidity) for the presence of this organism. Recommendations to clients to maintain the cleanliness of their pet's substrate (eg, removal of fecal material, replacing substrate regularly) should be provided when discussing husbandry and treatment. The potential for the organism to be associated with foodstuffs also needs to be evaluated and discussed. Reports of CANV infections in a variety of insectivorous reptiles (eg, geckos, bearded dragons, chameleons) suggest that a common source of exposure may be the diet, which is especially important to consider when comparing terrestrial species that live on a substrate (eg, bearded dragons) or are fossorial with arboreal species that have little/no contact with a substrate (eg, chameleons). Because CANV is keratophilic, it is possible that invertebrate food sources (eg, crickets) are serving as the source of infection for reptiles. Like many of the diseases encountered in captive reptiles, it is possible to diagnose and treat CANV, but little is known about how reptiles encounter or disseminate it. It is for this reason that future research endeavors should pursue characterizing the epidemiology of this pathogen so that more consistent methods for treatment and prevention of CANV infections can be developed.

Zoonotic Potential

Chrysosporium spp have been associated with disease in humans. Most cases are reported in immunocompromised individuals. Although osteomyelitis is a common finding, lesions in the brain have also been reported.[15,16] There is at least one case in which the infection was associated with CANV.[17] A middle-aged man seropositive for human immunodeficiency virus presented for mentation changes over an 8-month period. Magnetic resonance imaging confirmed the presence of 2 brain masses. The masses were aspirated and found to be fungal abscesses, confirmed by positive CANV culture. The patient responded to voriconazole treatment. It was not clear how the patient became exposed to the fungus. Although it is not expected that CANV will cause disease in healthy humans, individuals working around reptiles that are CANV positive should take precautions (eg, wear examination gloves) to minimize any risk of exposure.

SUMMARY

To date, CANV has been isolated from captive reptiles on at least 4 continents: Asia, Australia, Europe, and North America. In addition, the recent report of wild reptiles in North American developing clinical disease suggests that the relationship of this fungus with reptiles is evolving. Veterinarians working with captive or wild reptiles should consider CANV as a potential differential in cases presenting with dermatitis, especially cases characterized by necrosis and deforming osteomyelitis lesions.

REFERENCES

1. Pare JA, Sigler L, Hunter DB, et al. Cutaneous mycoses in chameleons caused by the *Chrysosporium* anamorph of *Nannizziopsis vriesii* (Apinis) Currah. J Zoo Wildl Med 1997;28(4):443–53.
2. Allender MC, Dreslik M, Wylie S, et al. *Chrysosporium* sp. infection in Eastern massasauga rattlesnakes. Emerg Infect Dis 2011;17(21):2383–4.
3. Pare JA, Sigler L, Rypien KL, et al. Cutaneous mycobiota of captive squamate reptiles with notes on the scarcity of *Chrysosporium* anamorph *Nannizziopsis vriesii*. J Herp Med Surg 2003;13:10–5.
4. Pare JA, Coyle KA, Sigler L, et al. Pathogenicity of the *Chrysosporium* anamorph *Nannizziopsis vriesii* for veiled chameleons (*Chamaeleo calyptratus*). Med Mycol 2006;44:25–31.
5. Bowman MR, Pare JA, Sigler L, et al. Deep fungal dermatitis in three inland bearded dragons (*Pogona vitticeps*) caused by the *Chrysosporium* anamorph of *Nannizziopsis vriesii*. Med Mycol 2007;45:371–6.
6. Johnson RS, Sangster CR, Sigler L, et al. Deep fungal dermatitis caused by the *Chrysosporium* anamorph of *Nannizziopsis vriesii* in captive coastal bearded dragons (*Pogona barbata*). Aust Vet J 2011;89(12):515–9.
7. Hellebuyck T, Baert K, Pasmans F, et al. Cutaneous hyalohyphomycosis in a girdled lizard (*Cordylus giganteus*) caused by *Chrysosporium* anamorph of *Nannizziopsis vriesii* and successful treatment with voriconazole. Vet Dermatol 2010;21:429–33.
8. Abarca ML, Martorel J, Castlella G, et al. Cutaneous hyalohyphomycosis caused by *Chrysosporium* species related to *Nannizziopsis vriesii* in two green iguanas (*Iguana iguana*). Med Mycol 2008;46:349–54.
9. Martel A, Fonteyne PA, Chiers K, et al. Nasal *Nannizziopsis vriesii* granuloma in an amevia lizard (*Amevia chaitzarni*). Vlaams Diergeneeskd Tijdschr 2006;75:306–7.
10. Bertelsen MF, Crawshaw GJ, Sigler L, et al. Fatal cutaneous mycosis in tentacle snakes (*Erpeton tentaculatum*) caused by *Chrysosporium* anamorph of *Nannizziopsis vriesii*. J Zoo Wildl Med 2005;36:82–7.
11. Eatwell K. Suspected *Chrysosporium* anamorph of *Nannizziopsis vriesii* (CANV) dermatitis in an albino boa constrictor (*Constrictor constrictor*). J Small Anim Pract 2010;51:290.
12. Nichols DK, Weyant RS, Lamirande BS, et al. Fatal mycotic dermatitis in captive brown tree snakes (*Boiga irregularis*). J Zoo Wildl Med 1999;30:111–8.
13. Thomas AD, Sigler L, Peuker S, et al. Nannizziopsis vriesii-like fungus associated with fatal cutaneous mycosis in the salt-water crocodile (*Crocodylus porosus*). Med Mycol 2002;40:143–51.
14. Van Waeyenbergh L, Baert K, Pasmans F, et al. Voriconazole, a safe alternative for treating infections caused by *Chrysosporium* anamorph *Nannizziopsis vriesii* in bearded dragons (*Pogona vitticeps*). Med Mycol 2010;48:880–5.
15. Stillwell WT, Rubin BD, Axelrod JL. *Chrysosporium*, a new causative agent in osteomyelitis. A case report. Clin Orthop 1994;28:443–53.
16. Warwick A, Ferrieri P, Burke B, et al. Presumptive invasive *Chrysosporium* infection in a bone marrow transplant recipient. Bone Marrow Transplant 1991;8:319–22.
17. Steninger C, van Lunzen J, Tintelnot K, et al. Mycotic brain abscess caused by opportunistic reptile pathogen. Emerg Infect Dis 2005;11(2):349–50.

Pathogenesis, Diagnosis, and Treatment of Amphibian Chytridiomycosis

Eric J. Baitchman, DVM, DACZM[a],*, Allan P. Pessier, DVM, DACVP[b]

KEYWORDS

- *Batrachochytrium dendrobatidis* • Chytridiomycosis • Amphibian • Treatment
- Diagnosis

KEY POINTS

- Chytridiomycosis causes death in amphibians by disrupting osmoregulatory function of the skin.
- Polymerase chain reaction testing is the diagnostic method of choice and should be used both to confirm infection and confirm negative status after treatment.
- Itraconazole is the most commonly used antifungal agent for treatment of chytridiomycosis.
- Successful treatment of amphibians that are clinically ill with chytridiomycosis requires supportive care, especially with electrolyte therapy.

INTRODUCTION

Amphibian chytridiomycosis, caused by the chytridiomycete fungus, *Batrachochytrium dendrobatidis* (Bd), is responsible for a global pandemic that has dramatically reduced global amphibian populations and diversity.[1–4] Species declines, extirpations, and extinctions attributed to chytridiomycosis have occurred in Australia, Europe, Latin America, and the United States.[5–8] The geographic origin of Bd is the subject of ongoing investigation. However, the spread of virulent Bd lineages to all continents (other than Antarctica) is largely believed to be caused by global trade in amphibians for food and research.[9–12] Global dissemination of this important

Disclosures: This project was supported by a National Leadership Program grant from the Institute for Museum and Library Services (IMLS). Any views, findings, conclusions, or recommendations expressed in this publication do not necessarily represent those of the IMLS.
^a Zoo New England, 1 Franklin Park Road, Boston, MA 02121, USA; ^b Amphibian Disease Laboratory, Wildlife Disease Laboratories, Institute for Conservation Research, San Diego Zoo Global, PO Box 120551, San Diego, CA 92112-0551, USA
* Corresponding author.
E-mail address: ebaitchman@zoonewengland.com

pathogen has led to its designation as an internationally notifiable disease by the World Organization for Animal Health (OIE), making it subject to OIE standards in international trade.[13]

Veterinarians are engaged in response to this crisis through assistance with treatment, research, and conservation programs taking place at zoos, aquaria, international ex situ assurance colonies, and private hobby and agricultural industry. There has been a proliferation of reports published recently that describe research on Bd, its pathogenesis, and treatment. This review focuses on recent advances in information concerning Bd, with emphasis on diagnosis, clinical response, and treatment.

Amphibian Skin Physiology

Understanding of normal skin physiology in amphibians is important in understanding the pathophysiology and treatment of chytridiomycosis as well as several other amphibian diseases.

Amphibian skin is highly adapted and arguably the most important organ in amphibian anatomy. Very permeable and well vascularized, the skin is a primary route of respiratory gas exchange and water and electrolyte balance.[14,15] In most species, the area of highest water uptake is the ventral pelvic region, also referred to as the pelvic or drink patch. Sodium, chloride, and calcium ions are actively transported from the environment in to the amphibian body through the skin via several mechanisms, including selective epithelial channels and ion pumps.[14] Potassium is passively regulated based on concentration differences across cell membranes.[14] Disruption of these processes can quickly lead to morbidity and mortality.[16,17]

CHYTRIDIOMYCOSIS
Life Cycle of Bd

The infective stage, a flagellated motile zoospore, encysts on the surface of stratified keratinizing epithelial cells of frog skin, the flagellum is resorbed, and a cell wall is formed. The cyst wall elongates to form a germination tube that penetrates a skin cell membrane within deeper cell layers beneath the stratum corneum.[18,19] Host cell cytoplasm is digested and the contents of the encysted zoospore migrate through the germ tube and develop into an intracellular thallus. The thallus matures from sporangium to zoosporangium, the contents of which divide to form more flagellated zoospores. As the zoosporangium is maturing, superficial stratum corneum cells are being shed, accelerated by effects of infection, and infected cells are brought to the skin surface.[18,20] Simultaneously, the thallus forms a discharge papilla that extends through the skin cell surface, from which the motile zoospores exit and disperse once sufficient moisture is present for zoospore migration. Established thalli can also directly infect deeper cells via projection of rhizoidlike structures that form new sporangia in a similar manner as described for the germination tube.[19]

Pathophysiology

Infection with Bd is limited to the keratinizing stratified squamous epithelium that comprises the skin of postmetamorphic amphibians and the mouthparts of larvae (tadpoles). The skin of larval amphibians begins to keratinize during metamorphosis, and mortality as a result of chytridiomycosis is often observed at this time as the fungus moves from the mouthparts to colonize the skin.[21] In susceptible species, as motile zoospores are released and spread out on the surface of the skin, local reinfection quickly leads to exponential increase in zoospore burden and infection intensity.[22] Initial infection in terrestrial amphibians is on those skin surfaces in contact with the ground, particularly the feet and ventrum. Zoospores then spread to cover other areas of the body. The histologic lesions of chytridiomycosis are primarily epidermal hyperplasia and hyperkeratosis, with myriad thalli of Bd present within cells of the stratum corneum (**Fig. 1**).[23] Inflammatory cell infiltrates are usually sparse unless there are secondary bacterial or fungal infections.

The cause of death from chytridiomycosis is suspected to be related to massive depletion of electrolytes caused by disruption of cutaneous epithelial function.[16,22] In experimental studies, all electrolyte transport across infected amphibian skin was decreased, with resulting decreases of all plasma electrolytes, especially sodium and potassium.[16,24] Significant decrease in plasma potassium in particular was proposed to be the main factor leading to death from asystolic cardiac arrest, similar to the mechanism in other vertebrates.[16] Naturally infected frogs in the wild did not show decreases in potassium relative to infection intensity, but both experimental and natural infection with Bd results in significant decreases in plasma sodium and chloride, which are negatively correlated to infection intensity.[17,22] The experimental studies used clinical signs as an indicator for sample collection in late-stage infection, when collection of wild frogs was not selective in that regard. It may be that wild infected frogs would also become hypokalemic, although it might occur at the end stage of infection, just before death.

Mechanisms of host defense against Bd are an area of active research. Although it seems that most amphibian species can probably become infected with Bd, not all go on to develop severe skin disease and lethal chytridiomycosis. These more resistant subclinically infected species can act as important reservoirs of infection for highly susceptible species.[25] Factors that may be involved in host resistance include innate cutaneous immunity (eg, antimicrobial peptides and symbiotic bacteria), acquired immunity, and inheritance of specific major histocompatibility complex type II alleles.[26]

Clinical Signs

The clinical signs of chytridiomycosis are referable to the skin or to metabolic derangements related to depletion of electrolytes. Typical signs can include lethargy, weakness, loss of righting reflex, cutaneous erythema particularly of the ventrum and feet, increased skin shedding, abnormal postures such as holding limbs away from the body or elevation of the ventrum from the substrate, and acute death without premonitory signs (**Fig. 2**).[22,27] Many of these clinical signs may have other causes as well. For instance, cutaneous erythema can be seen with differential diagnoses including bacterial sepsis or ranavirus infection.[28]

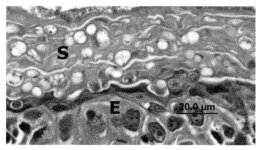

Fig. 1. Histologic section of the skin from a Wyoming toad (*Bufo baxteri*) with severe chytridiomycosis. The epidermis (E) is hyperplastic and the stratum corneum (S) is markedly thickened (hyperkeratosis) with numerous spherical thalli of Bd. Hematoxylin-eosin stain, original magnification ×60.

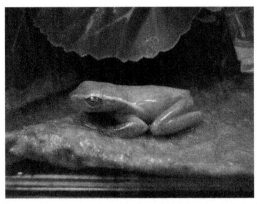

Fig. 2. A hylid tree frog, *Hyloscirtus colymba*, showing advanced clinical signs of chytridio-mycosis caused by a naturally acquired infection with Bd.

A lack of clinical signs is also seen with early low-intensity infections and in subclin-ically infected species that are less susceptible to disease. A lack of clinical signs should not equate with assumption of negative infection status. Clinical signs are generally absent in tadpoles; however, depigmentation of the mouthparts can be observed in heavy infections.[21]

DIAGNOSIS

The diagnosis of Bd infection can be made by either morphologic methods such as cytology or histopathology or by polymerase chain reaction (PCR)-based tests that detect Bd DNA.[29] The morphologic methods are most appropriate for clinically signif-icant infections that are associated with high numbers of organisms, whereas the greater test sensitivity of PCR is needed to diagnose low-intensity or subclinical infec-tions. PCR is essential for applications such as quarantine screening of new animals entering collections, detection of subclinically infected animals, evaluation of the suc-cess of antifungal treatment, and confirmation of diagnoses made by morphologic methods. Isolation of Bd requires specialized methods and therefore routine fungal culture is not helpful for diagnosis.

The morphologic methods of diagnosis depend on the microscopic observation of Bd thalli, which need to be differentiated from other potential inhabitants of amphibian skin such as protozoa or yeast forms of other fungi. The thalli of Bd are spherical to flask-shaped and can range from 7 to 20 µm in diameter. Features that can be useful for distinguishing Bd are: (1) thalli that contain numerous 1 to 2 µm basophilic zoo-spores (rare in cytologic preparations; see **Fig. 3**); (2) empty thalli, which have previ-ously discharged their zoospores (**Figs. 4** and **5**); and (3) colonial thalli, which have evidence of internal septation (**Fig. 6**). General sample collection guidelines for cytology and histopathology include:

- Suitable samples for cytology are gentle skin scrapings from the feet and ventral body or shed skin fragments, which are either examined as a wet mount or air-dried onto a microscope slide and routinely stained.
- Samples for histopathology are usually obtained at necropsy and should include at least 3 sections of skin from the ventral body (eg, pelvic patch, legs, and feet).
- Shed skin fragments collected from the animal or from the environment can also be fixed in formalin and examined by histopathology.

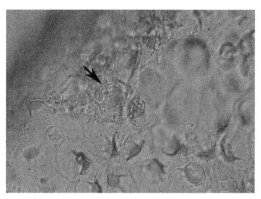

Fig. 3. A wet mount cytology preparation of amphibian skin infected with Bd, showing 2 thalli containing multiple zoospores (*arrow*), enlarged from 40×. In the living specimen, the zoospores can be seen moving within the thalli.

The increasing availability of both conventional and real-time Taqman PCR methods for detection of Bd infection has enabled the development of effective disease control programs for captive amphibian collections. The PCR techniques are exquisitely sensitive and under ideal laboratory conditions can detect as few as 1 to 10 Bd zoospores. This level of sensitivity allows for effective identification of most low-intensity infections and subclinical carriers of Bd. However, there are a few important points to keep in mind when interpreting the results of PCR testing:

- Because PCR can detect such small amounts of Bd DNA, a positive test result does not necessarily equate with disease. This caveat is important when investigating the cause of amphibian mortality events, in which another primary cause of death may be overlooked by Bd PCR testing alone.
- False-negative tests can occur under some circumstances. This finding is especially true with very-low-intensity Bd infections, situations in which it is difficult to obtain ideal samples for PCR testing (eg, very small wet frogs), and the presence

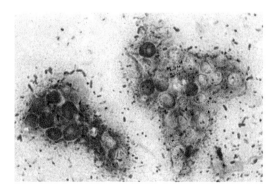

Fig. 4. Skin scraping from a blue poison dart frog (*Dendrobates azureus*) naturally infected with the amphibian chytrid fungus Bd. Thalli are both developing and degenerate in this case and may be difficult to distinguish from yeasts. Numerous empty thalli are present on the right side of the photomicrograph. Diff-Quik stain. (*From* Pessier AP. Cytologic diagnosis of disease in amphibians. Vet Clin North Am Exotic Anim Pract 2007;10(1):196; with permission.)

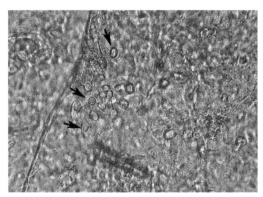

Fig. 5. A wet mount cytology preparation of amphibian skin infected with Bd, showing clusters of empty thalli (*arrows*), original magnification ×40.

of PCR reaction inhibitors in some samples. Although not always financially or logistically feasible, the use of up to 3 separate PCR tests collected over a 14-day period has been suggested to increase confidence in a negative test result in critical situations.[29–31]

- It is easy to cross-contaminate samples from different animals, resulting in false-positive test results. When sampling multiple animals, a fresh pair of gloves should be used for each individual and efforts made to avoid contact of swabs or instruments with work surfaces or substrates.

Skin swabs are the most practical and commonly used sample for Bd PCR testing. To obtain samples, a fine-tipped rayon swab is gently swept 3 to 5 times over the ventral surfaces of the feet, thighs, and abdomen (**Fig. 7**).[29,32] For Taqman PCR, samples are preferably air-dried before shipment to the laboratory; however, some laboratories may suggest preservation in ethanol, especially those using conventional

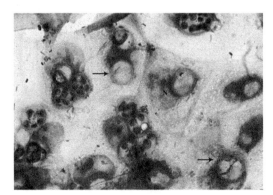

Fig. 6. Sheet of shed skin from a green and black poison dart frog (*Dendrobates auratus*) experimentally infected with the amphibian chytrid fungus Bd. There are numerous spherical intracellular chytrid thalli. Many thalli contain discrete basophilic zoospores and others are empty (*arrows*), having previously discharged zoospores. The empty thallus at the bottom right has evidence of internal septation (colonial thallus). N, nucleus of an epithelial cell. (*From* Pessier AP. Cytologic diagnosis of disease in amphibians. Vet Clin North Am Exotic Anim Pract 2007;10(1):195; with permission.)

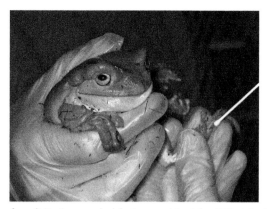

Fig. 7. White's tree frog (*Litoria caerulea*) being swabbed for PCR detection of Bd.

PCR techniques (contact specific laboratories for details: Amphibian Disease Laboratory, San Diego Zoo Global, San Diego, CA; Pisces Molecular LLC, Boulder, CO).

TREATMENT

There is no 1 treatment against chytridiomycosis that is effective in all species and at all life stages. Each treatment modality has its advantages and disadvantages, and there are relatively few reports describing controlled experiments of any 1 agent in more than a narrow range of species or life stages.[30] Further, many agents have been shown to cause adverse effects in certain species or life stages. Whenever possible, selection of a treatment protocol should be based on evidence of effectiveness and safety. If safety has not already been established for a specific protocol in certain species or life stages, it is advisable to evaluate the effect on a few animals first, before treating a large group.

General considerations to keep in mind with any treatments are as follows:

- Strict biosecurity practices are paramount for successful treatment.
- Bd is easily killed on equipment and in the environment with a wide range of disinfectants as well as heat and desiccation.[33]
- Bd organisms can survive and remain infective for long periods in a moist environment.[34]
- Because of persistence in the environment, including animal enclosures, it is important that treated animals are placed in a clean disinfected enclosure after each daily treatment until the full treatment course is completed. Relatively sparse, easily cleaned enclosures are recommended during the course of treatment. Inexpensive plastic containers work well and it is helpful to have 2 enclosures per animal, allowing 1 set to always be disinfected and ready for use.
- Permanent enclosures, including naturalistic vivaria or exhibits, should be completely broken down and all contents and components disinfected before an animal returns after treatments.
- Quarantine practices should be in place, such that untreated animals should not be brought close to animals undergoing treatment.
- Give careful attention to sequence of operations in relation to potential contamination. Do not touch clean equipment or enclosures, or freshly treated animals after touching used supplies, untreated animals, or water that has been in contact with either.

- Use a new pair of gloves for handling each animal and change gloves before moving between enclosures.
- No treatment course should be considered effective without confirmation via posttreatment PCR. As indicated earlier, highest level of confidence is achieved through 3 PCR tests over a 14-day period after treatment.[35]

Treatment Failure

If animals remain PCR positive after a complete course of treatment, it may be tempting to blame the medication as ineffective. It is important to first evaluate the treatment protocol. Biosecurity techniques should be examined for any potential breakdown in clean handling, disinfection, or quarantine procedures that might have allowed contamination and subsequent reinfection. A second treatment course should be attempted, using the same or different treatment agents, with continued focus on proper technique.

One large gap in studies evaluating clearance of infection is how infection intensity relates to treatment efficacy. It may be that some drugs are effective against low infection intensity, or low numbers of Bd zoospores, and treatment failures may occur in more heavily infected animals. For each drug, a dosage-dependent threshold might exist. Different concentrations or different drug combinations may be required against higher infection intensities. This finding is especially true in animals showing clinical signs. These animals require aggressive adjunctive supportive treatments in order to survive a full course of treatment, as is discussed in greater detail later. Treatment failure, in those cases defined by the death of the animal, might have more to do with the state of disease and timely supportive care than with efficacy or possible toxicity of treatment agent used.

Itraconazole

Itraconazole is widely used in a broad number of species, including some critically endangered, in zoos and amphibian conservation programs and is the most commonly used agent in experimental treatments.[31,36–43] It seems to be safe and effective in most instances. However, there are some reports of toxicity especially in tadpoles and newly emerged metamorphs. In other cases, groups of frogs such as the ranids have seemed especially sensitive to treatment through anecdotal and limited experimental reports.[30,32,37,39,40]

All itraconazole protocols are derived from the originally described method of using a 0.01% itraconazole bath solution diluted in 0.6% saline for 5 minutes a day for 11 consecutive days.[36] This original protocol has been empirically modified and many variations of concentration, diluting agent, timing, and length of treatments now exist. Lower concentrations have proved effective, down to 0.005% and 0.0025%.[31,40] Diluting agents described include purified water, 0.9% saline, and amphibian Ringer solution.

Recently published work with juvenile White's tree frogs (*Litoria caerulea*) and coastal plain toads (*Incilius nebulifer*) shows promise for effectiveness and increased safety at itraconazole concentration as low as 0.0025% for 5 minutes daily over as little as 6 days.[40] Further research and collective experience may find this to be a suitable protocol for a wide range of cases. In the meantime, we have the most experience with using 0.01% and 0.005% concentrations and feel comfortable recommending the 0.005% concentration at 5 minutes daily for 10 consecutive days for safe and effective treatment in most situations.[31] Use of the 0.01% concentration may still be required in certain species or with higher infection intensities, whereas the very low concentration protocols of 0.0025% may be considered for sensitive species or low-intensity infections.

The following protocol is recommended for most postmetamorphic animals:

1. Itraconazole 1% (10 mg/ml) solution (Sporanox Oral Solution, Centocor Ortho Biotech Products, L.P., Raritan, NJ) is diluted in amphibian Ringer solution (available commercially as stock solution: http://www.enasco.com, product number SA09708 (LM)M, or see published recipes[28]) to make a 0.005% treatment solution.
   • To make 100 ml of treatment solution, add 0.5 ml of 10 mg/ml itraconazole to 99.5 ml of amphibian Ringers solution.
2. The solution is applied as a bath treatment for 5 minutes daily for 10 consecutive days.
   • Appropriately sized, easily cleaned or disposable containers are recommended. Plastic bags with a sealable closure or small, lidded plastic cups or containers may be used (**Fig. 8**). Small containers reduce the volume of solution required and help to ensure the animal cannot avoid the solution. Plastic bags serve this purpose well and are more yielding to prevent trauma if an animal struggles during treatment.
   • If animals struggle excessively during treatment, recheck the concentration of solution or consider a lower concentration or an alternate drug.
   • Depth of solution should cover approximately midway up the animal's dorsum. Animals should not be completely immersed.
   • The bath solution should be agitated frequently, to ensure that all surfaces of the animal are covered with solution, and to keep medication evenly distributed through the bath.

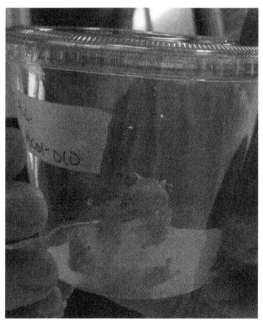

Fig. 8. A frog being treated with an itraconazole bath in a disposable plastic cup. The volume of the bath covers approximately midway up the dorsum, and the container is manipulated as necessary to ensure that the animal remains in the treatment solution.

- The investigators recommend rinsing animals once the bath is completed, using clean filtered water or fresh amphibian Ringer solution. This procedure can be accomplished by restraining the animal and showering it with a spray bottle, or if plastic bags are used as the bath container, the treatment solution can carefully be poured out and replaced with fresh rinse with the animal still inside.
- Return the animal to a clean enclosure after each treatment, as described earlier.

This protocol can easily be adapted for use in the field.[32] Amphibian conservation projects often collect target species from Bd-positive regions for return to ex situ assurance colonies.[42] Beginning treatment in the field can enhance survival by immediately reducing zoospore burdens before the onset of the potential stressors of transport and captivity. On long field expeditions, it can be multiple days from the time of capture until the return to the ex situ facility, and field application of the treatment protocol within the first 24 hours can be a valuable head start.

- Sealable disposable plastic bags or disposable plastic cups are lightweight and easily carried in to the field.
- Itraconazole stock solution can be carried, and filtered local water sources may be used to prepare the diluted treatment solution. Portable water filtration devices made for backpackers that include 0.5-µL filters or smaller can remove Bd organisms from the water.
- Carrying supportive medications, such as amphibian Ringer stock solution and antibiotics in to the field can also improve survival in animals that might already present clinically ill when collected. See additional information on supportive treatments later.

Itraconazole cannot be used at any of these concentrations for treating tadpoles because of high observed mortality. One study reports successful treatment of Mallorcan midwife toad (*Alytes muletensis*) tadpoles with a mere 0.5 to 1.5 mg itraconazole per liter (0.00005%–0.00015%) of treatment solution. However, there may have been toxic effects even at this very low concentration, because those tadpoles lost skin pigmentation after treatment, although the finding was not further investigated.[37]

Other Azole Antifungals

Voriconazole effectively treated Iberian midwife toad (*Alytes cisternasii*) juveniles and a few individual poison dart frogs (Dendrobatidae family) infected with low Bd zoospore burdens.[44]

- Voriconazole is mixed to a concentration of 1.25 µg/ml water and sprayed on to animals once a day for 7 days.

Voriconazole may also prove useful as a safe option for treatment of tadpoles. Tadpoles showed no toxic effect after exposure to voriconazole up to 12.5 µg/ml for 7 days, although treatment efficacy studies have not yet been reported.[44]

Miconazole may be an effective azole antifungal, although it has been only minimally described.[36] Fluconazole protocols have shown only marginal effectiveness.[30]

Chloramphenicol

Chloramphenicol is an antibiotic that acts by inhibiting protein synthesis.[45] Typically used against bacterial organisms, it has recently been found to also be active against Bd, although only reported in a few animals. Three clinically affected *L caerulea* with high zoospore burdens survived and were successfully cleared of Bd using chloramphenicol in conjunction with increased ambient temperature and isotonic fluid support.[46]

In humans and animals, bone marrow suppression and potentially aplastic anemia and leukemia can occur, including in amphibians.[46,47] Gloves should be worn when handling chloramphenicol, and prolonged exposure should be avoided.

The following protocol is described for use of chloramphenicol in treatment of Bd[46]:

1. Chloramphenicol stock solution is made by adding 200 mg of chloramphenicol powder (chloramphenicol C0378; Sigma-Aldrich, St Louis, MO) to 1 L of hot water. One part of the stock solution is diluted in 9 parts water to make a 0.002% treatment solution.
   - To make 100 ml of 0.002% chloramphenicol treatment solution, add 10 ml of 200 mg/L stock solution to 90 ml water.
2. Animals are placed into a shallow immersion bath of treatment solution with continuous exposure for 2 to 4 weeks.
   - Techniques for bath treatment are as described for itraconazole.
   - Treatment solution is changed daily.

Although this protocol was reported to be well tolerated in *L caerulea*, the prolonged immersion of several weeks seems best suited for aquatic species. Daily handling for up to 4 weeks and the logistics of husbandry and feeding in a continuous bath seems potentially stressful and impractical for terrestrial species. An anecdotal report within the same study does note that prolonged exposure had no ill effect in tadpoles, opening this as a potentially viable treatment of that difficult life stage.[46] More work should be carried out to determine efficacy and safety of chloramphenicol before wide use can be recommended. A related antibiotic, florfenicol, was not effective at treating Bd.[48]

Terbinafine

Terbinafine receives much attention in the private hobbyist trade, and terbinafine treatment protocols of various iterations are readily available online.[49] The popularity of its use is no doubt because of its ease of availability in the form of commercial over-the-counter athlete's foot preparations (Lamisil AT Spray, 1% terbinafine hydrochloride, Novartis Consumer Health, Parsippany, NJ). Although accounts are many, nearly all are anecdotal and none begins with PCR confirmation of Bd infection. There is only 1 peer-reviewed publication on the use of terbinafine,[50] which does report elimination of Bd infection in 5 anuran and 1 caudate species, although this was not a controlled experiment. Terbinafine dissolved in ethanol was diluted in distilled water to create solutions of 0.01% to 0.005% terbinafine and 1% to 0.5% ethanol, respectively. Animals were bathed for 5 minutes daily for 5 consecutive days. One experimental control that was not performed but might be interesting is bath solutions of the ethanol alone.

Chemical Treatments

Malachite green and formalin

- A colony of African clawed frogs (*Xenopus tropicalis*) was treated using malachite green 0.1 mg/L and formalin 25 ppm administered as a total tank treatment for 24 hours every other day for a total of 4 treatments.[51] Efficacy is unknown, because the study did not have appropriate follow-up available with PCR confirmation after treatment. Unknown effect and concerns with human and animal carcinogenesis leave this technique difficult to recommend.[30]

Benzalkonium chloride

- Benzalkonium chloride is another agent that is in use by private hobbyists with treatment protocols distributed on the Internet.[52] This chemical is a quaternary ammonium disinfectant occasionally used as an antifungal medication in fish and amphibians. Its use against chytrid is based on 1 early published report in dwarf African clawed frogs (*Hymenochirus curtipes*). Treatment did apparently reduce mortality, but did not eliminate Bd from the frogs.[53]
- Benzalkonium chloride treatment is not recommended.

Temperature

Optimum growth of Bd occurs between 17°C and 25°C. Higher than 25°C, growth slows, and at prolonged exposure to 30°C, Bd organisms begin to die.[54] Wild Panamanian golden frogs (*Atelopus zeteki*) have been documented to increase their body temperatures by altering thermoregulatory behavior in response to infection, with odds of infection decreasing as body temperature increases.[55] Experimentally infected *A zeteki* also survived longer at 23°C than did those kept at 17°C.[56] Natural microclimates with water temperature higher than 30°C was protective against Bd infection in wild lowland leopard frogs (*Lithobates yavapaiensis*).[57]

Increased temperature can be a useful adjunct to other treatment modalities and in some cases, increased temperature has been used exclusively to clear Bd infections. Naturally infected, subclinically affected wild bullfrogs (*Rana catesbeiana*) and cricket frogs (*Acris crepitans*) were nearly all (27 of 28) cleared of infection after being held at 30°C for 10 days. In other studies, chorus frogs (*Pseudacris triseriata*) cleared Bd infection after 5 days of exposure to 32°C, and green tree frogs (*Litoria chloris*) seemed to clear infection after only 2 8-hour exposures to temperatures of 37°C (although the latter study only used histopathology as a means to detect Bd organisms, a less sensitive method than PCR detection).[35,58,59]

- Given the expense, potential adverse effects, and various logistics of many of the described pharmaceutical and chemical treatments, increasing temperature as an easy form of treatment is an attractive option for appropriate species.
- Many amphibian species are adapted to cool temperatures and may not tolerate increases as high as described earlier. Finding tolerable temperature limits that do not overly stress a species, yet are still higher than ideal Bd growth ranges, may prove useful as an addition to other treatment methods.

Probiotics

The use of bacteria with anti-Bd properties has been researched to protect against Bd infection. *Janthinobacterium lividum*, a commensal bacterium isolated from redback salamanders (*Plethodon cinereus*) and other amphibians, produces an antifungal metabolite called violacein.[60] Inoculation of a Bd-susceptible amphibian, such as the mountain yellow-legged frog (*Rana muscosa*) with *J lividum* is protective against mortality from chytridiomycosis.[61] However, use of the probiotic technique may not be widely applicable. The microenvironment of amphibian skin has evolved with its own commensal assemblage of microbial flora, adapted for each species. It seems that the probiotic microorganism chosen should be one that might otherwise occur on the target species in natural circumstances. *J lividum*, for instance, has been found previously on *R muscosa* and was successfully used in that species to augment the protective flora.[61] *J lividum* has never been naturally isolated from *A zeteki*, on the other hand, and attempts to inoculate *A zeteki* with this bacteria result in only short-term persistence and no protective benefits.[62]

Supportive Treatments for Animals Clinically Ill with Chytridiomycosis

Animals showing clinical signs of chytridiomycosis, as described earlier, may have excessive skin shedding, lethargy, poor righting reflexes, hunched posture, or dermal hemorrhage. Prognosis for these animals is poor without supportive treatments to help keep them alive long enough for antifungal medications to clear the skin of Bd.

Fluid therapy

Critically low levels of electrolytes caused by loss of skin osmoregulatory function need to be addressed immediately.

- One of the authors has had good response by placing affected animals in an amphibian Ringer bath prepared at isotonic or slightly hypertonic concentration (1:9 vs 2:8 stock solution to water, respectively; sterile or distilled water can be used). Lethargic animals placed in these baths have been found to improve activity over time, with self-removal from the Ringer solution being a good indicator of positive response (Baitchman, personal experience). The bath is provided continuously throughout the course of Bd treatments, and replaced fresh daily.
- Experimental studies report recovery of moribund frogs with use of oral 12% Whitaker-Wright solution administered by stomach tube every 4 to 6 hours; or subcutaneous administration of injectable isotonic electrolyte solution every 8 hours.[16,46]
- Sodium chloride bath solutions alone reduced growth and motility of Bd and increased survival rates of Peron's tree frogs (*Litoria peronii*) infected with Bd, at concentrations greater than 3 ppt.[63]
- A review of amphibian fluid therapy and formulas for electrolyte solutions is available in Ref.[28]

Antibiotics

Empirical use of antibiotics is recommended for coverage against secondary bacterial invasion.

- Enrofloxacin is a good choice for first-line antibiotic use in amphibians, with excellent coverage of gram-negative organisms, including those typically associated with sepsis in amphibians.[64] pH of injectable enrofloxacin (Baytril 2.27%, Bayer Health Care, LLC, Shawnee Mission, KS) is greater than 11 and very caustic to amphibian tissues.[65] Dilution in sterile saline at a 1:1 ratio is recommended before use and can be administered topically or subcutaneously at 10 mg/kg once daily.[28]

Nutrition

Throughout the course of treating amphibians for chytridiomycosis, some attention should be given to the nutritional state of each animal. For many species, the process of treatments and repetitive handling is stressful. It is common for animals to become anorexic during this period. If an animal is not eating on its own after 5 to 7 days, consider providing nutrition through assist feeding or gavage tube. Body condition and disposition might also be assessed in terms of deciding need for these measures. If an animal is well conditioned and robust, it may have appropriate stores to neglect eating for a 7-day to 10-day treatment period. We offer no specific formula for these decisions, other than encouraging clinical judgment in each case relative to need for supplemental nutritional support.

Most amphibians that are bright and alert reflexively swallow items placed in the mouth. A relatively stress-free method of assist feeding an animal is to open its mouth with a soft, rigid speculum, place an appropriate crushed prey item (supplemented as appropriate with vitamin or calcium dusting or gut loading) in the oral cavity, and remove the speculum. Ideally, less digestible portions of the prey (eg, heads or legs of crickets) are removed before feeding.

Tube feeding may be performed with an appropriately sized ball-tipped gavage needle or similar feeding tube. The distance to the stomach is approximately one-third the body length, and the tube is placed cautiously a short way beyond the sphincter visible at the back of the pharyngeal cavity. Enteral feeding formulas made for carnivores, such as Lafeber's Emeraid Exotic Carnivore or Oxbow Animal Health Carnivore Care, approximate the nutritional needs of an amphibian. In calculating total volume to feed, metabolic requirements can be calculated exactly, although a rule of thumb is to not exceed 10% of the animal's weight per day.[28]

SUMMARY

Whichever modality is chosen for treatment of chytridiomycosis, attempt to make a selection based on previous evidence of safety and efficacy for the species you are working with. Careful attention to biosecurity and hygiene practices during treatment is necessary to ensure complete clearance of Bd organisms from the patient. Whenever possible, PCR should be used for confirmation of the diagnosis, as well as for posttreatment confirmation of clearance. Animals that are clinically ill with chytridiomycosis require additional supportive care to enhance survival during treatment.

REFERENCES

1. Longcore JE, Pessier A, Nichols DK. *Batrachochytrium dendrobatidis* gen. et sp. nov., a chytrid pathogenic to amphibians. Mycologia 1999;91(2):219–27.
2. Daszak P, Cunningham AA, Hyatt AD. Infectious disease and amphibian population declines. Diversity and Distributions 2003;9(2):141–50.
3. Lips KR, Brem F, Brenes R, et al. Emerging infectious disease and the loss of biodiversity in a neotropical amphibian community. Proc Natl Acad Sci U S A 2006;103(9):3165–70.
4. Fisher MC, Garner TW, Walker SF. Global emergence of *Batrachochytrium dendrobatidis* and amphibian chytridiomycosis. Annu Rev Microbiol 2009;63: 291–310.
5. Skerratt LF, Berger L, Speare R, et al. Spread of chytridiomycosis has caused the rapid global decline and extinction of frogs. Ecohealth 2007;4(2):125–34.
6. Lips KR, Diffendorfer J, Mendelson JR, et al. Riding the wave: reconciling the roles of disease and climate change in amphibian declines. PLoS Biol 2008; 6(3):e72.
7. Vredenburg VT, Knapp RA, Tunstall TS, et al. Dynamics of an emerging disease drive large-scale amphibian population extinctions. Proc Natl Acad Sci U S A 2010;107(21):9689–94.
8. Garner TW, Walker S, Bosch J, et al. Chytrid fungus in Europe. Emerg Infect Dis 2005;11(10):1639–41.
9. Weldon C, du Preez LH, Hyatt AD, et al. Origin of the amphibian chytrid fungus. Emerg Infect Dis 2004;10(12):2100–5.
10. Schloegel LM, Toledo LF, Longcore JE, et al. Novel, panzootic and hybrid genotypes of amphibian chytridiomycosis associated with the bullfrog trade. Mol Ecol 2012;21(21):5162–77.

11. Farrer RA, Weinert LA, Bielby J, et al. Multiple emergences of genetically diverse amphibian-infecting chytrids include a globalized hypervirulent recombinant lineage. Proc Natl Acad Sci U S A 2011;108(46):18732–6.
12. Goka K, Yokoyama J, Une Y, et al. Amphibian chytridiomycosis in Japan: distribution, haplotypes and possible route of entry into Japan. Mol Ecol 2009;18(23): 4757–74.
13. Schloegel LM, Daszak P, Cunningham AA, et al. Two amphibian diseases, chytridiomycosis and ranaviral disease, are now globally notifiable to the World Organization for Animal Health (OIE): an assessment. Dis Aquat Organ 2010; 92(2–3):101–8.
14. Hillman SS, Withers PC, Drewes RC, et al. Ecological and environmental physiology of amphibians. New York: Oxford University Press; 2009.
15. Duellman WE, Trueb L. Biology of amphibians. Baltimore (MD): Johns Hopkins University Press; 1994.
16. Voyles J, Young S, Berger L, et al. Pathogenesis of chytridiomycosis, a cause of catastrophic amphibian declines. Science 2009;326(5952):582–5.
17. Voyles J, Vredenburg VT, Tunstall TS, et al. Pathophysiology in mountain yellow-legged frogs (*Rana muscosa*) during a chytridiomycosis outbreak. PLoS One 2012;7(4):e35374.
18. Greenspan SE, Longcore JE, Calhoun AJ. Host invasion by *Batrachochytrium dendrobatidis*: fungal and epidermal ultrastructure in model anurans. Dis Aquat Organ 2012;100(3):201–10.
19. Van Rooij P, Martel A, D'Herde K, et al. Germ tube mediated invasion of *Batrachochytrium dendrobatidis* in amphibian skin is host dependent. PLoS One 2012;7(7):e41481.
20. Berger L, Hyatt AD, Speare R, et al. Life cycle stages of the amphibian chytrid *Batrachochytrium dendrobatidis*. Dis Aquat Organ 2005;68(1):51–63.
21. Rachowicz LJ, Vredenburg VT. Transmission of *Batrachochytrium dendrobatidis* within and between amphibian life. Dis Aquat Organ 2004;61(1–2): 75–83.
22. Voyles J, Rosenblum EB, Berger L. Interactions between *Batrachochytrium dendrobatidis* and its amphibian hosts: a review of pathogenesis and immunity. Microbes Infect 2011;13(1):25–32.
23. Pessier AP, Nichols DK, Longcore JE, et al. Cutaneous chytridiomycosis in poison dart frogs (*Dendrobates* spp.) and White's tree frogs (*Litoria caerulea*). J Vet Diagn Invest 1999;11(2):194–9.
24. Marcum RD, St-Hilaire S, Murphy PJ, et al. Effects of *Batrachochytrium dendrobatidis* infection on ion concentrations in the boreal toad *Anaxyrus (Bufo) boreas boreas*. Dis Aquat Organ 2010;91(1):17–21.
25. Reeder NM, Pessier AP, Vredenburg VT. A reservoir species for the emerging amphibian pathogen *Batrachochytrium*. PLoS One 2012;7(3):e33567.
26. Savage AE, Zamudio KR. MHC genotypes associate with resistance to a frog-killing fungus. Proc Natl Acad Sci U S A 2011;108(40):16705–10.
27. Pessier AP. Amphibian chytridiomycosis. In: Miller RE, Fowler ME, editors. Zoo and wild animal medicine: current therapy, vol. 6. St Louis (MO): Elsevier Saunders; 2008. p. 137–43.
28. Wright KM, Whitaker BR. Amphibian medicine and captive husbandry. Malabar (FL): Krieger; 2001.
29. Hyatt AD, Boyle DG, Olsen V, et al. Diagnostic assays and sampling protocols for the detection of *Batrachochytrium dendrobatidis*. Dis Aquat Organ 2007; 73(3):175–92.

30. Berger L, Speare R, Pessier A, et al. Treatment of chytridiomycosis requires urgent clinical trials. Dis Aquat Organ 2010;92(2–3):165–74.
31. Jones ME, Paddock D, Bender L, et al. Treatment of chytridiomycosis with reduced-dose itraconazole. Dis Aquat Organ 2012;99(3):243–9.
32. A manual for control of infectious diseases in amphibian survival assurance colonies and reintroduction programs. In: Pessier AP, Medelson JR, editors. IUCN/SSC Conservation Breeding Specialist Group. Apple Valley (MN). Available at: http://www.amphibianark.org/pdf/Amphibian_Disease_Manual.pdf. Accessed June 29, 2013.
33. Young S, Berger L, Speare R. Amphibian chytridiomycosis: strategies for captive management and conservation. Int Zoo Yearbk 2007;41(1):85–95.
34. Johnson ML, Speare R. Survival of *Batrachochytrium dendrobatidis* in water: quarantine and disease control implications. Emerg Infect Dis 2003;9(8):922–5.
35. Pessier AP. Diagnosis and control of amphibian chytridiomycosis. In: Miller RE, Fowler ME, editors. Zoo and wild animal medicine: current therapy, vol. 7. St Louis (MO): Elsevier Saunders; 2012. p. 217–23.
36. Nichols DK, Lamirande EW, Pessier A, et al. Experimental transmission and treatment of cutaneous chytridiomycosis in poison dart frogs (*Dendrobates auratus* and *Dendrobates tinctorius*). Paper presented at: American Association of Zoo Veterinarians. New Orleans (LA), September 17–21, 2000.
37. Garner TW, Garcia G, Carroll B, et al. Using itraconazole to clear *Batrachochytrium dendrobatidis* infection, and subsequent depigmentation of *Alytes muletensis* tadpoles. Dis Aquat Organ 2009;83(3):257–60.
38. Tamukai K, Une Y, Tominaga A, et al. Treatment of spontaneous chytridiomycosis in captive amphibians using itraconazole. J Vet Med Sci 2011;73(2):155–9.
39. Woodhams DC, Geiger CC, Reinert LK, et al. Treatment of amphibians infected with chytrid fungus: learning from failed trials with itraconazole, antimicrobial peptides, bacteria, and heat therapy. Dis Aquat Organ 2012;98(1):11–25.
40. Brannelly LA, Richards-Zawacki CL, Pessier AP. Clinical trials with itraconazole as a treatment for chytrid fungal infections in amphibians. Dis Aquat Organ 2012;101(2):95–104.
41. Pessier AP. Management of disease as a threat to amphibian conservation. Int Zoo Yearbk 2008;42(1):30–9.
42. Gagliardo R, Crump P, Griffith E, et al. The principles of rapid response for amphibian conservation, using the programmes in Panama as an example. Int Zoo Yearbk 2008;42(1):125–35.
43. Forzán MJ, Gunn H, Scott P. Chytridiomycosis in an aquarium collection of frogs: diagnosis, treatment, and control. J Zoo Wildl Med 2008;39(3):406–11.
44. Martel A, Van Rooij P, Vercauteren G, et al. Developing a safe antifungal treatment protocol to eliminate *Batrachochytrium dendrobatidis* from amphibians. Med Mycol 2011;49(2):143–9.
45. Neu HC, Gootz TD. Antimicrobial chemotherapy. In: Baron S, editor. Medical microbiology. 4th edition. Galveston (TX): The University of Texas Medical Branch at Galveston; 1996. Chapter 11. Available at: http://www.ncbi.nlm.nih.gov/books/NBK7986/. Accessed June 29, 2013.
46. Young S, Speare R, Berger L, et al. Chloramphenicol with fluid and electrolyte therapy cures terminally ill green tree frogs (*Litoria caerulea*) with chytridiomycosis. J Zoo Wildl Med 2012;43(2):330–7.
47. el-Mofty MM, Abdelmeguid NE, Sadek IA, et al. Induction of leukaemia in chloramphenicol-treated toads. East Mediterr Health J 2000;6(5–6):1026–34.

48. Muijsers M, Martel A, Van Rooij P, et al. Antibacterial therapeutics for the treatment of chytrid infection in amphibians: Columbus's egg? BMC Vet Res 2012;8:175.
49. Chytrid fungus. Available at: http://www.theaquariumwiki.com/Chytrid_fungus. Accessed December 18, 2012.
50. Bowerman J, Rombough C, Weinstock SR, et al. Terbinafine hydrochloride in ethanol effectively clears *Batrachochytrium dendrobatidis* in amphibians. J Herpetol Med Surg 2010;20(1):24–8.
51. Parker JM, Mikaelian I, Hahn N, et al. Clinical diagnosis and treatment of epidermal chytridiomycosis in African clawed frogs (Xenopus tropicalis). Comp Med 2002;52(3):265–8.
52. Benzalkonium chloride procedure for treating chytridiomycosis in African dwarf frogs. Available at: http://www.flippersandfins.net/ChytridBCTreatment.htm. Accessed December 18, 2012.
53. Groff JM, Mughannam A, McDowell TS, et al. An epizootic of cutaneous zygomycosis in cultured dwarf African clawed frogs (*Hymenochirus curtipes*) due to *Basidiobolus ranarum*. J Med Vet Mycol 1991;29(4):215–23.
54. Piotrowski JS, Annis SL, Longcore JE. Physiology of *Batrachochytrium dendrobatidis*, a chytrid pathogen of amphibians. Mycologia 2004;96(1):9.
55. Richards-Zawacki CL. Thermoregulatory behaviour affects prevalence of chytrid fungal infection in a wild population of Panamanian golden frogs. Proc Biol Sci 2010;277(1681):519–28.
56. Bustamante HM, Livo LJ, Carey C. Effects of temperature and hydric environment on survival of the Panamanian golden frog infected with a pathogenic chytrid fungus. Integr Zool 2010;5(2):143–53.
57. Forrest MJ, Schlaepfer MA. Nothing a hot bath won't cure: infection rates of amphibian chytrid fungus correlate negatively with water temperature under natural field settings. PLoS One 2011;6(12):e28444.
58. Retallick RW, Miera V. Strain differences in the amphibian chytrid *Batrachochytrium dendrobatidis* and non-permanent, sub-lethal effects of infection. Dis Aquat Organ 2007;75(3):201–7.
59. Woodhams DC, Alford RA, Marantelli G. Emerging disease of amphibians cured by elevated body temperature. Dis Aquat Organ 2003;55(1):65–7.
60. Becker MH, Brucker RM, Schwantes CR, et al. The bacterially produced metabolite violacein is associated with survival of amphibians infected with a lethal fungus. Appl Environ Microbiol 2009;75(21):6635–8.
61. Harris RN, Brucker RM, Walke JB, et al. Skin microbes on frogs prevent morbidity and mortality caused by a lethal skin fungus. ISME J 2009;3(7):818–24.
62. Becker MH, Harris RN, Minbiole KP, et al. Towards a better understanding of the use of probiotics for preventing chytridiomycosis in Panamanian golden frogs. Ecohealth 2011;8(4):501–6.
63. Stockwell MP, Clulow J, Mahony MJ. Sodium chloride inhibits the growth and infective capacity of the amphibian chytrid fungus and increases host survival rates. PLoS One 2012;7(5):e36942.
64. Schadich E, Cole AL. Pathogenicity of *Aeromonas hydrophila*, *Klebsiella pneumoniae*, and *Proteus mirabilis* to brown tree frogs (*Litoria ewingii*). Comp Med 2010;60(2):114–7.
65. Plumb DC. Plumb's veterinary drug handbook. 7th edition. Stockholm (WI): PharmaVet; 2011.

Itchy Fish and Viral Dermatopathies
Sampling, Diagnosis, and Management of Common Viral Diseases

E.P. Scott Weber III, VMD, MSc

KEYWORDS

- Virus • Fish • Herpesvirus • Iridovirus • CyHV1 • Lymphocystis • Quarantine

KEY POINTS

- Fish commonly succumb to a variety of dermatologic problems from poor handling, inappropriate husbandry, environmental conditions of suboptimal quality, interspecific and intraspecific aggression, and infectious disease.
- Several viruses can lead to primary or secondary dermatopathies.
- Nonlethal diagnostic skin scrapes, fin biopsies, skin cultures, and full-thickness skin biopsies can be readily taken from fish patients.
- There are currently no treatments available for viral diseases diagnosed in fish.
- Incorporation of appropriate quarantine, husbandry, and sanitation is the key to avoiding and preventing viral outbreaks in the home aquarium, public display, or aquaculture facility.

INTRODUCTION

From a taxonomic perspective, fish are the largest and most species-rich group of vertebrates, numbering 60,229 described species and subspecies, with 32,590 species scientifically validated.[1-3] More than 458 new species were described in 2012 alone, and it is estimated that 340 species are added annually.[1-3] This taxon includes 3 extant classes including the jawless fishes (Agnatha), bony fishes (Osteichthyes), and cartilaginous fishes (Chondrichthyes). With such a great number of species, fish have adapted to a wide range of aquatic environs from Arctic and Southern oceans, to desert puddles, and from deep-sea hydrothermal vents, to glacial mountain lakes

Disclosures: The author has nothing to disclose.
VM: Medicine and Epidemiology, University of California, Davis, 2108 Tupper Hall, Davis, CA 95616, USA
E-mail address: epweber@ucdavis.edu

Vet Clin Exot Anim 16 (2013) 687–703
http://dx.doi.org/10.1016/j.cvex.2013.05.012
1094-9194/13/$ – see front matter © 2013 Elsevier Inc. All rights reserved.

and streams.[1] The dispersal and abundance of fish have led to their use by humans in numerous ways.

- The Romans kept pet fish such as moray eels or lampreys 2000 years ago[4]; fish were described as being kept in ponds in the Middle East for food nearly 4500 years ago[5,6]; the Chinese raised carp and began selective breeding as early as 960 to 1279 AD during the Song Dynasty; and pet cichlids or other fish species kept at temples were depicted in wall paintings by Egyptians 1400 years ago.[7]
- In the United States the numbers of fish kept as pets are 151.1 million freshwater fish and 8.61 million saltwater fish, as reported in 2012 by the American Pet Products Association 2011/2012 National Pet Owners Survey.[8]
- The zebrafish has become one of the most common laboratory animal models for a variety of toxicologic and biomedical research.
- Aquatic animals are taking a center stage in public aquaria and zoos, with a Global Aquarium Strategy for Conservation and Sustainability being initiated by the World Association of Zoos and Aquariums drafted in 2009.[9]
- Fish are sentinel species for evaluation of marine and freshwater ecosystems, habitat assessment, conservation medicine, and ecological health.
- Several species are commonly stocked for recreational sport fishing and as game fish from private, state, federal, and tribal hatcheries.

Regardless of whether fish are for consumption or admiration, their aesthetic appearance is a driving factor for live whole food fish markets as well as ornamental pet and garden markets. The most expensive koi recorded was bought for roughly $450,000, although animals have been rumored to sell at prices exceeding $1.4 million to $2.2 million. The value of these animals is based on genetics, body confirmation, coloration, and external appearance. Everything from stress, trauma, toxins, and cancer to a variety of pathogens including metazoans, protozoans, algae, fungi, bacteria, and viruses can initially manifest as dermatopathies.[9,10] Some of these pathogens are well recognized, such as the protozoan cryptocaryon that causes white spot in marine tropical fish (**Fig. 1**), whereas other pathogens, such as several pigmented fungi, are newly emerging diseases such as *Exophiala angulospora*, isolated from several species including weedy (*Phyllopteryx taeniolatus*) and leafy seadragons (*Phycodurus eques*) in 2001 (**Fig. 2**), *Veronaea botryosa* from white sturgeon (*Acipenser transmontanus*) (Gary Marty, personal communication, 1997 to present), and *Aureobasidium*

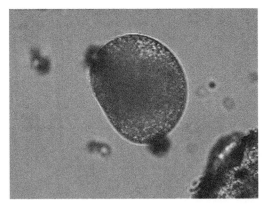

Fig. 1. Tomont stage of protozoan *Cryptocaryon irritans* from a blue tang *Paracanthurus hepatus* taken from a freshly mounted skin scrape (original magnification ×40).

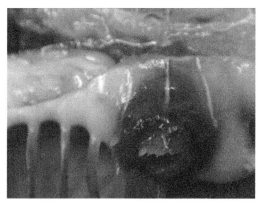

Fig. 2. Missing fin ray of a leafy seadragon *Phycodurus eques* infected by pigmented fungus *Exophiala angulospora.*

pullulans and *Cladosporium cladosporioides* complex identified in white sea bass (*Atractoscion nobilis*) in 2012 (Clinical case submitted by California Department of Fish and Wildlife).[11] Dermatologic lesions are often the first clinical signs of disease noted in fish by their owners. If undiagnosed and untreated, dermatologic lesions can lead to high morbidity and mortality for both the individual and collection animals, manifesting as a primary or secondary illness depending on the etiology, duration, and amount of integument infected. A hallmark of many fish diseases is a lack of pathognomonic signs that can aid with diagnosis in many outbreaks. Viral dermatopathies of fish are no exception, bearing many clinical signs similar to those in dermatopathies from other causes. This article offers an overview to approaching dermatologic presentations in fish, with an emphasis on sampling, diagnosis, and management of viral dermatopathies, building on previous publications.[12]

PISCINE INTEGUMENT

Fish integument is described in detail in various pathology and physiology text resources.[13–16] The skin in fish serves many of the same properties as in other vertebrates, but, unlike most vertebrates, fish integument is largely lacking in keratin. It serves as a protective barrier, physically as an external covering including skin and/or scales, and biologically and chemically as an active mucous membrane containing immune mediators.[12] The skin is involved heavily in osmoregulation through active transport of ions, and by its ability to tighten and loosen cell junctions and alter cell permeability. The outermost layer is the epidermis, composed of epithelial cells and a mucous membrane that covers the dermis; the dermis, in turn, has scales aiding in protection and movement, mucous glands, chloride cells, and chromatophores providing color. Scales in fish are embedded and derived from the mesoderm layer of dermis, which differ from the epidermal-derived scales found in reptiles. The dermal matrix consists of fibroblasts, collagen, blood vessels, and sensory organs. Scales help convey information regarding the natural history and habitat of the various species by the type (placoid: Heterodontidae; ganoid: Acipenseridae; cycloid: Salmonidae; ctenoid: Percidae; scutes: Monocentridae), size, color, and number, and evolved independently in both bony and cartilaginous fishes. Scales are produced by genes similar to those required for tooth and hair development in mammals.[17] Chromatophores in the dermis are of various colors, and include melanophores (melanin), erythrophores (reddish carotenoid pigments), xanthophores (yellowish pteridine pigments), and iridophores (guanine pigment that reflects light and appears metallic). By the movement of melanin granules within these cells, fish can change color, lighten, and darken.

COMMON CLINICAL SIGNS OF DERMATOPATHIES IN FISH

Several common nonspecific signs can be seen in fish with dermatopathies:

1. Pruritus, exhibited as "flashing." Fish with external irritation appear to rapidly shake or twist, sometimes scraping their sides, ventrum, or dorsum against hard surfaces such as driftwood, tank sides, filter-intake pipes, rocks, gravel, or other fish/invertebrates. An increase of frequency and duration of this behavior may indicate worsening irritation of the skin caused by a variety of factors, but most commonly is associated with increased protozoan or metazoan infections
2. Increased mucus production of the skin and gills
3. Darkening or lightening of the skin
4. Light- or dark-colored patches on the skin
5. Raised areas on the skin
6. Appearance of white spots, raised white patches, or nodules
7. Scale loss
8. Hemorrhage and ulceration, petechial hemorrhages increased or prominently appearing vascularization at skin surface
9. Dermal necrosis

DIAGNOSTIC OVERVIEW

The components of a basic fish workup and the concomitant environmental testing have been covered in a variety of peer-reviewed and academic-based textbooks.[18–24] After acquiring a comprehensive history including natural history of the species being maintained, husbandry, life-support system design and maintenance, and nonveterinary medical treatments and water conditioning administered, the basic components of the physical examination of the fish will help to narrow down a differential list using the following steps.

- A comprehensive water-quality analysis that may include general parameters, chlorine, and testing for heavy metals
- A general physical examination looking at body condition, including an ocular and oral examination of an individual or several representatives from a large school of animals
- Diagnostic sampling taken for fresh mounts such as a skin scrape, fin biopsy, gill biopsy, and impression smears from organs at necropsy
- Blood drawn for hematology, serum chemistry, heavy-metal testing, or nutrient analysis (taurine)
- An anal swab taken for a direct smear to look for fecal parasites, or acid-fast staining of the slide to see if the animal is passing acid-fast organisms; if a fecal sample is obtained, a direct smear and fecal float may be performed
- In some species bladder catheterization may be performed to obtain a urine sample, and ovarian or seminal fluid sampled[19,24]

When approaching a fish patient, the appearance of the integument should be observed, preferably while the animal is still in water. Changes that are noted include variations in coloration; changes in skin texture; missing scales; abrasions, lacerations, or ulcerations; excessive mucus; white, black, yellow, or red spots; the appearance of cotton-like material attached to skin or fins; and external parasites. The clinician can use a light or magnifying glass to examine the external integument when the fish is sedated. To investigate damage to the integument, fluorescein ophthalmic stain can be used externally on the skin in a similar manner as when used to stain vertebrate corneas to better highlight breaches in fish epidermis.[25]

Although most dermatologic problems in fish are directly related to external parasites, inappropriate husbandry, poor handling, trauma, and specific issues concerning poor water quality, several types of cancer and microbial infectious agents can cause primary and secondary skin lesions.[22,23]

Another challenge faced in diagnosing disease in aquatic patients is finding a laboratory that works with these species-specific pathogens, especially for fish microbiology. Aquatic organisms require specialized agars with or without salt, and lower incubation temperatures than traditional pathogens from terrestrial animals. Interpretation of microbiologic results requires knowledge of aquatic pathogens to help distinguish common environmental skin contamination from primary or secondary fish pathogens. To establish expertise in fish virology, most aquatic animal health diagnostic laboratories maintain fish-specific cell lines. For example, at the University of California Davis Laboratory for Aquatic Animal Health, more than 120 fish cell lines are maintained including those for cold water, temperate, and tropical marine and freshwater species, even including a cell line for elasmobranchs (great white shark *Carcharodon carcharias*). Once one identifies a suitable laboratory, the laboratory personnel may use 1 or multiple methods to obtain an accurate diagnosis. These diagnostic tests include direct microscopic examination and morphologic descriptions; culture and sensitivity via automated or manual methods; serologic testing such as serum agglutination, immunofluorescent antibody staining, immunohistochemistry staining, and serum neutralization assays; and/or enzyme-linked immunosorbent assay (ELISA) for measuring antigen or antibody against a specific pathogen. Although the polymerase chain reaction (PCR) is a valuable tool, diagnostic results using PCR should be interpreted with caution. Rather than be used as an exclusive diagnostic tool to determine infection with a specific agent, PCR should be used in conjunction with traditional culture techniques and/or histopathology to identify pathogens, which helps to ensure that molecular PCR findings corroborate directly with the disease problem being investigated rather than simply identifying and amplifying DNA. PCR can be used to sequence the genome of previously undescribed pathogens.

Many diagnostic samples taken from fish help to identify live external pathogens. A few procedures are described here for obtaining both a skin scrape for a fresh mount and a skin biopsy. It is always recommended to wear powder-free latex or vinyl gloves when performing this diagnostic sampling to protect the animal's external mucous layer and prevent the transfer of potential zoonotic diseases from the affected fish to the veterinarian or veterinary staff. Although skin scrapes are sometimes obtained with brief manual restraint, more invasive procedures should be done using sedation or anesthesia.[24] Once the animal is sedated one can begin to gather diagnostics, which may include a skin scrape, fin biopsy, and or skin biopsy and culture.

A skin scrape is performed as part of the routine physical examination of every fish. Skin scrapes can be performed without sedation in routine screening of healthy fish for quarantine examinations. As a word of caution before interpreting biopsy and scrape results as negative, some anesthetics commonly used as bath treatments for fish may also have an effect on external fish parasites. This procedure commonly detects bacteria, fungi, algae, and protozoan and metazoan parasites, but can also be valuable for diagnosing a few viral pathogens. A coverslip (or glass slide) is held at a 45° angle to the integument and, with mild pressure, is moved along the skin in a cranial to caudal direction. The best places to sample the epidermis are along the lateral flank, from the base of the pectoral fins, under the mandible and along the ventrum, or at the base of the dorsal fin: anywhere the hydrodynamic forces on the fish are minimal, thus allowing parasites to adhere most effectively. Epidermal cells, mucus, and parasites will be present on the edge of the coverslip or slide if performed correctly. The pressure used should not dislodge numerous scales or create hemorrhage. Because many of these external pathogens are more readily detected while alive and moving, before setting the coverslip a drop of fresh water or saline can be added to the slide corresponding with the environment the patient lives in. Slides should be viewed immediately and done in a methodical method to review the entire area, by starting at 100× magnification using a grid pattern and finishing by observing under 200× to 400× magnification. If the slide dries out, the diagnostic value is greatly reduced. Light-field and dark-field condensers can be used to help detect subtle movements of certain parasites. When carrying out routine fish health inspections for interstate export, small fin biopsies are taken and examined as described.[19]

If common clinical signs of dermatopathies are observed, a skin culture and full-thickness biopsy can be obtained and submitted for diagnostic evaluation. Obtaining diagnostic samples from fish integument for microbiological evaluation can be difficult because of environmental contamination of the skin and lesion site. Handling and chemicals can readily damage the epithelial layer and mucous coat of the fish, and/or dislodge scales embedded in the fish dermis. For this reason, physically scrubbing fish integument is detrimental to these patients, and many undiluted surgical scrubs can damage fish skin and predispose these patients to secondary bacterial, fungal, and protozoan infections. Although a true sterile area is difficult to attain for fish patients, based on the author's experience and unpublished data from more than 100 cases of ornamental fish, substerile areas can generally be prepared to obtain valuable diagnostic data. The fish should be appropriately anesthetized or sedated as previously suggested.[18] Microbiological cultures can be obtained for bacterial and viral pathogens from either standard swabs or small tissue biopsies. Rinsing the area with sterile water or saline for 5 minutes with a 12-mL curved-tip syringe will clean the area of interest. Culture and cytology samples can be obtained, making sure to procure tissue from the leading edge of the lesions or culturing just under the leading edge at the border between the lesion and healthy skin. This material can be obtained using standard culturettes or other sterile instruments. For tropical fish, Gram stain, acid-fast stain, and any standard in-clinic cytology stain such as eosin and hematoxylin can be used on impression smears, as gram-negative bacteria, fungi, and acid-fast organisms are common fish pathogens. Should the lesion require more thorough evaluation, a skin biopsy can be obtained. The area is prepped as previously described for culture but then is also rinsed with a dilute surgical scrub, such as with a povidone-iodine solution or chlorhexidine at 1:10 dilution with sterile water/saline, or Virkon solution 0.2% (Dupont Animal Health). Fish scales are often surrounded by a pocket of epithelial tissue extending into the dermis. To obtain a better biopsy, loose scales are removed using surgical forceps, pulling at a 45° angle, to remove the scale in its entirety and leave this tissue pocket intact to allow for new scales to grow back normally. A biopsy or multiple biopsies can be obtained. In simple cases, all that may be required is to excise affected tissue from between the fin rays using sharp scissors. Dermal punch biopsies or a small surgical instrument pack using scalpel, scissors, and forceps are used for larger full-thickness skin biopsies that include both a healthy edge of tissue and an affected area. Taking multiple samples is preferable to help obtain an accurate diagnosis. Often the biopsy site can be left open to heal or can be sutured using a simple interrupted throw of synthetic monofilament suture material.[26] If the affected area and biopsy sites are deep or expansive, analgesics should be given.[24] Dissolvable sutures need to be rechecked and removed after 2 to 3 weeks. To help improve the chances of an accurate diagnosis, it is best to split samples into a fresh sample, a formalin-fixed sample, and a 90% ethanol or frozen sample. Fresh tissue can be submitted for viral culture, bacterial culture, and/or cytology, while fixed tissues can be submitted for histopathology. The frozen or ethanol fixed tissues can be used for molecular diagnostic testing. The best course of action is to take all 3 samples and submit the most critical fresh tissue kept refrigerated for diagnosis with 24 to 48 hours. Should a diagnosis be elusive or further diagnostics are required, one can then submit the remaining fixed or frozen tissues for advanced diagnostics.

FISH VIROLOGY

The greatest challenge in the diagnosis of viral dermatopathies is the isolation and identification of the putative virus. Once the diagnostic tissue is obtained, sample processing begins for this laborious technique. Isolation begins with selection of appropriate fish cell culture lines based on the genus of fish affected. The infected tissue may be placed on multiple cell lines from a single case to improve the isolation process. Fish cell lines are derived from a variety of healthy fish tissues maintained in a monolayer culture, then incubated at appropriate temperatures dependent on the species of origin. Culturing requires holding samples for a minimum of 4 weeks in an attempt to rule out the presence of virus. When viable virus is added to these cell lines the virus will replicate, and can be isolated and further characterized. Often the virus will cause cytopathic effects in specific patterns or will affect healthy cells with specific cellular features (apoptosis, hypertrophy, nuclear or cytoplasmic inclusions) unique to certain virus families. Once isolated, a virus can be definitively identified using a variety of serologic and molecular methods including electron microscopy, antigen/antibody approaches, serum neutralization, fluorescent and immunofluorescent antibody tests (FAT and IFAT), immunostaining, PCR, dot blot (antigen and nucleic acid), nucleic acid analyses, sequence homologies, and inhibitor studies.

It is important that viral diseases and viral dermatopathies are diagnosed in fish, because currently there are no therapeutic treatments available. Avoidance and prevention are the most powerful tools for managing viral disease outbreaks, which must take into account understanding the biology and ecology of the viruses and may involve broodstock screening and egg treatments in breeding or hatchery populations, and includes water supply considerations and water disinfection for both supply and discharge.

Most currently identified virus families have been isolated from fish, with more than 80 agents implicated as pathogens. These families are[27]:

- Herpesviridae
- Adenoviridae
- Iridoviridae
  - Ranavirus
  - Megalocytivirus
  - Lymphocystis virus
- Poxviridae
- Retroviridae
- Birnaviridae
  - Aquabirnavirus
  - Blosnavirus

- Paramyxoviridae
- Orthomyxoviridae
- Rhabdoviridae
- Togaviridae
  - Alphaviruses
- Caliciviridae
- Reoviridae
  - Aquareoviridae
- Nodaviridae
  - Betanodavirus
- Nidovirales (order)
  - Coroniviridae, Roniviridae, Aterviridae

Although viral pathogens have been isolated from all of these families, the most common and problematic viral agents come from 4 of these families: Herpesviridae, Iridoviridae, Rhabdoviridae, and Birnaviridae. The first 2 of these families consist of double-stranded DNA viruses that are epitheliotropic, but may result in localized dermatopathies and/or systemic disease. The latter 2 are represented by single-stranded or double-stranded RNA viruses, respectively, and through infection of hematopoietic tissue can have skin-associated clinical signs such as petechial hemorrhages. Other families, Retroviridae and Poxviridae, include pathogens known to cause viral dermatopathies. Epithelial tropic viruses target epithelial cells of the skin and/or gills, and these cells, once infected, can respond by uncontrolled hyperplasia causing tumor-like growths or cell death and necrosis resulting in hyperemic-appearing blisters. The symptoms caused by these viruses can be self-limiting or can cause erosions and ulcerations, leading to mortality from the primary viral disease or by secondary parasitic or microbial infections. Viruses from several families have been identified with an epitheliotropic predilection, including the Herpesviridae, Iridoviridae, Poxviridae, and Retroviridae, and are discussed further.

Herpesviridae

Herpesviruses infect a wide range of commercially important fish species, causing localized infections of the skin and gills or systemic infections. In the ornamental fish trade, 3 cyprinid herpesviruses (CyHV 1, 2, and 3) are economically important, as they have been identified as causing disease in koi, common carp, and goldfish. CyHV1 is epitheliotropic and can infect koi and common carp (*Cyprinus carpio*), resulting in lesions characterized by epidermal hyperplasia.[28–30] This disease is commonly referred to as (and mistakenly called) "carp pox," although the virus is not from the family Poxviridae. As alluded to in the introduction, skin lesions can cause a disfiguring appearance, devaluing show and prize-winning animals. Clinically these infected cells are best described as appearing like melted candle wax on the skin of infected individuals (**Fig. 3**).[31,32] Systemic infection can occur in young fish with branchial, hepatic, renal, and splenic involvement. Fish are believed to be lifelong carriers of the virus, with the virus remaining dormant in nerve cells. Diagnosis is based on histopathology of lesions and/or viral cell culture with electron microscopy.

CyHV1 virus is self-limiting, and clinical signs are typically observed at water temperatures lower than 17° to 20°C. There have been clinical cases of affected fish having lesions year-round despite increases in temperature to above 25°C.[31] There is no commercial diagnostic testing or screening for infected fish or populations of animals. Because most koi are sold during warmer months, hobbyists may not become acutely aware that they have purchased an asymptomatic carrier until the

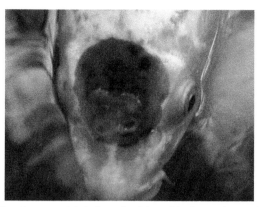

Fig. 3. Koi carp (*Cyprinus carpio*) infected with epitheliotropic cyprinid herpesvirus 1. (*Courtesy of* Lori Campbell, DVM, PhD, Davis, CA.)

autumn and winter months, when water temperatures drop below the critical threshold in their ponds. There is no treatment, and control may involve culling or removing known infected stock from the population regularly, quarantining new animals for longer periods of time and at cooler temperatures during this quarantine time, and/or purchasing koi in late autumn or early winter and avoiding animals that have any clinical signs of disease.[32]

Additional epitheliotropic herpesviruses include smooth dogfish herpesvirus, smelt virus, percid (walleye) herpesvirus, and white sturgeon herpesvirus type 2 (WSHV-2) (**Figs. 4** and **5**). WSHV-2 infects animals naturally or experimentally in the family Acipenseridae, including white, Russian, shovelnose, and lake sturgeon.[33] This disease is endemic in white sturgeon populations in the Northwestern United States from northern California, Oregon, and Idaho. In white sturgeon this disease can present differently in juvenile and older fish stocks. The typical disease presentation in juvenile animals is an absence of most clinical signs except slight discoloration and some reddening around the fins, fin bases, and scutes.[34] In older fish, clinical signs associated with recurrence of disease can include reddened skin lesions that progress to erosive white to gray necrotic areas on the nonscaled skin of the ventrum or lower lateral body walls. The head and gills in these older fish can also have lesions.[34] On histopathology there is marked hyperplasia of the epithelial layer with involvement of the Malpighian cells.[35] Diagnosis requires the observation of gross signs (generally

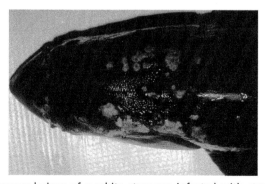

Fig. 4. Gross cutaneous lesions of a white sturgeon infected with sturgeon herpesvirus. (*Courtesy of* Joseph Groff, VMD, PhD, Davis, CA.)

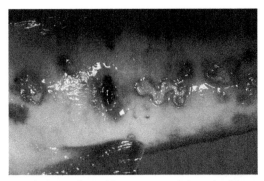

Fig. 5. Gross cutaneous lesions of a white sturgeon infected with sturgeon herpesvirus. (*Courtesy of* Joseph Groff, VMD, PhD, Davis, CA.)

at water temperature of 17°–20°C), histopathology, and viral cell culture on sturgeon cell lines, and can be confirmed using PCR. Transmission is thought to be both vertical and horizontal.[35] As with other viruses, there is no known treatment. Avoidance and prevention is the only way to limit outbreaks.

Other important systemic herpesviruses that may manifest with skin involvement include CyHV2 in goldfish and CyHV3 in koi and common carp. Both of these viruses cause serious disease of all goldfish (*Carassius auratus auratus*) varieties and koi or common carp, respectively, with acute mortalities as high as 100%.[36,37] Temperature is a key factor in disease outbreaks with both viruses: typically infection generally occurs from 17° to 28°C.[38] Although the exact origins for these viruses are unknown, the first reported outbreaks of CyHV3 were in Israel, the United Kingdom, and the United States in 1998.[37] Koi herpes virus disease (KHVd), caused by CyHV3, is reportable to the World Animal Health Organization (OIE) and in the United States to the US Department of Agriculture (USDA), thus requiring reporting to the appropriate authorities when shipping or accepting international fish shipments and/or diagnosing cases of KHVd infection, respectively.[39] As with other herpesviruses, fish exposed to CyHV3 can become asymptomatic carriers. Clinical signs caused by infections with either CyHV2 or CyHV3 include gill necrosis, enophthalmia, raised pale areas of skin (**Fig. 6**), dermal blisters, anorexia, and lethargy. Diagnosis is based on clinical

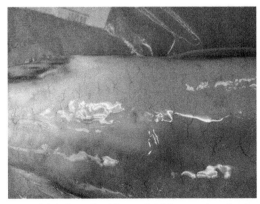

Fig. 6. Koi (*Cyprinus carpio*) infected with cyprinid herpesvirus 3, showing raised dermal lesions. (*Courtesy of* Lori Campbell, Davis, DVM, PhD, CA.)

observations, virus culture, and molecular diagnostics, including CyHV3 Taq-man PCR[40] and an ELISA for identifying CyHV3 antibody in asymptomatic carriers.[41]

At present there is no treatment available for these systemic diseases, and there is widespread misinformation and mischaracterization of them throughout the koi hobbyist population. A lack of appropriate viral screening at the time of sale has allowed carrier fish and this disease to become endemic in wild and captive United States populations of koi and common carp. Avoidance and prevention is best achieved through the development of protocols requiring retailers and wholesalers to screen stock using PCR on morbid or fresh mortalities, and by regular serum-screening of newly imported stock for KHV antibodies using ELISA to detect asymptomatic carriers. In 2005 a modified live vaccine was developed in Israel to prevent KHVd and was approved for use in the United States in spring 2012.[42]

Iridoviridae

Iridoviruses may be epitheliotropic and/or systemic, and can infect temperate and tropical fish species. Unlike the herpesviruses, iridoviruses seem to be less species-specific and have been identified from invertebrates, amphibians, reptiles and fish.[43–45] Fish can be infected with ranaviruses, lymphocystis viruses, and megalocytiviruses.[46]

The most commonly associated epitheliotropic iridovirus is fish lymphocystis virus disease (FLDV).[47] The host range for this virus includes freshwater and marine animals from temperate and tropical environments, with isolates obtained from more than 125 species in 42 families worldwide and new hosts being discovered regularly, such as the whitespotted puffer *Arothron hispidus*.[48,49] FLDV causes significant economic losses in both food and ornamental fish stocks, especially in marine flatfish raised for food in China.[47,50–52]

The most prevalent clinical sign is the appearance of small white to gray raised skin lesions described as pearls or grains of rice and referred to as lymphocysts. Lymphocysts may also develop internally in the kidney, spleen, and other organs. This virus causes a pathognomonic, histopathologic cellular hypertrophy characterized by continued cell growth without cellular division, resulting in extremely large hypertrophied cells up to 100,000 times the normal cell size with aberrant nuclei and intracytoplasmic inclusions (**Fig. 7**).[50–53] Diagnosis has been based on clinical signs and histopathology. The virus has been difficult to culture from marine fish, although

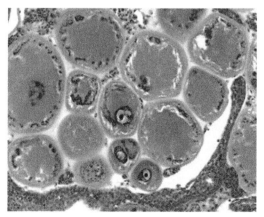

Fig. 7. Hypertrophied Malpighian cells of a fish infected with lymphocystis disease virus 1. (*Courtesy of* Ron Hedrick, PhD, Davis, CA.)

isolates have been obtained from freshwater species infected with virus.[54] New molecular tests are being developed, such as using a colloidal gold immunochromatographic test strip.[55] There are currently no definitive treatments available for this disease. However, because of the economic importance to the food fish being raised in mariculture, probiotics and chemotherapeutics are being researched to help decrease clinical signs.[56,57]

Systemic infections in both marine and freshwater fish, amphibians, and turtles are linked to both megalocytiviruses and ranaviruses.[58,59] The morbidity and mortality of these infections can be as high as 100%, as observed from imported marine ornamental Banggai cardinalfish (*Pterapogon kauderni*).[60] Having species specificity is characteristic of many viruses for infection, but megalocytiviruses and ranaviruses do not require a species-specific host, and it has been demonstrated that the same virus isolated from an animal can infect multiple taxa from either freshwater or saltwater animals, causing major impacts and threats to ornamental and food fish aquaculture.[61]

Clinical signs associated with other systemic iridoviruses, such as epizootic hematopoietic necrosis virus (EHNV) and EHNV-like agents, include petechial hemorrhages and darkening of the skin at the fin bases, skin ulceration, and gill hemorrhage.[62] Diagnosis is based on clinical signs, histopathology, and virus isolation and identification. On histopathology infected cells are characteristically hypertrophied, similarly to other viruses in this family. PCR has been developed for detection of some systemic iridoviral diseases such as EHNV in both symptomatic and asymptomatic carriers.[63] There are no treatments available for these infections. Transmission is thought to be horizontal, and avoidance is the best prevention. Vaccines against systemic iridoviruses are being investigated. In field trials, a vaccine developed against iridoviral disease in red sea bream was shown to offer protection against challenge with wild-type virus.[64]

Other Viruses

Several proliferative skin lesions have been identified in wild caught walleye. Walleye dermal sarcoma appears as clustered, sometimes coalescing, spherical nodules, 2 to 5 mm in diameter, with a smooth, often ulcerated surface of the dermis (**Fig. 8**).[65] These nodules do not metastasize, seasonally regress, and are associated with a retrovirus.[65] When lesions are observed seasonally, inflammation is seen histologically in sarcoma lesions during the spring but not from similar lesions biopsied in the fall.[66]

Poxvirus-like lesions have also been identified in seahorses and koi, but little information is available apart from a few isolated histopathology cases (Groff, UC Davis, personal communication, 2011). In farmed Atlantic salmon, a poxvirus has been associated with a proliferative gill disease.[67]

As more veterinarians work with fish patients, a greater contribution of clinical material will help to solve many uncharacterized diseases in aquatic animals, leading to the discovery of more viral pathogens.

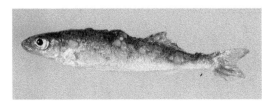

Fig. 8. Gross cutaneous lesions associated with walleye dermal sarcoma virus. (*Courtesy of* P. Bowser, PhD, Ithaca, NY.)

PREVENTION

To begin an effective preventive aquatic animal health program, one must understand basic husbandry requirements for the needs of the animals being maintained. One must also have a thorough understanding of the biology of the most common pathogens and of environmental issues that may exacerbate morbidity or mortality in affected fish. The first step in raising aquatic animals is to obtain and ensure a reliable and clean water source. Water isolated from other aquatic animals and wild stock is preferable to water from natural sources such as ponds, lakes, streams, bays, and estuaries. If water is used from ground sources, it should be purified using standards similar to those required for potable drinking water to eliminate potential toxins, contaminants, and pathogens.

All animals should be quarantined before being allocated to collections or stocked for aquaculture; this can be done at the hobbyist to commercial level, provided proper sanitation and separation can be achieved and maintained. New stock should be placed in an area separated and contained from other animals. The best results are obtained when age classes and animals from specific geographic regions, farms, or facilities are separated. All quarantine areas require dedicated equipment used only for that designated area, and both source and discharge water should be managed appropriately to ensure that quarantine animals receive healthy water and to prevent the spread of potential diseases from these animals to others via wastewater discharge. All equipment should be cleaned and disinfected regularly, and the tanks and life-support systems for quarantine should be cleaned and disinfected between new groups of animals. Personal hygiene is also important in the quarantine facility and between quarantine and nonquarantine areas; this requires proper hand washing, and footbaths to be appropriately placed, maintained, and used.

Quarantine duration should be ample to allow for ill individuals to break with disease, and a traditional 30 day quarantine is reasonable for most temperate and tropical fish species, although cold water fish may require longer time periods. For many viruses incubation to disease onset is 14 to 21 days. Quarantine is temperature dependent. Fish should be quarantined at optimum temperatures established for those species: for example, koi and goldfish at 21° to 24°C, and 24° to 30°C for many marine and freshwater tropical fish. Quarantine allows time for the aquarist or hobbyist to become familiar with the individual animal, group of stock, or new species. The goals of quarantine are to acclimatize new animals, understand their habits and nutritional requirements, and allow them to become healthy and strong so as to best compete in their new habitat, whether it be a community tank at one's home or public aquarium display, or stocked in a hatchery or grow-out facility. In commercial and some hobbyist situations, animals may undergo health examinations including skin scrapes and gill biopsies and some nonlethal disease testing, such as serologic testing of koi for KHVd and/or screening of broodstock for the listed reportable diseases. For large groups of fish, the aquarist may elect to sacrifice some animals for full health examinations that include histopathology, microbiology, and viral culture while awaiting final results from diagnostic testing, before releasing animals from quarantine into their next environment. During quarantine, animals may undergo prophylactic treatments and vaccination, depending on species or final disposition of the animals.

SUMMARY

Although recognized by fisheries biologists for decades, the intrinsic and extrinsic properties of fish mucus and the immunologic properties of fish integument are becoming important models for understanding innate immunity and investigating human-related models of dermatopathies.[67–69] With greater funding, fish researchers may be better able to understand how these defenses aid fish in protection against and prevention of a variety of pathogens including viruses.

It is vital to recognize clinical signs associated with viral dermatopathies because there are currently no treatments available. Avoidance and prevention are the key to controlling fish viral diseases. Optimizing husbandry practices and incorporating effective quarantine can help to prevent disease outbreaks in hobbyist and display collections as well as aquaculture stocks.

Vaccines that have been developed for some of these diseases have recently been approved for use in the United States. As with terrestrial animals, as these vaccines are made available they will become valuable tools in the aquatic veterinary arsenal in helping to prevent and control viral infections.

REFERENCES

1. Eschmeyer WN, editor. Catalog of fishes. California Academy of Sciences. Available at: http://research.calacademy.org/research/ichthyology/catalog/fishcatmain.asp. Accessed March 2, 2013.
2. Fricke R, editor. Catalog of fishes. Literature. Available at: http://research. calacademy.org/research/ichthyology/catalog/fishcatmain.asp.   Accessed March 2, 2013.
3. Eschmeyer WN, Fricke R, Fong JD, et al. Marine fish diversity: history of knowledge and discovery (Pisces). Zootaxa 2010;2525:19–50.
4. Banister K, Adams T. Aquarial fish. London: Frederich Müller Limited; 1977. p. 59.
5. Fosså SA. Fisk i det gamle Egypt. Akvariet, Gothenburg 1981;55(2):64–6.
6. Higginbotham J. Piscinae: artificial fishponds in Roman Italy. Chapel Hill (NC): The University of North Carolina Press; 1997. p. 312.
7. 2011/2012 APPA National Pet Owners Survey. Available at: http://www.prweb. com/releases/prweb2011/4/prweb8252684.htm. Accessed March 2, 2013.
8. Penning M, Reid G, Koldewey H, et al, editors. Turning the tide: a global aquarium strategy for conservation and sustainability. Bern (Switzerland): World Association of Zoos and Aquariums; 2009.
9. Noga EJ, Botts S, Yang S, et al. Acute stress causes skin ulceration in striped bass and hybrid bass (Morone). Vet Pathol 1998;35:102–7.
10. Noga EJ, Udomkusonsri P. The acute ulceration response (AUR): a potentially widespread and serious cause of skin infection in fish. Aquaculture 2005; 246(1):63–77.
11. Nyaoke A, Weber ES, Innis C, et al. Disseminated phaeohyphomycosis in weedy seadragons (Phyllopteryx taeniolatus) and leafy seadragons (Phycodurus eques) caused by species of Exophiala, including a novel species. J Vet Diagn Invest 2009;21(1):69–79.
12. Groff JM. Cutaneous biology and diseases of fish. Vet Clin North Am Exot Anim Pract 2001;4(2):321–411, v–vi.
13. Bullock AM, Roberts RJ. The dermatology of marine teleost fish: the normal integument. Oceanogr Mar Biol Ann Rev 1974;13:383–411.
14. Evans DH, Claiborne JB, editors. The physiology of fishes. 3rd edition. Boca Raton (FL): CRC Press; 2006. p. 601.
15. Ferguson H, Bjerkas E, Evensen O, editors. Systemic pathology of fish: a text and atlas of normal tissue responses in teleosts and their responses in disease. 2nd edition. London: Scotian Press; 2006. p. 368.

16. Roberts RJ, editor. Fish pathology. 4th edition. Oxford (UK): Wiley-Blackwell; 2012. p. 590.
17. Sharpe PT. Fish scale development: hair today, teeth and scales yesterday? Curr Biol 2001;11(18):R751–2.
18. Weber EP, Weisse C, Schwarz T, et al. Anesthesia, diagnostic imaging, and surgery of fish. Compend Contin Educ Vet 2009;31(2):E1–9.
19. Weber EP, Govett P. Parasitology and necropsy of fish. Compend Contin Educ Vet 2009;31(2):E1–7.
20. Harms CA. Fish. In: Fowler ME, Miller RE, editors. Zoo & wild animal medicine: current therapy 4. Philadelphia: W.B. Saunders; 1999. p. 158–63.
21. Noga EJ. Fish disease: diagnosis and treatment. Ames (IA): Iowa State University Press; 2010. p. 536.
22. Citino SB. Basic ornamental fish medicine. In: Kirk RW, Bonagura JD, editors. Current veterinary therapy X. Philadelphia: W.B. Saunders; 1989. p. 703–21.
23. Lewbart GA. Medical management of disorders of freshwater tropical fish. In: Rosenthal K, editor. Practical exotic animal medicine. Trenton (NJ): Veterinary Learning Systems Co., Inc; 1997. p. 250–7.
24. Weber ES, Innis C. Piscine patients: basic diagnostics. Compend Contin Educ Vet 2007;29(5):276–7, 280, 282–6; [quiz: 286, 288].
25. Noga EJ, Udomkusonsri P. Fluorescein: a rapid, sensitive, nonlethal method for detecting skin ulceration in fish. Vet Pathol 2002;39(6):726–31.
26. Hurty CA, Brazic DC, Law JM, et al. Evaluation of the tissue reactions in the skin and body wall of koi (*Cyprinus carpio*) to five suture materials. Vet Rec 2002; 151:324–8.
27. Crane M, Hyatt A. Viruses of fish: an overview of significant pathogens. Viruses 2011;3:2025–46.
28. Schubert GH. The infective agent in carp pox. Bull Off Int Epizoot 1966;65(7): 1011–22.
29. Sano T, Fukada H, Furukawa M. A herpesvirus isolated from carp papilloma in Japan. In: Elis AE, editor. Fish and shellfish pathology. London: Academic Press; 1985. p. 307–41.
30. Sano T, Fukada H, Furukawa M. *Herpesvirus cyprini*: biological and oncogenic properties. Fish Pathol 1985;20:381–8.
31. Hedrick RP, Sano T. Herpesviruses of fishes. In: Ahne W, Kurstak E, editors. Viruses of lower vertebrates. New York: Springer-Verlag, University of CA; 1989. p. 161–70.
32. Calle PP, McNamara T, Kress Y. Herpesvirus-associated papillomas in koi Carp (*Cyprinus carpio*). J Zoo Wildl Med 1999;30(1):165–9.
33. Hedrick RP, Groff JM, McDowell T, et al. An iridovirus infection of the integument of the white sturgeon *Acipenser transmontanus*. Dis Aquat Organ 1990;8: 39–44.
34. Hedrick RP, McDowell TS, Groff JM, et al. Isolation of an epitheliotropic herpesvirus from white sturgeon. Dis Aquat Organ 1991;11:49–56.
35. Hedrick RP, McDowell TS, Groff JM, et al. Isolation and properties of an iridovirus-like agent from white sturgeon *Acipenser transmontanus*. Dis Aquat Organ 1992;12:75–81.
36. Goodwin AE, Merry GE, Sadler J. Detection of the herpesviral haematopoietic necrosis disease agent Cyprinid herpesvirus 2 in moribund and healthy goldfish: validation of a quantitative PCR diagnostic method. Dis Aquat Organ 2006;69:137–43.

37. Hedrick RP, Marty GD, Nordhausen RW, et al. A herpesvirus associated with mass mortality of juvenile and adult koi *Cyprinus carpio*. Fish Health Newsletter 1999;27:7.

38. Gilad O, Yun S, Adkison MA, et al. Molecular comparison of isolates of an emerging fish pathogen, koi herpesvirus, and the effect of water temperature on mortality of experimentally infected koi. J Gen Virol 2003;84:2661–8.

39. Way K. Koi herpesvirus and goldfish herpesvirus: an update of current knowledge and research at CEFAS. Fish Vet J 2008;10:62–73.

40. Gilad O, Yun S, Andree KB, et al. Initial characteristics of koi herpesvirus and development of a polymerase chain reaction assay to detect the virus in koi, *Cyprinus carpio* koi. Dis Aquat Organ 2002;48:101–8.

41. Adkison MA, Gilad O, Hedrick RP. An enzyme linked immunosorbent assay (ELISA) for detection of antibodies to the koi herpesvirus in the serum of koi, *Cyprinus carpio*. Fish Pathol 2005;40(2):53–62.

42. Ronen A, Perelberg A, Abramowitz J, et al. Efficient vaccine against the virus causing a lethal disease in cultured *Cyprinus carpio*. Vaccine 2003;21:4677–84.

43. Chinchar VG. Ranaviruses (family *Iridoviridae*): emerging cold-blooded killers. Arch Virol 2002;147:447–70.

44. Daszak P, Berger L, Cunningham AA, et al. Emerging infectious diseases and amphibian population declines. Emerg Infect Dis 1999;5:735–48.

45. Delhon G, Tulman ER, Afonso CL, et al. Genome of invertebrate iridescent virus type 3 (mosquito iridescent virus). J Virol 2006;80:8439–49.

46. Chinchar VG, Essbauer S, He JG, et al. Iridoviridae. In: Fauquet CM, Mayo MA, Maniloff J, et al, editors. Virus taxonomy: 8th report of the International Committee on the Taxonomy of Viruses. London: Elsevier; 2005. p. 163–75.

47. Walker R. Fine structure of lymphocystis disease virus in fish. Virology 1962;18: 503–5.

48. Sheng XZ, Zhan WB, Wang Y. Whitespotted puffer *Arothron hispidus*, a new host for lymphocystis in Qingdao Aquarium of China. Dis Aquat Organ 2007; 75:23–8.

49. Xu HT, Piao CA, Jiang ZL, et al. Study on the causative agent of lymphocystic disease in cultured flounder *Paralichthys olivaceus*, in Mainland China. China J Virol 2000;16:223–6.

50. Hossain M, Kim SR, Oh MJ. The lymphocystis diseases in the Olive flounder, *Paralichthys olivaceus*. Univ J Zool Rajshahi Univ 2007;26:59–62.

51. Hossain M. Lymphocystis disease virus persists in the epidermal tissues of olive flounder, *Paralichthys olivaceus* (Temminch & Schlegel), at low temperatures. J Fish Dis 2009;32:699–703.

52. Zwillenberg LD, Wolf K. Ultrastructure of lymphocystis virus. J Virol 1968;2: 393–9.

53. Hossain M, Oh MJ. Histopathology of marine and freshwater fish lymphocystis disease virus (LCDV). Sains Malays 2011;40(10):1049–52.

54. Berthiaume L, Alain R, Robin J. Morphology and ultrastructure of lymphocystis disease virus a fish iridovirus, grown in tissue culture. Virology 1984;135: 10–9.

55. Sheng XZ, Song JL, Zhan WB. Development of a colloidal gold immunochromatographic test strip for detection of lymphocystis disease virus in fish. J Appl Microbiol 2012;113(4):737–44.

56. Harikrishnan R. Immune enhancement of chemotherapeutants on lymphocystis disease virus (LDV) infected *Paralichthys olivaceus*. Fish Shellfish Immunol 2010;29:862–7.

57. Harikrishnan R. Effect of probiotics enriched diet on *Paralichthys olivaceus* infected with lymphocystis disease virus (LCDV). Fish Shellfish Immunol 2010; 29:868–74.
58. Hedrick RP, McDowell TS, Ahne W, et al. Properties of three iridovirus-like agents associated with systemic infections of fish. Dis Aquat Organ 1992; 13(3):203–9.
59. Daszak P, Cunningham AA, Hyatt AD. Infectious disease and amphibian population declines. Divers. Distrib 2003;9:141–50.
60. Weber ES, Waltzek TB, Young DA, et al. Systemic iridovirus infection in the Banggai cardinalfish (*Pterapogon kauderni* Koumans 1933). J Vet Diagn Invest 2009;21:306–20.
61. Whittington RJ, Chong R. Global trade in ornamental fish from an Australian perspective: the case for revised import risk analysis and management strategies. Prev Vet Med 2007;81:92–116.
62. Ariel E. Challenge studies of European stocks of redfin perch, *Perca fluviatilis* L., and rainbow trout, *Oncorhynchus mykiss* (Walbaum), with epizootic haematopoietic necrosis virus. J Fish Dis 2009;32:1017–25.
63. Kurobe T, Marcquenski S, Hedrick RP. PCR assay for improved diagnostics of epitheliotropic disease virus (EEDV) in lake trout *Salvelinus namaycush*. Dis Aquat Organ 2009;84(1):17–24.
64. Nakajima K, Maeno Y, Honda A, et al. Effectiveness of a vaccine against red sea bream iridoviral disease in a field trial test. Dis Aquat Organ 1999;36(1):73.
65. Martineau D, Bowser PR, Wooster G, et al. Histologic and ultrastructural studies of dermal sarcoma of walleye (Pisces: *Stizostedion vitreum*). Vet Pathol 1990;27: 340.
66. Bowser PR, Wolfe MJ, Forney JL, et al. Seasonal prevalence of skin tumors from walleye (*Stizostedion vitreum*) from Oneida lake, New York. J Wildl Dis 1988; 24(2):292–8.
67. Nylund A. Morphogenesis of salmonid gill poxvirus associated with proliferative gill disease in farmed Atlantic salmon (*Salmo salar*) in Norway. Arch Virol 2008; 153:1299–309.
68. Rakers S, Niklasson L, Steinhagen D, et al. Antimicrobial peptides (AMPs) from fish epidermis: perspectives for investigative dermatology. J Invest Dermatol 2013. http://dx.doi.org/10.1038/jid.2012.503.
69. Esteban MA. An overview of the immunological defenses in fish skin. ISRN Immunol 2012;(8534700):1–29. http://dx.doi.org/10.5402/2012/853470.

Viral Skin Diseases of the Rabbit

Anna L. Meredith, MA, VetMB, PhD, CertLAS, DZooMed, MRCVS

KEYWORDS

- Viral skin disease • Rabbit • Myxomatosis • Myxoma virus • Shope papilloma virus
- Shope fibroma virus • Rabbitpox

KEY POINTS

- Myxomatosis is the most important viral skin disease of the domestic rabbit.
- Severity of myxomatosis is determined by the strain of the virus and the immune status of the host.
- Clinical signs are usually severe and death occurs within 10 to 12 days; euthanasia is frequently indicated, although rabbits with milder signs, including those suffering from the amyxomatous form or that have been previously vaccinated, may survive with nursing care.
- Prevention is by vaccination, control of insect vectors, and prevention of contact with wild rabbit reservoirs.
- Other viral skin diseases less commonly seen in North America, but not in Europe or other parts of the world, are Shope papilloma virus and Shope fibroma virus.
- Rabbitpox has not been reported in wild or pet domestic rabbits.

MYXOMATOSIS
Introduction and History

Myxomatosis is caused by the myxoma virus, a poxvirus. The natural hosts are wild jungle rabbits, or tapeti (*Sylvilagus brasiliensis*), in South and Central America, and wild brush rabbits (*Sylvilagus bachmani*) in California. In these species of rabbits, myxoma virus causes a mild, self-limiting cutaneous fibroma, and no systemic disease.

However, in the European wild rabbit, which includes the domestic rabbit (*Oryctolagus cuniculi*), myxomatosis is a severe and almost invariably fatal systemic disease. Myxomatosis is probably the best known example of what occurs when a novel pathogen makes a species jump into a naïve host, and its high pathogenicity in European wild rabbits has been exploited in attempts at biologic control of wild populations.

Disclosures: The author has nothing to disclose.
Department of Veterinary Clinical Studies, Royal (Dick) School of Veterinary Studies and The Roslin Institute, Easter Bush Veterinary Centre, University of Edinburgh, Roslin, Midlothian, Scotland EH25 9RG, UK
E-mail address: Anna.Meredith@ed.ac.uk

The disease originated in the New World and was first described in laboratory rabbits in Uruguay in 1896. However, myxoma viruses are now endemic in Europe and Australia in addition to South and North America. In 1950 a Brazilian strain of the virus was released into Australia as a means of controlling introduced wild rabbits (O cuniculi) that had reached pest proportions. It was initially highly effective (>90% mortality) but subsequent emergence of attenuated strains and genetically resistant rabbits have reduced its impact (<50% mortality).[1,2] In the 1930s attempts were made to use myxomatosis as biologic control of rabbits in the United Kingdom, Denmark, and Sweden, but these were not successful, presumably because of the lack of appropriate vectors.[3,4] In 1951 the disease was introduced to France to control rabbits, and it spread rapidly across continental Europe and to the United Kingdom. It has not been reported in Asia, Southern Africa, or New Zealand.

In wild European rabbits, introduction of the disease killed more than 99% of infected animals, but over time a degree of immunity and less virulent strains emerged.[1,2] Although overall mortality in wild populations has decreased over time, outbreaks continue to occur with more virulent strains, and the disease still has an important regulatory effect on wild rabbit populations (Ross and colleagues 1989,[5] Calvete and colleagues 2002[6]). Myxomatosis outbreaks are reportable to the World Organization for Animal Health.

Wild rabbits act as a reservoir of the disease in domestic rabbits, where it is an important cause of morbidity and high mortality in many areas, particularly in Western Europe. Most cases in domestic pet rabbits are a result of direct or indirect contact with wild rabbits rather than domestic rabbit spread. Myxomatosis is enzootic in the western United States and, although outbreaks are not seen as commonly in domestic rabbits as in Europe, they have been described, particularly in California and Oregon.[7]

Cause

The myxoma virus is in the genus *Leporipoxvirus* (family Poxviridae; subfamily Chordopoxvirinae). Like other poxviruses, myxoma viruses are large DNA viruses with linear double-stranded DNA. Virus replication occurs in the cytoplasm of the cell. There are different strains of the virus, and the severity of the disease in rabbits depends on the strain and on host resistance.

Transmission

The virus is transmitted primarily by insect vectors, although direct transmission can occur. It is transmitted passively by biting arthropods, usually the rabbit flea (in the United Kingdom and Europe *Spillopsysliis cuniclui* and *Echidnopaga gallinacean*—the "stick-tight" fleas; in the United States the Eastern rabbit flea [*Cediopsylla simplex*] and giant Eastern rabbit flea [*Odontopsyllus multispinous*]), and the mosquito (*Aedes*/*Anopheles* spp). However, a wide variety of other parasitic arthropods can also act as vectors, such as cat and dog fleas (*Ctenocephalides* spp.), fur mites (*Cheyletiella parasitovorax*), harvest mites (*Trombicula autumnalis*), biting flies, and lice.

The virus sticks to the mouthparts of biting arthropods when they probe through virus-infected epidermis (usually around the face and ears) and does not replicate within the vector. It is then passively inoculated intradermally into a new host at a subsequent feed. Any virus ingested in a blood meal is just excreted in the insect feces. Myxoma virus is also capable of transmission by fomites such as spiny thistles or birds' feet.[8] As well as being present in the skin lesions, the virus is also shed in discharges and can be found in high titers in ocular and nasal secretions, and transmission by close contact also occurs. Direct and air-borne contact are important routes of transmission for the rarer amyxomatous form of the disease.[9]

Clinical Signs

The clinical signs depend on the strain of virus, the route of inoculation, and the immune status of the host. Clinical signs of the classic nodular form of the disease are a primary subcutaneous mass, swelling and edema of the eyelids (**Fig. 1**) and genitals (**Fig. 2**), a milky or purulent ocular discharge, pyrexia, lethargy, depression, and anorexia (**Fig. 3**). More generalized swelling of the face and ears can then occur (**Fig. 4**) and multiple secondary skin nodules up to 1 cm in diameter may be found on the face, ears, and body (**Fig. 5**).

The typical time course of disease is as follows:

- Swelling at inoculation site: days 2–4
- Pyrexia: day 4
- Swelling of eyelids, face, base of ears, and anogenital area: day 6
- Secondary skin lesions: from day 6, often initially red pinpoint lesions on eyelids, cutaneous lesions over body
- Serous conjunctival and nasal discharge: days 6–8, becoming mucopurulent and crusting (**Fig. 6**)
- Respiratory distress: days 7–8
- Hypothermia: days 8–9
- Complete closure of eyes due to swelling: day 10 (**Fig. 7**)
- Death: days 10–12

In peracute disease with a highly virulent strain, death may occur within 5 to 6 days of infection with minimal clinical signs other than the blepharoconjunctivitis. More usually death usually occurs between days 10 and 12.

In rabbits infected with attenuated, less virulent strains of the virus, the lesions seen can be similar to those described above, but are more variable and generally milder and the time course may be delayed and prolonged. Many rabbits will survive and the cutaneous lesions gradually scab and slough, leaving scarring.

A milder form of the disease is also seen in previously vaccinated domestic rabbits that have partial immunity.[10] These previously vaccinated domestic rabbits often present with a localized scabbing lesion, frequently on the bridge of the nose (**Fig. 8**) and around the eyes, or multiple cutaneous masses over the body. They are often still quite bright and survive with nursing care.

The exact cause of death caused by myxoma virus infection is unclear and is often thought to be due to overwhelming secondary gram-negative bacterial infection and

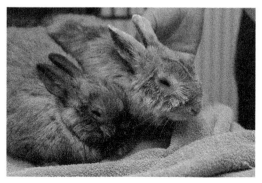

Fig. 1. Myxomatosis in 2 companion rabbits—initial swelling and edema of the eyelids. (*Courtesy of* MSD Animal Health, Hertfordshire, United Kingdom; with permission.)

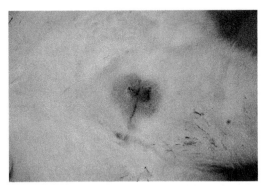

Fig. 2. Myxomatosis—genital swelling in a female rabbit. (*Courtesy of* Exotic Animal and Wildlife Service, Royal (Dick) School of Veterinary Studies, Midlothian, United Kingdom; with permission.)

septicemia due to viral-induced immunosuppression. However, in acute and hyperacute forms of the disease, there is often little evidence of bacterial infection, and antibiotic treatment has little effect on the outcome of acute infection. Secondary bacterial infection is more likely to be a significant factor in rabbits affected with more attenuated or amyxomatous forms of the virus. Pulmonary edema, massive destruction of lymphoid cells, and widespread skin tissue damage triggering a septic shock have been suggested as a cause of death in acute and peracute infections.[9,11,12]

Amyxomatous or respiratory myxomatosis

Since the 1970s an amyxomatous form of the disease has been reported that differs from the classic nodular form. The amyxomatous form is clinically milder and generally nonlethal.[13,14] Fewer and smaller cutaneous lesions develop and respiratory signs are prominent, such as a serous or purulent rhinitis.[15] However, perineal edema, swollen eyelids, and purulent blepharoconjunctivitis may also be seen. This form has been observed in wild rabbits, but is significant mainly in farmed rabbits. It has been suggested that it emerged as an adaptation to the absence of vectors and is largely spread by direct contact, but there is inconclusive evidence to support this. Use of

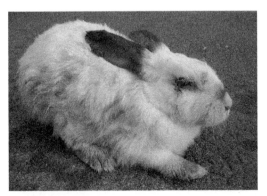

Fig. 3. Myxomatosis—affected rabbit exhibiting typical clinical signs of ocular discharge and crusting, lethargy, depression, and lack of grooming. (*Courtesy of* MSD Animal Health, Hertfordshire, United Kingdom; with permission.)

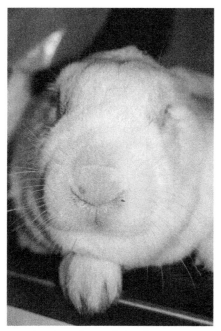

Fig. 4. Myxomatosis—generalized swelling of the face. (*Courtesy of* Exotic Animal and Wildlife Service, Royal (Dick) School of Veterinary Studies, Midlothian, United Kingdom; with permission.)

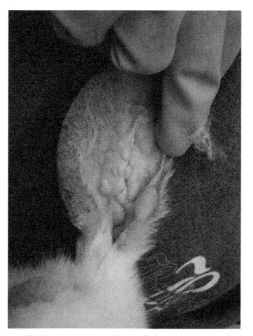

Fig. 5. Myxomatosis—multiple secondary skin nodules on the medial aspect of the pinna. (*Courtesy of* MSD Animal Health, Hertfordshire, United Kingdom; with permission.)

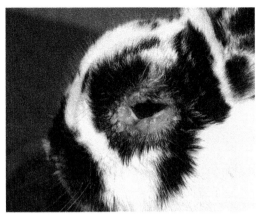

Fig. 6. Myxomatosis—mucopurulent ocular discharge and crusting. (*Courtesy of* MSD Animal Health, Hertfordshire, United Kingdom; with permission.)

vaccines giving partial protection and interactions with other pathogens such as *Pasteurella multocida* in farm situations may have led to different selection pressures on the virus, resulting in these amyxomatous strains.

Pathology and Immunity

Following skin inoculation, the virus replicates at the inoculation site in major histocompatibility complex class II positive cells at the dermal/epidermal junction and then spreads within leukocytes to the regional lymph node within 24 hours, where it replicates further (mainly in T lymphocytes) and disseminates to the skin, spleen, other lymph nodes, mucosal surfaces and mucocutaneous junctions, testes, lungs, and liver. A primary mucoid subcutaneous mass (*myxoma* = Greek for mucus) forms at the initial site of infection 3 to 5 days after virus inoculation.

The mucoid subcutaneous swellings contain large stellate mesenchymal cells within a seromucinous matrix, with few inflammatory cells. The epidermis overlying the swellings is hyperplastic and both epidermal and conjunctival cells may contain intracytoplasmic inclusions. Hypertrophy of endothelial cells can result in narrowing of blood

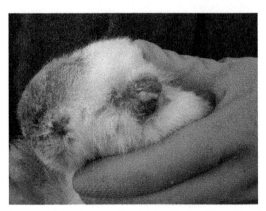

Fig. 7. Myxomoatosis—complete closure of eyes due to swelling. (*Courtesy of* MSD Animal Health, Hertfordshire, United Kingdom; with permission.)

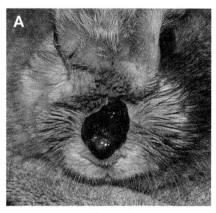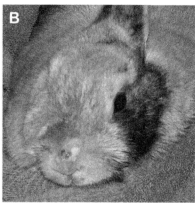

Fig. 8. (*A, B*) Atypical form of myxomatosis in a previously vaccinated rabbit where the only clinical sign was a scabbing lesion developing on the bridge of the nose, which eventually sloughed. (*Courtesy of* MSD Animal Health, Hertfordshire, United Kingdom; with permission.)

capillaries and necrosis of lesions in severe disease. At postmortem examination there are few gross lesions in internal organs, but consolidated areas of lung, splenomegaly, and enlarged lymph nodes may be noted. Lymphoid depletion of the spleen is commonly seen, and additional histologic findings may include alveolar epithelial proliferation, hypertrophy/hyperplasia of reticulum cells in lymph nodes and spleen, and focal necrosis, hemorrhage, and proliferative vasculitis.

Myxoma virus produces several immunomodulatory and immunosuppressive factors and infection increases susceptibility to other viral and bacterial pathogens.[2,3,16] Both humoral and cellular immune responses are important in mediating immunity. Despite the viral-associated immunosuppression, antibodies are developed and immunoglobulin M can be detected from days 6 to 10 and immunoglobulin G can be detected by day 10. These antibodies can persist for at least 2 years in rabbits that survive infection. Maternal immunoglobulin G crosses the placenta but disappears in the kits by 6 to 9 weeks of age. Antibodies are believed to provide some but not complete protection from natural infection. Cell-mediated immunity is believed to be essential for clearing virus and providing long-term protection from re-infection.

Diagnosis

Diagnosis is largely based on the typical clinical signs. Histopathology and virus isolation can confirm the diagnosis. PCR is also useful for rapid diagnosis.

Treatment

Given the severe and distressing nature of the classic form of myxomatosis, the high rate of mortality, and generally poor prognosis, euthanasia is often indicated on humane grounds. However, carefully selected cases may respond to treatment and survive. These carefully selected cases include rabbits that have received previous vaccination and those suffering from the amyxomatous or respiratory form. Rabbits affected by attenuated, less virulent forms of the virus may also survive with nursing care, but in the early stages of disease, it can be difficult to determine clinically the likely outcome.

Affected animals should be housed away from other rabbits. Antibiotics, nonsteroidal anti-inflammatory agents, high ambient temperature (28°C), and good nursing care, including fluid therapy and assisted feeding, are indicated. Opioid analgesics such as buprenorphine do not seem to reduce pain in affected rabbits.[17] Corticosteroids are contraindicated due to their profound immunosuppressive effects in rabbits.

Close monitoring, severity and progression of lesions and clinical signs, response to treatment, and, above all, animal welfare should be assessed continually when making therapeutic or euthanasia decisions.

Prevention and Control

Vector control

Insect vectors can be controlled using physical means, such as insect screens and netting, ultraviolet fly killers, keeping rabbits indoors, and preventing contact with wild rabbits, domestic cats, and dogs. Insecticidal treatments include ivermectin, selamectin, imidocloprid, and permethrin.

Vaccination

Control of myxomatosis is mainly by vaccination and a variety of vaccines are available depending on the country. All vaccines are live and based either on attenuated myxoma virus strain or on the closely related Shope fibroma virus, which provides cross-immunity. The attenuated myxoma virus vaccines may be immunosuppressive, especially on younger rabbits, and the Shope fibroma virus–based vaccines can be poorly immunogenic and provide only short-lived and incomplete protection. Recently, in the United Kingdom and Europe a novel bivalent vectored vaccine has become available for protection against both myxomatosis and rabbit hemorrhagic disease.[18] This vaccine has been shown to provide 100% protection for at least 1 year in rabbits from 5 weeks of age.

It is recommended that all rabbits in areas of the world where myxomatosis is reported in wild rabbits be routinely vaccinated, even if kept indoors, because of the ability of the virus to be carried inside by vectors or fomites. In group situations where rabbits are not routinely vaccinated, vaccination in the face of an outbreak is beneficial in limiting morbidity and mortality.

Myxomatosis in North America

Myxomatosis is endemic in the wild rabbit population on the west coast of North America. It causes little illness in wild rabbits but has an estimated 99% mortality rate in domesticated rabbits. In southern California the peracute and acute forms are seen. In the peracute form, rabbits die within 5 to 7 days of infection, with infected rabbits showing minimal clinical signs, most commonly unilateral or bilateral periocular edematous swelling, or no signs at all. In the acute form, the rabbits initially present with periocular edema and inflamed conjunctiva and subsequently develop perineal edema and lethargy. Skin hemorrhages may occur shortly before death, which occurs within 7 to 10 days. These clinical presentations caused by the California strain of the myxoma virus are somewhat different from the typical, more chronic signs usually described and seen in Europe and elsewhere, so it is important that veterinary practitioners recognize that myxomatosis is a differential diagnosis. Definitive diagnosis is made by histopathology of affected tissues. The California Department of Food and Agriculture Animal Health branch lists myxomatosis as a monitored disease in commercial rabbits.

SHOPE PAPILLOMA VIRUS

The Shope papilloma virus (family Papovaviradae) occurs in wild California brush rabbits (S bachmani) and cottontail rabbits (Sylvilagus floridanus). It is an oncogenic

DNA virus, mechanically transmitted by biting arthropods, including ticks. Infection of domestic rabbits (*O cuniculus*) is rare but has been reported, causing multiple hyper-keratotic hornlike lesions mainly around the ears, eyelids, neck, and shoulders. Manual removal results in healing in wild rabbits, but in domestic rabbits experimental infection resulted in approximately 75% of inoculation sites undergoing malignant transformation to squamous cell carcinoma.[19] Papillomas typically undergo immune-mediated resolution if they do not progress to carcinomas.[20] Host immunity has been shown to have 2 distinct targets: viral structural antigens, invoking protection against virus reinfection, and tumor antigens, invoking papilloma regression.[20] Diagnosis is by histopathology and surgical treatment to remove the papillomas can be successful. Insect control is also important in preventing spread of the disease.

SHOPE FIBROMA VIRUS

The Shope fibroma virus is a naturally occurring *Leporipoxvirus* of North and South American wild rabbits (*Sylvilagus* spp). The natural host is the Eastern cottontail (*S floridanus*) and transmission is via biting arthropod vectors. It is considered a benign, self-limiting disease in the wildlife population.[20] Domestic rabbits are occasionally infected via mosquito vectors and develop fibromas that slough away about 30 days postinoculation. These fibromas are variable is size, typically occurring on legs, feet, and at times involving the muzzle periorbital, and perineal regions. Newborn and young animals develop more extensive lesions. Diagnosis is by histopathology and virus isolation. Affected animals can be treated supportively and given antibiotics to control any secondary infection. A live-attenuated Shope fibroma virus is used as a myxomatosis vaccine because it provides some cross-immunity against the related myxomavirus.

RABBITPOX

Rabbitpox virus is a large DNA virus within the family Poxviridae and the genus *Orthopoxvirus*. Rabbitpox was first described after outbreaks in laboratory rabbits in the United States between 1930 and 1933. It was highly contagious and the mortality rate was high (up to 50%). Clinical signs included fever, lymphadenitis, poxlike eruptions in the skin and mucous membranes, keratitis, and orchitis, very similar to smallpox in humans. Several subsequent outbreaks of rabbitpox occurred in Europe and the United States but with rabbits primarily showing respiratory signs rather than skin lesions. All reported rabbitpox outbreaks have occurred in laboratory rabbit colonies, with no reports since the 1960s, and it has not been recognized in wild rabbit populations.[21]

ACKNOWLEDGMENTS

The author would like to thank Sari Kanfer, DVM of Pasadena, California for sharing her experience with Myxomatosis disease.

REFERENCES

1. Hayes RA, Richardson BJ. Biological control of the rabbit in Australia: lessons not learned? Trends Microbiol 2001;9(9):459–60.
2. Kerr PJ. Myxomatosis in Australia and Europe: a model for emerging infectious diseases. Antiviral Res 2012;93(3):387–415.

3. Fenner F, Ratcliffe FN. Myxomatosis. Cambridge (United Kingdom): Cambridge University Press; 1965.
4. Lockley RM. Failure of myxomatosis on Skokholm Island. Nature 1955;175:906–7.
5. Ross J, Tittensor AM, Fox AP, et al. Myxomatosis in farmland rabbit populations in England and Wales. Epidem Infect 1989;103(2):333–57.
6. Calvete C, Estrada R, Villafuerte R, et al. Epidemiology of viral haemorrhagic disease and myxomatosis in a free-living population of wild rabbits. Vet Rec 2002; 150:776–82.
7. Kerr PJ, Best SM. Myxoma virus in rabbits. Rev Sci Tech 1998;17(1):256–68.
8. Dyce AL. Transmission of myxomatosis on the spines of thistles, Cirsium vulgare (savi) Ten. CSIRO. Wildl Res 1969;6:88.
9. Psikal I, Smid B, Rodak L, et al. Atypical myxomatosis–virus isolation, experimental infection of rabbits and restriction endonuclease analysis of the isolate. J Vet Med B Infect Dis Vet Public Health 2003;50(6):259–64.
10. Meredith A. Dermatoses. In: Meredith A, Flecknell P, editors. BSAVA manual of rabbit medicine and surgery. 2nd edition. Gloucester (United Kingdom): BSAVA; 2006. p. 129–36.
11. Silvers L, Inglis B, Labudovic A, et al. Virulence and pathogenesis of the MSW and MSD strains of Californian myxoma virus in European rabbits with genetic resistance to myxomatosis compared to rabbits with no genetic resistance. Virology 2006;348(1):72–83.
12. Stanford MM, Werden SJ, McFadden G. Myxoma virus in the European rabbit: interactions between the virus and its susceptible host. Vet Res 2007;38(2): 299–318.
13. Marlier D, Mainil J, Linde A, et al. Infectious agents associated with rabbit pneumonia: isolation of amyxomatous myxoma virus strains. Vet J 2000;159(2):171–8.
14. Marlier D, Mainil J, Sulon J, et al. Study of the virulence of five strains of amyxomatous myxoma virus in crossbred New Zealand White/Californian conventional rabbits, with evidence of long-term testicular infection in recovered animals. J Comp Pathol 2000;122(2–3):101–13.
15. Farsang A, Makranszki L, Dobos-Kovacs M, et al. Occurrence of atypical myxomatosis in Central Europe: clinical and virological examinations. Acta Vet Hung 2003;51(4):493–501.
16. Kerr P, McFadden G. Immune responses to myxoma virus. Viral Immunol 2002; 15(2):229–46.
17. Robinson AJ, Muller WJ, Braid AL, et al. The effect of buprenorphine on the course of disease in laboratory rabbits infected with myxoma virus. Lab Anim 1999;33(3):252–7.
18. Spibey N, McCabe VJ, Greenwood NM, et al. Novel bivalent vectored vaccine for control of myxomatosis and rabbit haemorrhagic disease. Vet Rec 2012;170(12): 309.
19. Rous P, Beard JW. The progression to carcinoma of virus-induced rabbit papillomas (Shope). J Exp Med 1935;62:523–48.
20. Percy DH, Barthold SW. Rabbits. In: Pathology of laboratory rodents and rabbits. 3rd edition. Ames (IA): Blackwell; 2007. p. 253–307.
21. Nalca A, Nichols DK. Rabbitpox: a model of airborne transmission of smallpox. J Gen Virol 2011;92(Pt 1):31–5.

Bumblefoot

A Comparison of Clinical Presentation and Treatment of Pododermatitis in Rabbits, Rodents, and Birds

Jennifer Blair, DVM

KEYWORDS

- Bumblefoot • Pododermatitis • Bird • Avian • Rabbit • Guinea pig • Rat

KEY POINTS

- Pododermatitis is a common condition encountered in birds, rabbits, and rodents in clinical practice.
- Pododermatitis is a condition of the foot that encompasses a range of clinical presentations including mild erythema, superficial to deep ulcerations, and deep ulcerations with concurrent osteomyelitis.
- Predisposing factors include excess body weight, lack of activity, improper substrate or perches, anatomic or conformational abnormalities, poor husbandry, improper nutrition, trauma, and behavioral conditions.
- Diagnostics may include a history, physical examination, minimum database, culture & sensitivity, and imaging.
- Medical therapy may include wound care, bandaging, topical medications, systemic antibiotics, and analgesics. Surgical therapy, and natural remedies, therapeutic laser, and acupuncture, may also be used.
- Management of pododermatitis must always include correction of the underlying causes.
- Patients with mild pododermatitis can have a good prognosis. Many cases of pododermatitis are incurable and progress despite aggressive multimodal therapy.

INTRODUCTION

Pododermatitis describes a condition of the foot that encompasses a range of clinical presentations, including mild erythema, superficial to deep ulcerations, and deep ulcerations with concurrent osteomyelitis. It is a common condition in rabbits, guinea pigs, rats, and many avian species. In rabbits and rodents, *ulcerative pododermatitis* or *sore hocks* are the terms used to describe ulcerated infected areas of skin on the

Disclosures: The author has nothing to disclose.
St Francis Animal & Bird Hospital, 1227 Larpenteur Avenue West, Roseville, MN 55113, USA
E-mail address: jenblair25@me.com

caudal aspect of the tarsus and metatarsus and occasionally the metacarpus and phalangeal region of the front limbs.[1] Avascular necrosis of the plantar (or palmar) aspect of the feet may be a more accurate term to describe this condition.[1] In birds, pododermatitis is defined as a degenerative, inflammatory condition of the plantar surface of the foot, either the plantar metatarsal pad or plantar digital pads, that can progress to deeper infections, including tendon necrosis and osteomyelitis of the digital bones.[2,3] Some authors prefer to call this condition *bumblefoot* to encompass the frequent involvement of tissues other than the skin.[3]

Numerous articles and chapters are dedicated to this condition, but few encourage a multimodal approach to management. This article explores the anatomy and physiology of the foot, lists the most common predisposing factors, and discusses the diagnostics recommended for this condition. Therapeutics, including medical, surgical, and alternative therapies, are explored.

ANATOMY AND PHYSIOLOGY OF THE FOOT
Avian

Avian skin is composed of the epidermis and the dermis. The avian epidermis is avascular and thin, usually only measuring 3 to 5 cells thick, although it is thicker over the areas of the body that lack feathers, such as the face and feet.[4] The dermis is made up of a superficial layer, which includes capillaries, and the deep layer, which consists of adipose tissue, vessels, lymphatics, nerves, smooth muscle, and the base of feather follicles.[4] The plantar aspect of the foot has a rough surface consisting of numerous tiny protuberances called *papillae*. It is anatomically divided into the metatarsal pad and multiple digital pads. Each pad contains underlying fibrous connective tissue and fat that bridge the area between the dermis and the underlying tendons.[5] Despite these pads, very little tissue exists between the perching surface and the deeper structures, such as bone and tendons.

Rabbit

Compared with dogs and cats, rabbits are unique in that they lack footpads. Instead, the skin in rabbits is thin and firmly attached to the underlying tissues forming a tarsometatarsal skin pad.[1] Thick fur also protects the plantar aspect of the metatarsus. During locomotion on proper substrate, the claws bear most of the weight, whereas during rest, the weight is distributed between the hind claws and the plantar aspect of the metatarsus.[1] Improper substrate or excessive body weight leads to alterations in this normal weight-bearing physiology.

The normal hindlimb stance in rabbits is digitigrade. In healthy rabbits, the superficial digital flexor tendon is constantly under tension, which allows the rabbit to spring rapidly into action.[1] However, with the development of advanced pododermatitis, erosion of the ligaments of the hock joint leads to medial displacement of the superficial digital flexor tendon. This process, in turn, leads to further redistribution of weight, progression of disease, and loss of mobility.[1]

Rodents: Guinea Pigs and Rats

Guinea pigs and rats lack hair on their feet and metatarsal region. As in rabbits, their skin is relatively thin and adhered to the underlying tissues, so they are very susceptible to local injury, ischemia, and pressure necrosis on the plantar (and palmar) surfaces of their feet. Guinea pigs have a plantigrade stance at rest. The forefoot has a 3-lobed palmar pad with a caudal carpal pad, whereas the hindfoot has a bilobed plantar pad with a large tarsal pad.[6] Rats also have a plantigrade stance at rest.

They have heavily keratinized pads. The front feet have 5 digital pads, 3 metacarpal pads, and 2 carpal pads, whereas the hind feet have 5 digital pads, 4 metatarsal pads, and 2 tarsal pads.[7] Sweat glands embedded in the fat deposits of the subcutis in rats function to maintain adhesive friction between the foot and surfaces.[7]

PATHOGENESIS

Avascular necrosis is a term that describes the pathogenesis of pododermatitis in many patients. The primary pathologic changes that occur are ischemia and necrosis of the soft tissues that are compressed between the bony structures of the foot and the substrate or resting surface.[1] Ischemia and necrosis lead to biochemical changes, release of inflammatory mediators, and intermittent reperfusion injury to the area, which, in turn, lead to further damage of the tissues and thrombosis of the small vessels.[1] The owner or veterinarian may notice mild to severe inflammation, erythema, thinning of the skin, a dry crusty scab, or a callous-like swelling in this early stage.[2,8]

Chronic inflammation leads to hyperkeratosis of the epithelium or dermal thickening, followed by superficial ulceration.[1,2,8] Without treatment, the ulceration may extend into the subcutaneous tissues and erode underlying vasculature, leading to hemorrhage.[1] Secondary bacterial infection may occur and extend to deeper tissues, including bone and synovial structures. The most common bacteria identified in association with pododermatitis include:

- *Staphylococcus aureus*: guinea pigs[9]
- *S aureus* and *Pasteurella multocida*: rabbits[1]
- *S aureus* and *Escherichia coli*: raptors[3]
- *Staphylococcus* spp: psittacines[10]

Other bacterial organisms may also invade the area. Invasion of fungal organisms has been reported,[11] but is rare. Cellulitis and abscess formation may occur. Primary injury to the foot may also serve as a source for infection, leading to the same cascade of inflammatory events.

In late stages, erosion of the bone and ligaments of the hock results in displacement of tendons.[1] Secondary osteomyelitis, tenosynovitis, and arthritis cause additional disability to the animal, abnormal weight-bearing, and further disease progression. By this stage, prognosis for recovery of normal use and function is very poor in all species.

Advanced pododermatitis may also lead to systemic disease such as vegetative endocarditis or polyarthritis. Evidence shows that chronic inflammation and infection from pododermatitis can lead to systemic amyloidosis of the kidney, liver, spleen, adrenal glands, and pancreas, especially in guinea pigs.[8,9] This condition has also been reported in other species, including cattle with inflammatory diseases.[12]

CLASSIFICATION

In raptors, the disorder has been graded into 5 classifications depending on extent, severity, and prognosis. This classification scheme was described in *Raptor Bumblefoot: A New Treatment Technique* by J. David Remple, DVM,[13] and is currently used to classify this condition at The Raptor Center at the University of Minnesota (Dr Pat Redig, The Raptor Center, personal communication, 2012).

1. Type I: early lesion of the plantar surface involving integument only, with no secondary infection of deeper tissues. A loss of papilla and early erythema is usually present. Prognosis is excellent (**Fig. 1**).

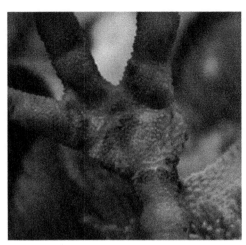

Fig. 1. Type I pododermatitis in a raptor. (*Courtesy of* The Raptor Center, St Paul, MN; with permission.)

2. Type II: infection of the subcutaneous tissues with no gross swelling of affected feet. Prognosis is good (**Fig. 2**).
3. Type III: infected, swollen, painful feet without apparent damage to deep vital structures. Prognosis is good to guarded (**Fig. 3**).
4. Type IV: infection of deep vital structures such as tendons and bones, though patient still retains pedal function. Patients with this type may have tenosynovitis, arthritis, and/or osteomyelitis. Prognosis is guarded to poor (**Fig. 4**).
5. Type V: end-stage disease with osteomyelitis, crippling deformity, and loss of pedal function. Prognosis is grave and euthanasia is often performed (**Figs. 5** and **6**).

Jenkins[14] has classified pododermatitis in rabbits into 3 groups based on the tissues involved and the severity of the infection.

1. Type I: mild localized lesion of one metatarsal surface. Plantar fur pad may be thin or missing and skin is inflamed. Skin may be necrotic, but surface is intact with no ulceration. The prognosis is favorable to good.

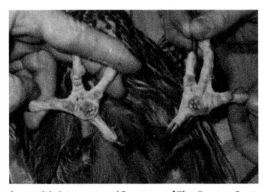

Fig. 2. Type II pododermatitis in a raptor. (*Courtesy of* The Raptor Center, St Paul, MN; with permission.)

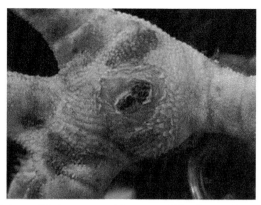

Fig. 3. Type III pododermatitis in a raptor. (*Courtesy of* The Raptor Center, St Paul, MN; with permission.)

2. Type II: extensive lesion with well-established infection and inflammation causing pain. Skin is necrotic and a scab or open ulceration is present (**Fig. 7**). Lesion bleeds easily and purulent exudate is beginning to accumulate. Infection may begin to spread to other tissue planes including tendons. New lesions may develop on the other hind foot or on the volar metacarpal or digital surfaces of the front foot. Patients with type II pododermatitis have a fair to guarded prognosis requiring an aggressive multimodal approach to therapy.
3. Type III: chronic lesions that follow type II lesions. Fibrous connective tissue begins to encapsulate the infection, the central portion of lesion may become necrotic, cellulitis develops, and an abscess may form. Tendons, joints, and bone are involved at this point, the patient is painful, and function is limited. The prognosis is poor to grave for patients with type III pododermatitis.

PREDISPOSING FACTORS AND PREVENTION

Many factors may play a role in the development of pododermatitis, and avoiding them is essential in preventing this condition in all species.

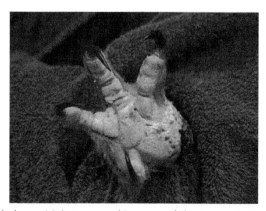

Fig. 4. Type IV pododermatitis in a raptor. (*Courtesy of* The Raptor Center, St Paul, MN; with permission.)

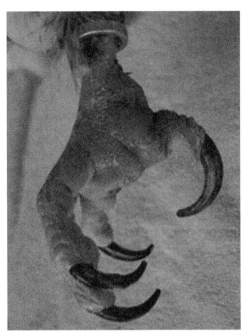

Fig. 5. Type V pododermatitis in a raptor. (*Courtesy of* The Raptor Center, St Paul, MN; with permission.)

Weight

Obesity and pregnancy both lead to increased pressure on the weight-bearing surfaces. The additional weight also likely affects the weight distribution and normal stance of the animal, further placing pressure on surfaces that would not normally bear weight. Larger species or breeds may be particularly susceptible. For example, large-breed rabbits, falcons, penguins, large anseriformes, and heavy-bodied psittacine birds such as Amazon parrots[10] may be predisposed.

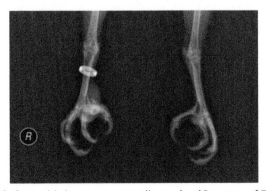

Fig. 6. Type V pododermatitis in a raptor – radiographs. (*Courtesy of* The Raptor Center, St Paul, MN; with permission.)

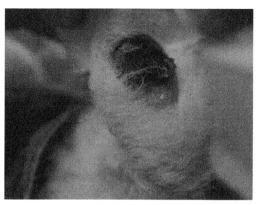

Fig. 7. Type II pododermatitis in a rabbit. (*Courtesy of* Peter G. Fisher, DVM, Virginia Beach, VA.)

Lack of Activity

Lack of activity or confinement to a small space or cage predisposes an animal to developing pododermatitis. This practice creates a vicious cycle, because lack of activity or confinement often leads to weight gain, which in turn leads to a further lack of activity. Providing environmental enrichment through encouraging play and exercise outside the cage for all species is important. Providing access to pools for swimming is essential for waterfowl. **Fig. 8** shows a duck that developed pododermatitis after being housed in an enclosure with inadequate access to swimming. Raptors kept in small enclosures tend to jump from perch to perch instead of flying, which is a common cause of damage to the plantar surface of the foot in these species.[5]

Substrate or Perches

For rabbits and rodents, the type of flooring or substrate can affect the distribution of weight between the metatarsus and claws.[1] Wire flooring forces the animal to walk or rest entirely on the hock and metatarsus. Hard flooring, such as tile or cement, may lead to abnormal weight-bearing on the hock and metatarsus. Abrasive substrate, such as carpet, can also lead to pododermatitis from increased friction and irritation of the skin. It is best to provide deep soft substrate, such as hay, straw, or recycled paper, to prevent pododermatitis in these species.

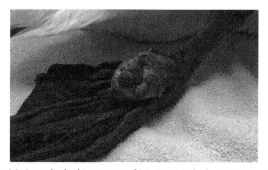

Fig. 8. Pododermatitis in a duck. (*Courtesy of* M. Scott Echols, DVM, Centerville, UT.)

For birds, poor perches, perching surfaces, or flooring substrate can all predispose to pododermatitis. Perches or platforms that are too large or too small can lead to abnormal weight-bearing. Rough abrasive perches (such as those composed of sandpaper or cement) cause increased friction and irritation of the skin (**Fig. 9**).

Anatomic or Conformational Abnormalities

Certain breeds of rabbits, such as the Rex, have fine sparse hair on the metatarsus that offers little protection to the feet.[1] Clipping hair from the metatarsal or metacarpal surfaces in rabbits also decreases the protection to the foot. In all species, physical conditions that alter the normal stance of an animal can lead to abnormal forces on the weight-bearing surfaces. For example, animals with spondylosis, arthritis, painful joints, neurologic disease, or conformational deformities may be predisposed to developing pododermatitis (**Fig. 10**).

Poor Husbandry

Dirty, wet bedding or fecal contamination of perches and cage floors increases the risk of pododermatitis and secondary bacterial infection in both birds and mammals. Cages and perches should be cleaned and bedding should be changed regularly for all species. Overcrowding should be avoided, because this can contribute to poor husbandry.

Nutritional

In guinea pigs, vitamin C deficiency may be an important predisposing factor (**Fig. 11**).[8] Lack of vitamin C results in defective type IV collagen, laminin, and elastin, leading to abnormalities in skin and hair coat, loose teeth, gastrointestinal

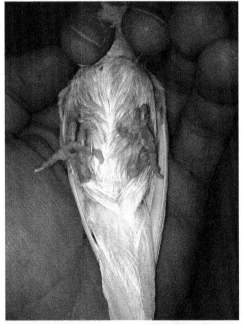

Fig. 9. Pododermatitis in a budgerigar on poor perches. (*Courtesy of* M. Scott Echols, DVM, Centerville, UT.)

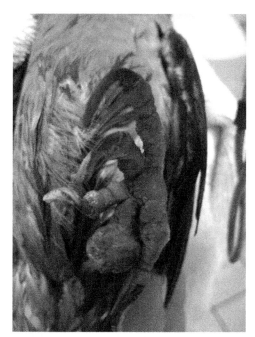

Fig. 10. Pododermatitis in a rose-breasted cockatoo with neurologic disease. (*Courtesy of* Andrew Bean, DVM, El Cajon, CA.)

disturbances, joint abnormalities, increased susceptibility to infections, and hemorrhage.[8] In birds, malnutrition can predispose to secondary skin abnormalities. Seed diets are generally deficient in many nutrients including vitamins, minerals, amino acids, fiber, and omega 3 fatty acids.[15] Psittacines ingesting a seed diet may develop hypovitaminosis A, which may lead to hyperkeratosis, dry flaky skin, loss of skin elasticity, and other skin abnormalities.[15] The stability of the diet should also be evaluated, because prolonged storage may lead to reduction of available vitamin C in guinea pig pellets and possible rancidity in formulated avian diets.[15] Biotin deficiency has been cited as a possible cause of pododermatitis in turkeys.[16]

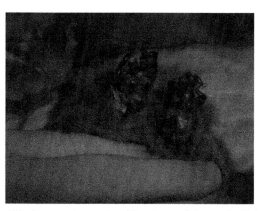

Fig. 11. Pododermatitis in a guinea pig. (*Courtesy of* Peter G. Fisher, DVM, Virginia Beach, VA.)

Trauma and Other Medical Diseases

In raptors, trauma to the bottom of the foot, such as from puncture with a sharp talon (**Fig. 12**) or other penetrating object, a bite wound, or a thermal or chemical burn, can lead to pododermatitis. Bacterial infection may occur secondary to the trauma. In other species of birds or small mammals, sharp wire in the cage or puncture from straw, hay, or sticks may cause similar injuries, leading to secondary infection.

Other pathologic conditions, such as injury to the other leg or foot, concurrent infections (ie, poxvirus in raptors and poultry), *Knemidokoptes* in budgerigars, or frostbite in animals housed outdoors can also predispose to this condition.[2]

Behavioral

Nervous rabbits that stamp and thump repeatedly and raptors that repeatedly bate against the jesses may have an increased risk for developing pododermatitis.[1,5] Reducing stress, providing exercise, and improving environmental enrichment for these patients may help lessen these behaviors.

DIAGNOSTICS
History and Physical Examination

A complete medical history should be obtained for every patient, but especially for small mammal and avian patients. History should include information about diet (both offered and ingested), treats, cage/housing, bedding, litter box substrate (if applicable), and exercise. Any supplements, herbal medications, or topical therapies should be noted in the medical record.

A systematic approach to the physical examination is important to discover concurrent diseases or predisposing causes of the pododermatitis. One should begin by observing the patient in the cage or enclosure, noting any changes in gait or abnormalities at rest or while perching. A weight and body condition score should be noted in the medical record and compared with previous values.

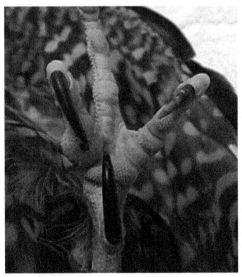

Fig. 12. Puncture wound in a hawk. (*Courtesy of* The Raptor Center, St Paul, MN; with permission.)

Clinical signs and physical examination findings may include pedal alopecia (if applicable), erythema, erosions or ulcerations, swelling, lameness, reluctance or inability to move, and pain on palpation. Lesions are generally more common on the plantar footpad surfaces in small mammals, but may also occur on the palmar surfaces. In birds, lesions may be noted on the metatarsal pad or digital pads. Severely affected animals may lay down in sternal recumbency to relieve pressure on their feet.

Minimum Database

A minimum database should be obtained for all patients. A complete blood cell (CBC) count, serum chemistry panel, and urinalysis (if applicable) will identify any concurrent diseases or predisposing factors. In birds, bile acids should also be evaluated.

Culture and Sensitivity

A culture and sensitivity should be performed to guide the choice of antibiotic therapy. In all species, the best results are obtained through culturing a deep portion of the lesion or a piece of infected tissue.

Imaging

If the ulceration has extended into the underlying tissues, imaging is recommended to identify whether underlying bone is involved (ie, osteomyelitis). Radiographs are easily performed in most clinical settings. Computed tomography (CT) or magnetic resonance imaging (MRI) may detect more subtle abnormalities of bone and soft tissue.

THERAPEUTICS

Treatment of pododermatitis in all species is aimed at correcting the underlying causes, relieving pressure on the affected areas, reducing swelling, establishing drainage (if applicable), treating any secondary infection, and addressing the associated pain and inflammation. Treatment will depend on the severity of the lesions. Concurrent disease conditions, nutritional deficiencies, and pain, stress, and anxiety levels should also be addressed.

A multimodal approach to treatment should be used to manage patients with pododermatitis. A combination of medical and surgical options and alternative options, such as natural remedies, herbal therapy, therapeutic laser, and acupuncture, should be used when feasible.

Correcting Underlying Causes

Any underlying causes should be corrected if possible. For rabbits and rodents, the cage floor should have adequate padding and bedding to reduce pressure on the feet. Foam rubber or a thick towel placed under newspaper with an overlying layer of hay provides a soft compliant bed.[1] Fleece, hay, artificial sheepskin, recycled paper products, or cellulose fiber bedding (CareFRESH, Absorption Corp, Ferndale, WA, USA)[17] may also be used for small mammals as long as they are not ingesting the material. Bedding should be changed frequently.

In perching birds, perches of varying sizes and types should be offered. For psittacines, perches consisting of wood, rope, and rubber should be provided. In most cases, small wooden dowels should be avoided. Perches should be rotated frequently to encourage the bird to perch on different surfaces. Rotating the location of the perches is also important, because many birds will choose their perch based on its location. During management of pododermatitis, perches may be wrapped in safe, soft material such as cotton padding or foam covered with Vetrap Bandaging Tape

(3M, St Paul, MN, USA). For raptors, the proper shape and configuration of the perch varies with major raptor groups. For example, falcons prefer flat perches, such as a shelf covered with artificial turf, whereas eagles, hawks, and owls should be provided with round or elliptical perches made of hemp or sisal rope.[3] Surfaces should be kept clean and dry, and perches and covering materials should be rotated frequently. For free-lofted birds, adequate maneuvering space must be provided to allow space to land normally.[3]

For waterfowl, proper access to water for swimming is essential. For most species, a large pond should be provided with a minimum depth of 2 ft for most species and 4 ft for diving species.[18] The enclosure should contain areas of shade and sunlight, gradual slopes in and out of the water, and islands for resting. Water must be kept clean and free of organic matter. For hospitalized patients, soft flooring or mats and a pool with gradual slopes should be provided.[18]

Improving environmental enrichment for captive species is also essential. Providing enclosures, toys, and feeding stations that foster movement, exercise, and activity more closely resembling natural activity may help to reduce the risk of pododermatitis. For parrots, foot toys, foraging toys, and a foraging tree encourage the bird to move around the enclosure and actively use its feet for activities other than perching. Tunnels, solid wheels (for rats), and toys made of hay offer similar benefits for small mammals.

Correction of the diet is important in all species, and for overweight animals a weight loss program should be instituted. For rabbits and guinea pigs, hay and fresh greens should constitute the primary diet. Reducing the amount of pellets offered is especially important for overweight animals. Guinea pigs should have vitamin C supplementation in the form of tablets or foods such as cabbage, red peppers, kale, oranges, and strawberries. Nonbreeding, healthy adult guinea pigs require 10 to 25 mg/kg of vitamin C daily, whereas pregnant or growing guinea pigs should have 30 mg/kg daily.[8] Guinea pigs with suspected vitamin C deficiency should be supplemented with parenteral vitamin C at a dose of 50 to 100 mg/d.[8] Rats should be fed a rodent block and limited amounts of fresh foods. For psittacines, gradual transition from a seed diet to a formulated diet with additional fresh vegetables is recommended. Addition of foods high in beta-carotene, such as peppers, carrots, squash, and sweet potatoes, is important for production of vitamin A. Waterfowl and poultry, under most circumstances, should be fed a maintenance ration appropriate for the individual species, whereas raptors should be fed a varied whole-prey diet if possible. Animals undergoing any diet change should be monitored closely to prevent rapid weight loss and other secondary problems, such as hepatic lipidosis. If the animal is able to exercise, a daily exercise program should also be instituted.

Medical

Wound care

Ulcerated areas should be kept clean and dry. Depending on the species and the extent of the lesion, recommendations may vary. For small mammals, long hair surrounding the lesion may be trimmed to prevent matting and contamination of the area. If possible, the hair should not be shaved down to the skin, because this will further decrease the protection of the thin skin on this area. The wound should be thoroughly cleaned. In the initial phases of therapy, 0.05% chlorhexidine or 1% povidone iodine solutions may be used, but these should not be used in later stages because they can be cytotoxic to fibroblasts and may reduce white blood cell viability and phagocytic efficiency, leading to delayed wound healing.[9] Hydrotherapy or soaking in a warm saline solution or lactated Ringer solution may be used in later stages of treatment.

Bandaging

With early pododermatitis lesions, such as flattening of the papilla in birds or thinning of the epidermis in small mammals, liquid bandages (New-Skin, Prestige Brands Holdings, Inc., Irvington, NY, USA),[17] cyanoacrylate skin protectants (Marathon Liquid Skin Protectant, Medline Industries, Inc., Mundelein, IL, USA),[17] or skin tougheners (camphor and benzoin)[3] may be painted on the lesions.

Bandages are necessary in all but mild cases. They should be designed to protect the wound against further pressure and trauma, prevent desiccation of the tissue, and shield the wound from contamination. Bandages are generally composed of 3 layers: (1) a primary layer that contacts the wound; (2) a secondary layer that has absorptive properties; and (3) a tertiary layer to hold the other layers in place.[19,20]

The primary layer consists of a dressing in direct contact with the dermal lesion. The dressing should deliver medication, encourage drainage of exudate, protect the wound, and debride necrotic tissue if present. In the initial phases of wound healing, the primary layer may be an adherent dressing, such as gauze or wet-to-dry gauze, to aid in debridement. A seton (sterile strip of gauze, umbilical tape, or a latex drain) may be placed within the wound after preparation of the site and before bandaging to encourage continued drainage.[3] In later stages of wound healing (development of granulation tissue), nonadherent dressings should be used. Nonadherent dressings protect the healing wound bed and prevent desiccation, and may be divided into either occlusive or semiocclusive dressings (**Table 1**).[19,20] Semiocclusive dressings allow excess fluid to enter the secondary bandage layer.[19]

Petrolatum-impregnated sponges/gauze and polyethylene pads are also acceptable semiocclusive dressings.[19,20] For advanced lesions, hydrocolloid or hydrogel wound dressings are best. Topical hydrogel dressings with acemannan, such as CarraVet Wound Gel (Veterinary Products Laboratories, Phoenix, AZ, USA), may also be useful as a primary nonadherent dressing.[19] Acemannan is thought to enhance healing by increasing cytokine production, which in turn stimulates fibroblast proliferation and epidermal growth.[19]

The secondary layer is usually composed of an absorptive material, such as cast padding or cotton padding.[20] The tertiary layer keeps the bandage in place and usually consists of Vetrap Bandaging Tape (3M) or a similar product. Additional protection may be applied along with the tertiary layer, depending on the species and type of lesion present. Interdigital bandages (**Fig. 13**), dental acrylic shoes, polypropylene foam shoes (**Fig. 14**),[3] styrene plastic polymer foot casts,[13] and ball bandages in birds (**Fig. 15**), doughnut-shaped bandages in small mammals, and other forms of protective bandages may be used if the patient will tolerate them. These bandages are

Table 1	
Nonadherent wound dressings	
Semiocclusive	**Occlusive**
Cotton nonadherent bandages • Telfa "Ouchless" Non-Adherent Pads, Covidien, Mansfield, MA, USA	Hydrogel dressings • Tegagel, 3M, St Paul, MN, USA
Polyurethane foam dressing • Hydrasorb, Covidien, Mansfield, MA, USA	Hydrocolloid dressings • Tegasorb, 3M, St Paul, MN, USA
Moisture/vapor permeable dressings • Tegaderm, 3M, St Paul, MN, USA	Calcium alginate dressing • Curasorb, Covidien, Mansfield, MA, USA

Adapted from Refs.[9,19,20]

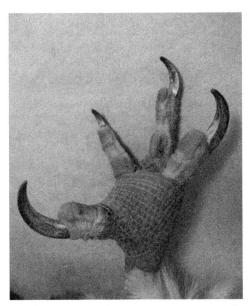

Fig. 13. Interdigital bandage. (*Courtesy of* The Raptor Center, St Paul, MN; with permission.)

designed to relieve pressure on prominent weight-bearing surfaces and redistribute body weight and pressure onto other surfaces.

The choice of bandage often changes depending on the stage of healing. For example, a wet-to-dry bandage or the use of a seton with a ball bandage may be used in the initial drainage stage, followed by a ball bandage without the seton in the granulation stage, polypropylene shoes in the early healing stage, and an interdigital bandage in the later stages of healing.[21] Regardless of the type of dressing and bandage chosen, bandages must be changed regularly, usually daily in the initial stages then every 3 to 7 days thereafter, by either the veterinary staff or an educated owner in select cases. One must be cautious with bandaging, however, because soiled, wet bandages or bandages that have slipped out of position may actually worsen the condition. In addition, one must be cautious when bandaging small exotic mammals, because self-mutilation of the exposed toes may occur.[22] In raptors,

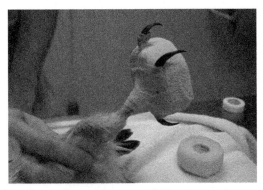

Fig. 14. Polypropylene foam shoes. (*Courtesy of* The Raptor Center, St Paul, MN; with permission.)

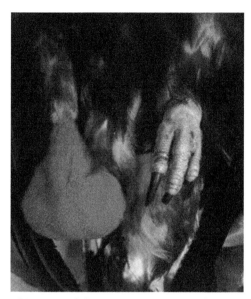

Fig. 15. Ball bandage. (*Courtesy of* The Raptor Center, St Paul, MN; with permission.)

however, the recommended bandaging techniques (ie, acrylic shoes) allow the toes to be exposed to encourage perching and normal pedal function.

Topical medications

Topical medications may be used with or without a bandage. Many products have been used for this purpose, but very little scientific evidence promotes one product over another. Silver sulfadiazine 1%,[5,9,19,20] HEALx Soother Plus (Zoological Education Network, West Palm Beach, FL, USA),[23] Collasate Postoperative Dressing (PRN Pharmacal, Pensacola, FL, USA) (Dr Leslie Reed, Wildlife Rehabilitation Center, personal communication, 2012), and nontoxic antimicrobial products such as triple-antibiotic ointment (Neosporin, Johnson & Johnson Consumer Companies, Inc., New Brunswick, NJ, USA)[5,19] have been successfully used for this condition. Zymox Otic (Pet King Brands, Inc., Westmont, IL, USA), a topical product containing the enzymes lactoperoxidase, lysozyme, and lactoferrin, has been successfully used in a rat.[24] Care must be taken if using topical antibiotics, because ingestion or prolonged absorption can lead to toxicity in many species, and oil-based products may damage avian feather quality and impair thermoregulation. In general, topical corticosteroids are avoided in birds and small mammals, because they may cause severe immunosuppression and delayed wound healing.[17] However, in raptors, a single local treatment with a combination of dimethyl sulfoxide, dexamethasone, and an antibiotic such as ticarcillin, enrofloxacin, or cefazolin has been used successfully (Drs Julia Ponder and Pat Redig, The Raptor Center, personal communication, 2012) (**Table 2**).

Systemic antibiotics

Systemic antibiotics may be indicated in cases of pododermatitis showing evidence of persistent or deep infection. Choice of antibiotic is ideally based on a culture and sensitivity. If a culture is unavailable, the best choice is a broad-spectrum antibiotic that has both a gram-positive and gram-negative spectrum. In advanced cases, an antibiotic that can penetrate deep tissues such as tendons and bones should be

Table 2 Topical therapy in raptors: single-use treatment[25]	
Dimethyl sulfoxide (DMSO)	0.5 mL
Dexamethasone	0.2 mL
Antibiotic (ticarcillin, enrofloxacin, or cefazolin)	0.3 mL

Courtesy of Drs Julia Ponder and Pat Redig, The Raptor Center, University of Minnesota, St Paul, MN.

chosen. Trimethoprim-sulfamethoxazole (TMS) and enrofloxacin are good choices in all species. In birds, oral clindamycin and parenteral cefotaxime, piperacillin/tazobactam, ticarcillin, and amikacin have been used, although potentiated penicillins are often ineffective in raptors.[3] Azithromycin has been used successfully in rabbits at a dose of 40 mg/kg every 24 hours for 5 days, then every 48 hours for 10 days, then twice weekly (Dr Jeffrey Jenkins, Avian & Exotic Animal Hospital, personal communication, 2012). Oral amoxicillin-clavulanic acid has been used successfully in a rat.[24] Treatment may be necessary for an extended period.

Analgesia
Analgesics are essential, because most animals with this condition experience pain, even those with superficial lesions. Meloxicam can be used in rabbits, rodents, and avian patients. All nonsteroidal anti-inflammatory medications (NSAIDs) have the potential for gastrointestinal, liver, or renal side effects, and therefore patients should be monitored accordingly, especially with long-term therapy. In addition to NSAIDs, opioids may be used for multimodal pain control. Buprenorphine, especially in the initial stages, has been used in small mammals, and butorphanol is recommended in birds. Opioid medications may cause sedation in some patients. Various papers have been published on the use of analgesics in exotic species. Dosages vary by species, and the reader should consult a drug formulary for dosages for individual patients. More information on dosing and specific references is available in the *Exotic Animal Formulary, 4th Edition*.[26]

Surgical
Debriding devitalized and infected tissue and establishing drainage, especially if an abscess is present, is necessary in many cases. The goal of surgical debridement is to remove infected or necrotic tissue, relieve pressure, stimulate the formation of granulation tissue, and improve circulation to the area. This will only be successful, however, if it can be combined with other therapies to reduce pressure on the weight-bearing surface and address the underlying causes.

After the lesion is debrided surgically, antibiotic-impregnated polymethylmethacrylate (AIPMMA) beads are a consideration for implantation into the lesion. Choice of antibiotic depends on culture and sensitivity of the lesion, but assuming the organism is susceptible, the local antibiotic concentrations with beads generally far exceed the minimum inhibitory concentration (MIC) for most pathogens.[27] The most common categories of antibiotics used in avian medicine for AIPMMA include aminoglycosides, cephalosporins, penicillins, fluoroquinolones, and clindamycin.[27] The reader should consult other sources for details on making AIPMMA beads. Beads must be sufficiently small (2–4 mm) to implant in this region. After placement, soft padded bandages should be applied, and bandages should be changed daily initially, then every 2 to 3 days thereafter.[28] Removal of the beads is indicated if the beads cause abnormal pressure to the area.

In raptors, closure of the wound may be attempted after the development of a well-formed granulation bed if the wound edges can be approximated.[3] One article described the successful use of an advancement flap to treat a previously unresponsive bumblefoot lesion in a red-tailed hawk.[29]

In general, however, these advanced surgical techniques are not recommended. In rabbits, guinea pigs, rats, and birds, there is usually insufficient skin in this region to allow the use of skin flaps or other reconstructive methods of correcting the defect as may be used in dogs or cats. In addition, the lesion often involves diffuse cellulitis that infiltrates the surrounding tissue, and severe bleeding occurs with any surgical manipulation.[9]

In severe cases, as a salvage procedure, limb amputation may be considered.[8] Amputation would not be recommended for raptors or other wild birds.

Alternative Therapies

Natural remedies

Honey has been shown to have many beneficial properties, including analgesia, anti-inflammatory, antimicrobial, antioxidant, and immunostimulant actions, and acceleration of wound healing.[30] Honey has been used for wound healing for thousands of years. Pure honey (*Leptospermum* spp, such as manuka honey) may be used, or commercial honey dressings can be purchased. A list of medical honey sources is available in "Use of Honey for Wound Management" by Signe E. Beebe.[30] The successful use of honey for wound healing requires that an adequate amount be kept in close contact with the wound.[30] The frequency of bandage changes will depend on the amount of exudation from the wound and generally ranges from daily to every 3 to 5 days.[30]

Several natural nontoxic products are available through the Zoological Education Network (www.HEALx.com) and may be beneficial in treating pododermatitis and for wound healing.[23] HEALx/AVIx Booster contains a combination of red palm fruit oil and a patented monolaurin. Red palm fruit oil originates from the fruit of the palm tree, *Elaeis guineensis*. It is an excellent source of carotenoids, including β-carotene, α-carotene, lycopene, and phytoene.[23] Both β-carotene and α-carotene can be converted to vitamin A. In addition, red palm fruit oil is rich in vitamin E.[23] Monolaurin is the glycerol ester derivative of lauric acid, similar to a fatty acid found in small quantities in coconut products. It has antiviral, antimicrobial, and antiprotozoal properties.[23] These natural ingredients may be beneficial during wound healing and management of pododermatitis. HEALx/AVIx Booster is usually dosed at 0.06 mL per 100 g of body weight by mouth daily (Dr Greg Harrison, Zoological Education Network, personal communication, 2012). HEALx Soother Plus is a topical therapy that has been used successfully in many cases of pododermatitis. This product contains a combination of monolaurin, a monoglyceride of a fatty acid, aloe vera juice and a patented quaternary ammonium solution. Together, these ingredients may provide anti-inflammatory, antibacterial, antifungal, antiviral, and immunoregulating properties.[23] HEALx Soother Plus may be used in combination with other medications, and has been used successfully for topical therapy in numerous patients.[23]

Dr. Tracy Bennett and Dr. Donna Kelleher report the use of a Wound Formula (**Box 1**) composed of herbs for topical management of pododermatitis (Dr. Tracy Bennett, Bird & Exotic Clinic of Seattle, Seattle WA, personal communication, Sep 2012 and Dr. Donna Kelleher, Whole Pet Vet, Bellingham WA, personal communication, Jan 2013).

Therapeutic laser

Low-level laser therapy (LLLT) or therapeutic laser may help with wound healing.[9,31] Lasers used for therapy are generally class IIIb lasers with 5 to 500 mW of power.

Box 1
Wound formula

3 quarts bottled or purified water

1/3 cup cut plantain leaf

1/3 cup cut comfrey leaf

1/3 cup packed calendula flowers (fresh is best)

1/3 cup chamomile flowers

1/3 cup packed yarrow flowers

2 tablespoons aloe vera gel (fresh is best)

2 tablespoons powdered Oregon grape or goldenseal root

Combine all ingredients in a large stainless steel or ceramic pot, cover, and simmer for 3 minutes. Remove from heat, uncover, and let cool. Strain the tea, discarding the solids, and save it in the refrigerator. Apply to skin either as an herbal soak or with a cotton ball. Allow tea to stay in contact with the skin for at least 5 minutes twice per day; leave tea on skin and do not rinse with water. This tea is safe to use daily, but as soon as the affected area improves, use may be discontinued.

Infusion may be kept for 3 weeks in the refrigerator if it does not become contaminated. It may also be aliquoted into smaller portions and frozen for 2 to 3 months. If the skin is red and inflamed, it is best to warm up the tea to room temperature before applying.

Courtesy of Dr Donna Kelleher, Whole Pet Vet, Bellingham WA and Dr Tracy Bennett, Bird & Exotic Clinic of Seattle, Seattle WA.

The benefits of LLLT in wound healing may include promoting fibroblast development, collagen production, and epithelialization; enhancing leukocyte infiltration and macrophage activity; promoting angiogenesis and stimulating vasodilation; increasing the concentration of growth factors to the region; and increasing lymphatic drainage.[9,31] Laser therapy may be contraindicated in areas with severe infection. Laser therapy has been used to encourage wound healing in a rabbit with pododermatitis at 5 W for 30 seconds for each foot (Dr Peter Fisher, Pet Care Veterinary Hospital, personal communication, 2012). Treatments were performed twice weekly for 6 treatments in conjunction with topical medications, bandages, and improvements in the rabbit's husbandry. Because LLLT is generally used in conjunction with other therapies, the significance of its role in the resolution of these cases is difficult to determine.

Acupuncture
Acupuncture may also be beneficial for managing pododermatitis. Acupuncture is the insertion of needles into specific points of the body to produce a desired response. Acupuncture may provide analgesia, reduce inflammation, improve circulation, and stimulate cells of tissue growth and repair.[32]

Eckermann-Ross has had great success in mammalian, reptilian, and avian species using acupuncture at *Ba feng*, ST-36, and other points as relevant for each case. Aquapuncture and moxibustion have also been used successfully (Dr Christine Eckermann-Ross, Avian & Exotic Animal Care, personal communication, 2012).

PROGNOSIS

Measuring the ulcerated areas and documenting the progress with digital photos at each follow-up visit are essential to evaluate success or failure of a treatment plan.

Medical progress examinations should be scheduled at least every 1 to 2 weeks, but in the initial stages, rechecks and bandage changes may need to be performed more frequently.

Patients with mild pododermatitis that is detected early can have a good prognosis, especially if underlying causes can be corrected. Treatment duration may be as long as 8 to 12 weeks, and in raptors, preventative use of padded perches may be necessary for up to 28 weeks.[2] Many cases of pododermatitis, however, are incurable and progress despite aggressive multimodal therapy. In severe cases, euthanasia should be considered.

SUMMARY

Pododermatitis, or bumblefoot, is a common condition encountered in birds, rabbits, and rodents in clinical practice. This article is intended to encourage practitioners to use a multimodal approach for the successful management of this disease in all species. Treatment should address the underlying causes and use medical, surgical, and alternative therapies to increase the likelihood of success in these patients.

REFERENCES

1. Harcourt-Brown F. Skin diseases. In: Harcourt-Brown F, editor. Textbook of rabbit medicine. Oxford (United Kingdom): Butterworth-Heinemann; 2002. p. 233–40.
2. McCluggage D. Bandaging. In: Altman R, Clubb S, Dorrestein G, et al, editors. Avian medicine and surgery. 1st edition. Philadelphia: WB Saunders; 1997. p. 830–2.
3. Redig P. Raptors: practical information every avian practitioner can use [abstract 640]. In: Association of Avian Veterinarians Proceedings. 2006. Veterinary Information Network Web site. Available at: http://www.vin.com/Members/Proceedings/Proceedings.plx?CID=aav2006&PID=pr16224&O=VIN. Accessed August 5, 2012.
4. Shivaprasad HL. Avian integument: anatomy and diseases [abstract 740]. In: Association of Avian Veterinarians Proceedings. 2009. Veterinary Information Network Web site. Available at: http://www.vin.com/Members/Proceedings/Proceedings.plx?CID=aav2009&PID=pr55154&O=VIN. Accessed August 5, 2012.
5. Ford S, Chitty J, Jones M. Raptor medicine master class [abstract 620]. In: Association of Avian Veterinarians Proceedings. 2008. Veterinary Information Network Web site. Available at: http://www.vin.com/Members/Proceedings/Proceedings.plx?CID=aav2008&PID=pr26597&O=VIN. Accessed August 5, 2012.
6. O'Malley B. Guinea pigs. In: O'Malley B, editor. Clinical anatomy and physiology of exotic species. New York: Elsevier; 2005. p. 197–208.
7. O'Malley B. Rats. In: O'Malley B, editor. Clinical anatomy and physiology of exotic species. New York: Elsevier; 2005. p. 209–25.
8. Hawkins MG, Bishop CR. Disease problems of guinea pigs: dermatologic diseases. In: Quesenberry K, Carpenter J, editors. Ferrets, rabbits, and rodents: clinical medicine and surgery. 3rd edition. St Louis (MO): Elsevier Saunders; 2012. p. 305–6.
9. Brown C, Donnelly T. Treatment of pododermatitis in the guinea pig. Lab Anim (NY) 2008;37(4):156–7.
10. Bauck L. Avian dermatology. In: Altman R, Clubb S, Dorrestein G, et al, editors. Avian medicine and surgery. 1st edition. Philadelphia: WB Saunders; 1997. p. 554–6.

11. Stoute ST, Bickford AA, Walker RL, et al. Mycotic pododermatitis and mycotic pneumonia in commercial turkey poults in Northern California. J Vet Diagn Invest 2009;21(4):554–7.

12. Elitok OM, Elitok B, Unver O. Renal amyloidosis in cattle with inflammatory diseases. J Vet Intern Med 2008;22(2):450–5.

13. Remple JD. Raptor bumblefoot: a new treatment technique. In: Redig PT, Cooper JE, Remple JD, et al, editors. Raptor biomedicine. Minneapolis (MN): University of Minnesota Press; 1993. p. 154–60.

14. Jenkins JR. Conditions of the feet of rabbits and rodents. In: British Small Animal Veterinary Congress Proceedings. 2006. Veterinary Information Network Web site. Available at: http://www.vin.com/Members/Proceedings/Proceedings.plx?CID=bsava2006&PID=pr12813&O=VIN. Accessed August 5, 2012.

15. Harrison GJ, McDonald D. Nutritional considerations section II: nutritional disorders. In: Harrison G, Lightfoot T, editors. Clinical avian medicine, vol. 1. Palm Beach (FL): Spix Publishing; 2006. p. 108–15.

16. Clark S, Hansen G, McLean P, et al. Pododermatitis in turkeys. Avian Dis 2002; 46(4):1038–44.

17. Hess L, Tater K. Dermatologic diseases. In: Quesenberry K, Carpenter J, editors. Ferrets, rabbits, and rodents: clinical medicine and surgery. 3rd edition. St Louis (MO): Elsevier Saunders; 2012. p. 235.

18. Hernandez-Divers S. Waterfowl husbandry and medicine. In: Atlantic Coast Veterinary Proceedings. 2007. Veterinary Information Network Web site. Available at: http://www.vin.com/Members/Proceedings/Proceedings.plx?CID=acvc2007&PID=pr19020&O=VIN. Accessed August 5, 2012.

19. Graham JE. Rabbit wound management. Vet Clin North Am Exot Anim Pract 2004;7:37–55.

20. Grunkemeyer V. Management of avian skin wounds [abstract 340]. In: Association of Avian Veterinarians Proceedings. 2009. Veterinary Information Network Web site. Available at: http://www.vin.com/Members/Proceedings/Proceedings.plx?CID=aav2009&PID=pr55127&O=VIN. Accessed August 5, 2012.

21. Bueno-Padilla I, Arent L, Ponder J. Tips for raptor bandaging. Exotic DVM 12(3):29–47.

22. Tully TN. Dermatologic disease of small mammals. In: Atlantic Coast Veterinary Proceedings. 2008. Veterinary Information Network Web site. Available at: http://www.vin.com/Members/Proceedings/Proceedings.plx?CID=acvc2008&PID=pr25850&O=VIN. Accessed August 5, 2012.

23. Bankstahl T. Clinical results with selected complementary therapies in birds [abstract 915]. In: Association of Avian Veterinarians Proceedings. 2007. Veterinary Information Network Web site. Available at: http://www.vin.com/Members/Proceedings/Proceedings.plx?CID=aav2007&PID=pr20002&O=VIN. Accessed August 5, 2012.

24. Fisher PG. Successful treatment of pododermatitis in a rat. Exotic DVM 6(5):3–4.

25. Redig P. Raptors. In: Altman R, Clubb S, Dorrestein G, et al, editors. Avian medicine and surgery. 1st edition. Philadelphia: WB Saunders; 1997. p. 927.

26. Carpenter JW. Exotic animal formulary. 4th edition. St. Louis (MO): Elsevier Saunders; 2013.

27. Remple JD. Antibiotic-impregnated polymethylmethacrylate beads: advantages, antibiotic choices, and production [abstract 640]. In: Association of Avian Veterinarians Proceedings. 2005. Veterinary Information Network Web site. Available

at: http://www.vin.com/Members/Proceedings/Proceedings.plx?CID=aav2005& PID=pr11655&O=VIN. Accessed August 5, 2012

28. Bennett A. Soft tissue surgery. In: Quesenberry K, Carpenter J, editors. Ferrets, rabbits, and rodents: clinical medicine and surgery. 3rd edition. St Louis (MO): Elsevier Saunders; 2012. p. 337.

29. Haskins S, Burgdorf-Moisuk A, Whittington JK, et al. Advancement flap treatment for pododermatitis in a hawk [abstract 1330]. In: Association of Avian Veterinarians Proceedings. 2011. Veterinary Information Network Web site. Available at: http://www.vin.com/Members/Proceedings/Proceedings.plx?CID=aav2011& PID=pr82898&O=VIN. Accessed August 5, 2012.

30. Beebe SE. Use of honey for wound management [abstract SA44]. In: Western Veterinary Conference Proceedings. 2011. Veterinary Information Network Web site. Available at: http://www.vin.com/Members/Proceedings/Proceedings.plx? CID=wvc2011&PID=pr82731&O=VIN. Accessed August 5, 2012.

31. Browning DC. Alternative therapies in veterinary wound management [abstract VT64]. In: Western Veterinary Conference Proceedings. 2012. Veterinary Information Network Web site. Available at: http://www.vin.com/Members/Proceedings/ Proceedings.plx?CID=wvc2012&PID=pr86408&O=VIN. Accessed December 9, 2012.

32. Marsden S. Evidence-based acupuncture. In: 62nd Convention of the Canadian Medical Association Proceedings. 2010. Veterinary Information Network Web site. Available at: http://www.vin.com/Members/Proceedings/Proceedings.plx? CID=cvma2010&PID=pr58252&O=VIN. Accessed December 9, 2012.

Vesicular, Ulcerative, and Necrotic Dermatitis of Reptiles

Adolf K. Maas III, DVM, DABVP (Reptile & Amphibian Practice)[a,b]

KEYWORDS

- Dermatitis • Reptile • Chelonia • Vesicle • Husbandry • Squamate • Skin • VUND

KEY POINTS

- Dermatitis of reptiles is most commonly a systemic disease.
- The underlying issue must be identified for resolution.
- Appropriate combinations of therapies are required; there is no "one size fits all."
- Husbandry is a factor in identifying cause, determining therapy, and creating a resolution.

INTRODUCTION

Dermatologic conditions of reptiles are common and often misunderstood. Traditionally, any time a reptilian patient presented to a veterinarian with a skin disease it was categorized as a "rot" (skin rot, scale rot, shell rot) and assumed to be primarily a bacterial dermatologic condition, somewhat analogous to a superficial dermatitis in a dog. As a result, the bulk of these conditions were treated topically, often to the detriment of the patient. Current research and analysis of effective therapies address these as systemic diseases that require the pursuit of appropriate diagnostics and therapies.

The skin is the delineation between the often contaminated, random outside world and the sterile, controlled environment of the body. As such, so long as this border is intact and healthy, the challenges posed by an animal's environment are much more defensible. Once this margin is damaged or broken, this barrier to invasion is lost, allowing for further damage or disease to enter into the system. There is loss of the immune system function of the epidermis against pathogen invasion and loss of fluid regulation function when the damage to the skin is extensive.[1]

Vesicular dermatitis is a not infrequent condition found in veterinary and human medicine, and most species of animals have been found to be susceptible to this condition. It is characterized by formation of fluid-filled blisters within the structure of the skin. Histologically, these blisters (vesicles and bullae) are identified by the dermal, epidermal, or intraepidermal separation of the skin, forming cutaneous fluid-filled

Disclosures: The author has nothing to disclose.
[a] Center for Bird and Exotic Animal Medicine, 11401 Northeast 195th Street, Bothell, WA 98011, USA; [b] ZooVet Consulting, PLLC, PO Box 1007, Bothell, WA 98041, USA
E-mail address: DrMaas@TheExoticVet.com

vesicles and necrosis of the elevated epidermis.[2] These vesicles can be formed by many causes, including infectious, thermal and chemical burns, trauma, and autoimmune. They often rupture, forming erosions and ulcers.[3] The open wounds created by these ruptured vesicles then provide a venue for secondary complications, such as infections and prolonged healing.[4]

Although categorized into vesicular, ulcerative, and necrotic dermatitis (VUND), these diseases are often different stages of the same pathophysiology and within the confines of this article are treated as a similar condition with different presentations based on the species affected and progression of disease.

CLINICAL ANATOMY AND PHYSIOLOGY

Reptile skin is neither simpler nor more complex than that of other vertebrates; it is only different. The general division of this tissue, like mammals, is that of a superficial keratinized epidermal layer supported by an underlying dermis. The epidermis of lepidosaurs is made up of multiple distinct layers that are cyclically replaced (ecdysis, discussed later). The layers from most superficial to deepest are as follows:

- *Oberhautchen*: a thin (1 μm) layer of mature, very tough keratinized cells overlaying the outermost portion of the β cellular layer
- β Stratum: an inelastic, tough, stratified epithelial layer composed primarily of β keratin (the hinge area between scales is lacking this layer)
- Mesos stratum: the transitional cells between the β and α layers
- α Stratum: a soft, flexible, stratified epithelium composed primarily of α keratin
- Lacunar stratum/clear layer: the inner-most strata of the outer-generation layer, tightly interdigitated with the newly forming *Oberhautchen*
- Inner-generation layer: a developing *Oberhautchen* layer and newly developing α and β layers
- Stratum germanativum: deepest basal layer of progenitor columnar epithelium (**Figs. 1** and **2**)

The superficial tissue layer of chelonia, in contrast to lepidosaurs, is constructed much like that of a mammal. The epidermis is superficial; tightly adhered to the dermis;

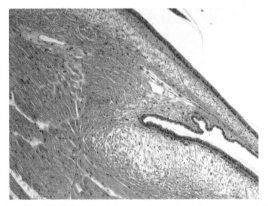

Fig. 1. Normal snake skin, *Lichanura trivirgata* (hematoxylin-eosin, original magnification ×10). The β and α keratin layers are seen as a thin pink layer, separated from the underlying cellular layers. The cellular epidermal layers are a more organized, defined superficial structure, whereas the dermis is looser, more disorganized in appearance. (*Courtesy of* Drury Reavill, DVM, DABVP, DACVP, West Sacramento, CA.)

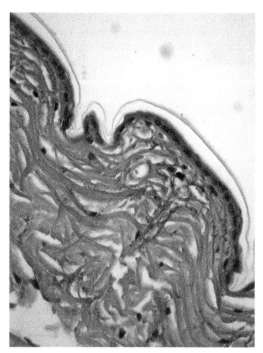

Fig. 2. Gecko skin, *Eublepharis macularius* (hematoxylin-eosin, original magnification ×40). The dense kearatin layers are lifted from the cellular layers at the *Oberhautchen* layer. The stratum germinativum is the best defined layer of the epidermis in this view, seen as a single layer of columnar epithelium overlying the thick dermal layer. (*Courtesy of* Drury Reavill, DVM, DABVP, DACVP, West Sacramento, CA.)

and constructed of pseudostratified to stratified epithelial cells that subsequently form either the horny scute (modified epidermal tissue mostly made up of β keratin) or the stratum corneum (consisting of many layers of flat keratinized cells).[5] Under the epidermis, the highly vascular and collagen-laden, deeper dermal layer overlays either the dermal bone or the subcutaneous adnexa.

The deep dermal layer is highly vascular; innervated; elastic; and intermixed with large numbers of immune cells and chromatophores (pigment cells). Osteoderms or osteoscutes found in some reptiles (eg, *Anguidae*, *Cordylus*, *Scincidae*, *Chelonia*) are anchored here, and form an external "skeleton" in these animals.[6] In *Chelonia*, the carapace and plastron arise from fusion of these with vertebrae and ribs dorsally, and the sternum ventrally.[7] In other groups (*Helodermatidae*, *Crocodylia*), the osteoderms fuse with the dorsal portions of the skull, fusing the combined structures into a solid "skull."[6]

In shelled and nonshelled portions of *Chelonia* and in *Crocodylia*, epidermal cell growth is continuous and is replaced and shed similar as to the same process in mammals.[2] The claws and horns of most reptilian species and the beak of *Chelonia* are formed as highly keratinized structures, often encasing underlying bony structures (terminal phalanges, mandible or maxilla). Hence, systemic disease or pathology of associated epidermis and dermis often effect any of these structures. Note, however, claws in Lepidosaurs do not undergo cyclic ecdysis as the rest of their keratinized ectodermal structures do.

In contrast to mammals, reptiles have few skin glands in general. Knowledge of the specific glands for a species is important to recognize normal from abnormal, but these glands are generally not associated with pathology related to VUND. Most chelonia (excluding *Testudinidae* and some *Emydidae*) have Rathke glands on each bridge between the carapace and plastron. Mental glands are found bilaterally on their lower jaw of male *Testudinidae* species. Many *Lacertilia* (including *Iguania*, *Scincomorpha*, and *Gekkota*) develop femoral and pubic scent glands with sexual maturity (often, but not only in, males). *Serpentes* have paired scent glands caudal to the vent. A few other species of reptiles that live in demanding environments have salt glands.[5]

ECDYSIS

The distinct layers of the epidermis allow for synchronized replacement on a regular basis (ecdysis) in Lepidosaurs. Ecdysis can be divided into four overlapping stages:

- During the first stage or rest cycle, the epidermis outer-generation layer is mature. The basal stratum germinativum is overlaid by the α layer and protected by the more superficial β layer.
- The growth cycle starts with the stratum germanativum undergoing hypertrophy and cellular migration to build a new epidermis deep to the superficial skin. The older outer-generation layer becomes distinct from the growing inner-generation layer.
- As development proceeds to the maturation cycle, these newly formed cells mature and differentiate into the new α layer, β layer, and the formation of a new *Oberhautchen*.
- The shed cycle finishes the process as enzymes cleave the cellular bonds between the clear and *Oberhautchen* layers, permitting release of the older skin layer and ecdysis.[8]

Disruptions during any of these stages may cause pathologies of the skin. Factors that influence ecdysis frequency include age, specific species, environmental ambient temperature and humidity, infections or health status, and parasite load.

NONINFECTIOUS CAUSES OF VUND

Thermal burns are well understood to cause vesicles and blisters, but they are usually localized to a specific area of exposure. Radiation burns have been discussed by practitioners[9] and suspect sunburns have been seen by the author in snakes and lizards overexposed to powerful UV bulbs, but are not well documented in the literature. These sunburns likely have UV and thermal components to their pathology, but anecdotally seem to be more common in nocturnal species and albinistic individuals that may lack sufficient endogenous protection. Cases involving only heat sources are reported and thermal burns are often implicated when a ventral vesicular or ulcerative dermatitis is seen in a snake. It seems to rarely be the case, based on measurements of the temperature of enclosure surfaces. Histopathologic examination of affected tissues rarely finds lesions typical of thermal injury and infectious cause must remain as a primary differential. However, sick reptiles are less active and may seek those areas of the cage where the highest heat is provided, thus increasing the risk of thermal injury. Nonetheless, careful evaluation and thermal measurements must be made to the animal's enclosure to assist in the diagnostic process.

Renal disease has been implicated in epidermal or dermal separation causing bullae in reptiles.[10] Metastatic mineralizations with the formation of dermal fluid pockets have been seen by the author and others (John Trupkiewicz, Northwest Zoo Path, Monroe, WA, and Drury Reavill, Zoo/Exotic Pathology Service, West Sacramento, CA, personal communication, 2010). These can be differentiated from vesicular dermatitis by biochemical profile analysis and histopathology of renal, skin, and other affected tissues.

Autoimmune disease should be considered as a differential in reptiles that develop separation of the epidermis from the dermis with the subsequent formation of vesicles. Pemphigus diseases are well described in the human and domestic veterinary literature and grossly produce the same lesion as vesicular dermatitis. Histologically, the lesions are similar with dermatoepithelial separation, but easily differentiated. Although not reported in reptiles, this has been suggested in other nontraditional species, such as the Korean fowl[11] and in Malayan tapirs.[12]

Suboptimal or inappropriate husbandry is the most common unifying issue in cases of VUND.[4] In all cases of reptile medicine, a thorough knowledge of appropriate housing and enclosure ventilation and humidity, ambient temperatures, lighting and night cycle, and diet is necessary for the accurate diagnosis of any condition in any species.[13]

Environmental moisture is believed to be a significant factor in the development of vesicular dermatitis, but not as the sole cause. Many cases are found to have excessive environmental humidity, wet bedding, or even standing water in their enclosures. Ventilation factors into humidity levels, in that poor air circulation holds moisture within the enclosure, moistens the bedding without appearing to be wet, and creates an environment that is conducive for bacterial growth. Furthermore, when ventilation is poor, general air quality is generally likewise so. Inhaled contaminants have been shown to effect mammalian immune systems,[14] are commonly believed to predispose reptiles to respiratory disease and generally are thought to be immunosuppressive.

The enclosure temperature must be considered in any reptilian condition, especially that of dermatologic diseases. Because reptiles are poikilothermic ectotherms,[15] their immune system function is highly dependent on their enclosure temperature, and suboptimal temperatures coupled with predisposing conditions (undigested meal in the stomach, parasite-induced skin wounds, excessive moisture, bacteria-laden bedding, poor air quality, and so forth) can allow for the development of bacterial infections and septicemia.

Environmental contamination with toxins has been implicated in necrotic shell disease of chelonians. This may be related to immunosuppression combined with substandard husbandry or environmental toxin exposure.[16] Further investigation into the role that environmental toxins may play is warranted but in any case of necrotic dermatitis or shell disease an evaluation of toxin exposure is warranted.

Nutritional dyscrasias are commonly considered to cause dermatologic disease in many species of reptiles. Hypovitaminosis E from high-fat diets is implicated in the development of sloughing, necrotic skin secondary to underlying steatitis.[17] Hypervitaminosis A, iatrogenically caused by subcutaneous injections of concentrated vitamin A, produces focal to generalized dermal necrosis with subsequent skin sloughing and secondary infections. Intradermal, subcutaneous, or superficial intramuscular injections of irritating medications (eg, enrofloxacin) are well documented to cause localized dermal necrosis and skin slough.

Neoplastic dermatologic conditions can resemble necrotic or ulcerative dermatitis caused by loss of the normal epithelial layer or the inability of the skin to repair. Cutaneous sarcomas (believed to be secondary to *Arenavirus* infection) have been reported that are similar in presentation to necrotic dermatitis. The author has seen a single case of chondrosarcoma in a corn snake (*Elaphe* [*Pantherophis*] *guttata*) whose initial presentation was similar to that of an ulcerative dermatitis. Paraneoplastic syndromes that cause the formation of epidermal-dermal vesicles have been reported in many domestic species,[18] but have not been reported in reptiles.

INFECTIOUS CAUSES OF VUND
Viral

Viral causes are not found to specifically result vesicular dermatitis, but references suggest that there may also be a viral cause associated with or underlying the bacterial or husbandry causes identified. Several viral infections in reptiles produce skin lesions (flavivirus, poxvirus, herpesvirus, papillomavirus), and could be considered as differentials, but there are no specific viral infections yet identified that commonly produce epidermal vesicles in their pathology.[19] Necrotic or ulcerative dermatitis is observed in association with pathogens that cause damage to the regenerative epidermal or underlying dermal layers. These lesions may be the primary presenting sign or may develop into secondary bacterial dermatitis.

The following is a summary of reptile viruses that are believed to cause dermatologic lesions, with species affected and a description of lesions observed[19,20]:

- Poxvirus: enveloped double-strand DNA virus.
  - Tegu (*Tupinambis* sp): disseminated brown papular lesions.
  - Hermann tortoise (*Testudo hermanii*): papular periocular lesions.
  - *Crocodylia* (worldwide, many species): gray-white, tan, or brown papular skin lesions, with or without superficial crusts. May be focal or disseminated.
- Iridovirus: enveloped and nonenveloped double-stranded DNA virus.
  - Frilled lizard (*Chlamydosaurus kingii*): "pox-like" lesions. It is unknown if this is a virus cross-over from invertebrates, or a primary infection.
- Herpesvirus: enveloped double-strand DNA virus.
  - Green sea turtles (*Chelonia mydas*): "gray patch disease" in individuals younger than 3 months old, starting as small, circular papular lesions that coalesce.
- Papillomavirus: nonenveloped double-strand DNA virus.
  - Bolivian side-necked turtles (*Platemys platycephala*): focal to coalescing papular skin lesions, developing into areas of necrosis.
- Arenavirus: enveloped single-stranded negative-sense RNA virus.
  - Ophidia (multiple species): putative cause of inclusion body disease,[21] which has been associated with undifferentiated cutaneous sarcomas that can resemble necrotic dermatitis.
- Paramyxovirus: enveloped single-stranded negative-sense RNA virus.
  - Hermann tortoise (*Testudo hermanii*): dermatitis.
- Flavivirus: enveloped, single-stranded positive-sense RNA virus.
  - American alligators (*Alligator mississippiensis*): lymphohistiocytic-proliferative cutaneous lesions, caused by West Nile virus.[22]

Fungal

Mycotic dermatitis of reptiles is well reported with multiple infectious agents implicated, including *Mucor*,[23] *Penicillium*, *Geotrichium*, and *Nannizziopsis*.[24] Fungal dermatitis rarely manifests with the formation of cutaneous vesicles; however, the cutaneous lesions typically seen in fungal dermatitis can grossly resemble the common presentation of denuded epithelia in vesicular or necrotic dermatitis.[25] Gross examination of many cases of fungal dermatitis is misinterpreted as ulcerative or necrotic dermatitis of bacterial origin.

Mycotic skin infections are often secondary infections and opportunistic to a predisposing condition. The underlying issue may be bacterial, parasitic, or viral infections or husbandry conditions (including environmental conditions, crowding, and malnutrition). Fungal nodular skin lesions progressing to necrotic epidermal lesions after stress of capture and captivity has been reported in healthy, wild-caught Marlborough green geckos (*Naultinus manukanus*).[26]

A proved exception to fungal dermatitis as a secondary infection is the pathogen, *Chrysosporium* anamorph of *Nannizziopsis vriesii*. In clinical trials, it has been shown to be a primary pathogen in veiled chameleons (*Chamaeleo calyptratus*) and to fulfill Koch postulates.[27] Although infection in this species is through dermal penetration and lesions are most readily seen in the skin, this dermatologic condition should be addressed as a systemic mycotic disease. Confirmed infection has been identified in many different species of squamate reptiles and has been shown to be pathogenic in most cases.[26,28–30] This pathogen is covered in much greater detail elsewhere in this issue.

Parasitic

External parasites may induce bacterial dermatitis, with ticks (*Aponnoma latus*)[31] and mites (*Ophionyssus natricus*) suspected as carriers of infectious agents through direct introduction by saliva or through environmental contamination of the bite wounds. Internal parasites, such as nematodes, cestodes, and other helminthes, may affect the frequency of ecdysis and have been found to migrate to subcutaneous tissues or infect circulatory and lymphatic systems resulting in cutaneous lesions.[32,33,34] However, there are no reported specific causes of primary parasitic VUND.

Bacterial

It is suggested that bacterial infections are the most common cause of disease in reptiles.[35] Bacterial vesicular dermatitis has been reported in many species of reptiles, including *Testudines*[36] and *Squamata*.[37] In caged snakes, it is possibly one of the most common presentations seen in practice.[4] Often, the vesicles are ruptured at the time of examination with sloughing of the overlying necrotic epidermis, and the patient presents with denuded lesions, representative of an ulcerative dermatitis. These lesions are often open and raw, covered by a pseudomembrane of fibrin, or caked with debris from their enclosure. If the scales are still present, they often appear thickened, rough, or brown and dilated blood vessels may be visible on adjacent skin and scales. There may be pockets of fluid subepidermally or areas covered with fibrin deposits, even with portions of scales missing from necrosis. Histologically, these lesions exhibit a loss of most or all of the superficial epidermis with exposed dermal layers and infiltrations of heterophils and monocytes, often with crusts overlying the lesions (**Figs. 3** and **4**).

Despite bacterial dermatitis being commonly seen in the practice setting, primary bacterial dermatitis in snakes and other reptiles has not been widely reported in the literature. Cultures of these lesions commonly identify a wide range of bacterial agents including gram-positive, gram-negative, and anaerobic bacteria. Because many of these lesions have broken skin or are exposed to the animal's environment, pure cultures of pathogens are rare and often contain a wide variety of environmental bacterial contaminates.[4,38] A clinician must be careful not to overdiagnose these results and should take precautions to minimize contamination when taking diagnostic samples to produce the most reliable results possible. In many of these animals, the cause of the bacterial agent is suggested to be secondary to systemic infections, rather than a primary bacterial dermatitis (**Fig. 5**). Many affected reptiles are septicemic and blood cultures may also identify a large variety of causative bacteria.

Vesicular disease has been reported in the chelonian, with chronic shell disease being the most common presentation. These turtles and tortoises present with defects in the carapaces and (more commonly) the plastron with varying degree of shell

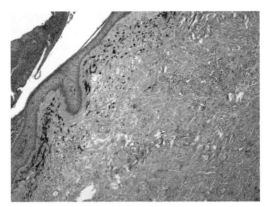

Fig. 3. Intact epithelium with an overlying inflammatory crust (*upper left*). In the dermis there are nodular proliferations of perivascular inflammatory cells, *Naja annulifera* (hematoxylin-eosin, original magnification ×4). (*Courtesy of* Drury Reavill, DVM, DABVP, DACVP, West Sacramento, CA.)

damage and necrosis. Apparently minor superficial lesions found on initial examination may underscore the severity of deeper lesions, which in many cases involve extensive damage through the entire shell that extends as caseous lesions and abscesses into the coelom and viscera. The underlying cause of bacterial shell disease may be a primary infectious agent,[39,40] but the origin can just as easily be that of systemic disease because it could be shell wounds with secondary contamination.[41]

One putative cause of necrotic dermatitis/shell disease is that superficial trauma damages the fine vasculature of the superficial osteoscutes resulting in an ischemic condition and devitalization of the dermis and bone. This tissue death and loss of the overlying protective tissue promotes secondary bacterial and fungal infection (L. Clayton, DVM, DABVP, National Aquarium, Baltimore, MD, personal communication, 2012). Further research is needed to elucidate the occurrence of these events, and if there are species predilections.

An example of bacterial-associated skin disease is the condition cutaneous dyskeratosis, which has been identified in desert tortoises (*Gopherus agassizii*), characterized

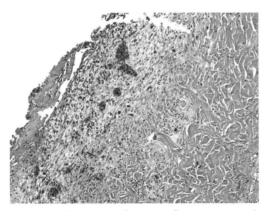

Fig. 4. Ulcerative dermatitis with a thin adherent inflammatory exudate, *Naja annulifera* (hematoxylin-eosin, original magnification ×10). (*Courtesy of* Drury Reavill, DVM, DABVP, DACVP, West Sacramento, CA.)

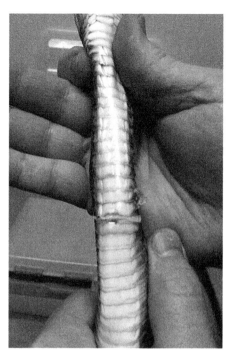

Fig. 5. Subadult indigo snake (*Drymarchon corais*) presenting with area on ventrum of vesicular dermatitis and 1-week history of anorexia. Husbandry considered to be very good. Blood culture for this individual was positive. Blood cultures are commonly positive for *Providencia rettgeri*, *Pseudomonas aeruginosa*, *Morganella morgannii*, *Enterococcus* species, *Clostridium* species, and *Salmonella* species. (*Courtesy of* Adolf K. Maas III, DVM, Bothell, WA.)

by a white discoloration of the superficial keratin, flaking and peeling of the scutes, and irregular foci of pitting and chipping of the keratin of the plastron and carapace. Environmental and cellular debris, with or without bacteria or fungal elements, was identified when examining between the horn layers of the scutes. Epithelial atrophic and hyperplastic changes were seen with histopathologic examination of some of these lesions along with deeper tissue pathology including osteopenia and osteoclastic resorption of the underlying bone.[42,43] Evidence of trauma was also seen in some of these animals found to have bacterial and fungal infections and it is not entirely clear as to the specific causal pattern.

Another example is ulcerative dermatitis of the feet of swamp tortoises, reported with *Pseudomonas* and unidentified fungal elements being present. Affected animals were treated topically and systemically because septicemia was determined to be the cause of death in many individuals. Improvement of husbandry and increased temperatures are believed to be the appropriate therapy.[44]

A chronologic order has been proposed for highly variable lesions seen in at least two species of water turtles.[45] Initially, the lesion starts as an area of focal acute epidermal necrosis. This then proceeds to loss of the overlying keratin and subsequent ulceration, then dermal necrosis with migration of inflammatory cells into the lesion. The blood supply to this area and the adjacent bone becomes compromised, causing osteotic necrosis and resorption. These lesions can then spread or coalesce because of further damage and infection.

DIAGNOSING REPTILE DERMATITIS

Diagnosis of VUND first requires identification of any deficiencies or incongruity in the patient's husbandry. Interviewing the client and obtaining a complete history should include the following:

- If the clinician is familiar with the correct husbandry for that species, that knowledge can be simply compared with the description of the animal's terrarium provided by the owner. In less common species, research to identify the species' natural history and range provides clues to possible husbandry factors, and there are well-researched published refereed articles (ie, www.ARAV.org, *Journal of Herpetological Medicine and Surgery*) on the care and keeping of many common species of snakes, lizards, and chelonians.
- Consultations with zookeepers, professional breeders, and other herpetologic veterinarians familiar with the species are very good resources.
- In many species, captive husbandry is not known; a review of the animal's natural history becomes the best source of information, followed by comparing that knowledge with other species' established captive husbandry. Many resources[46] are available for these data, but care must be taken to ensure that correct data are obtained.
- Use of the Internet as a resource for identifying appropriate husbandry must be with caution. Much of the content has not been assessed for accuracy, and thus may be fraught with errors.[47]

A full physical examination must be conducted to assess the overall condition of the patient, keeping in mind that many dermatologic conditions have underlying systemic causes. The skin itself can then be examined to assess its condition.

- Identify lesions and record for size, approximate depth of ulceration or vesicles, degree of erythema, and other superficial vascular changes.
- Determine the distribution pattern and the regional localization of affected areas.
- Evaluate the patient's nails for marks analogous to "stress bars" (a term used in avian species), changes in density, and color of keratin, and even overall shape or form of the keratinized structure itself.
- The chelonian shell and beak should be "picked," scraped, and tested for soundness and evaluated for color, texture, and density (compared with healthy tissue on the same animal).
- Be certain to evaluate the entire animal, rather than only the primary lesions, because subtle lesions or symptoms may be present elsewhere.

Diagnosing the specific condition and ruling in or out differentials requires a thorough and organized diagnostic plan, which may include the following:

- Blood biochemical and hematologic analysis to identify underlying or predisposing conditions, such as hepatic, renal, or other metabolic diseases.
- Bacterial and fungal cultures of vesicular fluid or cytologic analysis of deep skin scrapes after the superficial crusts and debris have been removed.
- Skin and shell biopsies (that include areas of lesion and normal skin) with histopathologic analysis.
- Radiographs have been shown to be very useful in determining the depth and severity of tissue damage in what grossly appear to be mild cases of shell disease (**Figs. 6** and **7**).
- A blood culture is indicated in virtually any reptile dermatitis, because the vesicular fluid is occasionally sterile, or organisms isolated from inside the lesion may

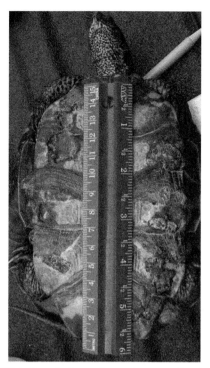

Fig. 6. Ulcerative dermatitis in the plastron of a western pond turtle (*Actinemys marmorata*). (*Courtesy of* T. Schmidt, Lakewood WA.)

be secondary or contaminants, whereas the causative agent can often be identified as a septicemia.[48]

- Electron microscopy, viral culture, and polymerase chain reaction sequencing in conjunction with or in addition to other diagnostics may be necessary to identify specific underlying or concurrent infectious causes.
- Further diagnostics, such as serum vitamin levels, hormone assays, or other specific tests, need to be considered on a case-by-case basis, depending on the specific presentation of the species and the results of the other diagnostic testing performed.

Because husbandry issues are identified (excessive surface moisture, fecal or urate material, malodorolus or ammonia smell to the enclosure, fungal or mold present, inappropriate bedding material) and are correlated to other diagnostic tests, a more thorough diagnosis and treatment plan can be generated (**Fig. 8**).

WOUND HEALING: REPAIR OF DAMAGE TO REPTILIAN SKIN

A discussion addressing the therapeutic management of reptilian VUND needs to begin with a discussion on wound healing. The healing of squamate skin lesions follows four stages[49]:

1. The first stage is that of the initial response to injury, the initiation of inflammatory responses in the injured tissue, and the migration of macrophages and heterophils into the wound. These leukocytes provide a local barrier against pathogens, remove debris and damaged tissue, and may stimulate fibroblast activation.

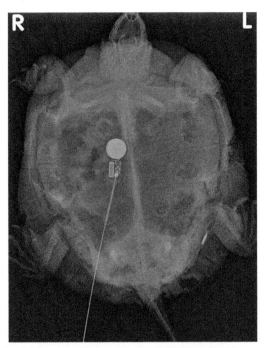

Fig. 7. A radiograph of the same individual as in **Fig. 3**. Note that the areas of bone lysis are much larger and more disseminated than what might be assumed from gross examination.

2. Fibroplasia, the migration and generation of mesodermal cells within the wound, dominates the second stage. This, coupled with angiogenesis and the formation of collagen, provides a structural bridge to the skin defect. To restore the integrity of the damaged skin and subsequently decrease fluid loss and protect against secondary pathogenic invasion, the surface of the defect is filled with fibrin. This repair is a migratory process, starting at the wound margins across the defect with the central and deeper layers (hypodermis) being repaired last.

3. The third stage of squamate wound healing involves the restoration of the epithelial layer, and is shown to be similar to how it occurs in mammals.[50] The epithelial cells migrate from the wound edges across the basement membrane of fibrin and granulation tissue, recently formed by the fibroblastic dermal layer.

4. The last stage of healing is the growth, reorganization, and maturation of the epithelial layer into a skin layer nearly identical to that of tissue adjacent to the damaged area. Ordered stratification and keratinization of the epidermis and a restructuring of the inner-generation layers occur at this point.

All of these stages of healing occur concurrently with normal ecdysis, although they are not reported to be in synchrony with the shed cycle. When the reptile's skin is at its resting phase, the generation of epithelial cells all but stops, with increases in regeneration and repair observed primarily during the renewal phases.[5] Wound regeneration rates mirror that of normal skin; however, differentiation is not complete until the structure and function of the regenerated dermis and epidermis match that of the rest of the surrounding tissue.[51]

Thyroid hormones play a role in the regeneration of squamate skin. The functional form is suspected to be T4, but T3 is also active in reptilian systems and further

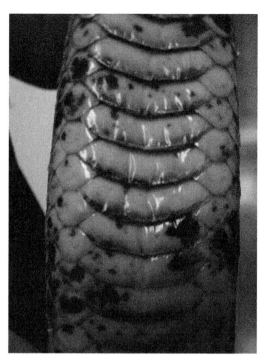

Fig. 8. Common presentation of early stages of vesicular and necrotic dermatitis in a common boa (boa constrictor). Note the raised ventral scales (scutes); edematous appearance to the scutes; and the dark, hemorrhagic caudal margination. Husbandry considered to be substandard. Blood culture for this individual was positive. Blood cultures are commonly positive for *Providencia rettgeri*, *Pseudomonas aeruginosa*, *Morganella morgannii*, *Enterococcus* species, *Clostridium* species, and *Salmonella* species. (*Courtesy of* Adolf K. Maas III, DVM, Bothell, WA.)

studies are needed for a greater understanding. In lizards, it has been found that increased thyroid hormone levels are a stimulator of the skin's regenerative phase and inhibitor of the resting phase, thus increasing ecdysis frequency. In contrast, increased thyroid hormones in the snake promotes the resting phase of ecdysis, whereas decreased serum thyroid hormone levels may bring on the renewal phase.[52–54] Another assessment of the role of thyroid hormones in the ecdysis cycle of *Sepentes* suggests that their epidermal regeneration is accelerated by hyperthyroidism.[55] These countering findings indicate that much more study is needed, but it is agreed that many factors can effect circulating thyroid levels, including systemic health and seasonal variation.[56]

In *Chelonia* and *Crocodylia* regeneration of skin is continuous and although the healing stages are the same as in squamates, there is no reported cyclic activity or any established hormonal control of skin replacement in these animals.

Regeneration of shell and osteoscutes seems to follow a specific pattern. Viable epidermis adjacent to necrotic foci become hyperplastic and the associated dermis becomes thickened and fibrotic. This tissue then undermines the necrotic bone and dermis, regenerating the tissue from deeper layers. This dermal-epidermal combination then extrudes the necrotic bone from the shell. Often seen in chronic cases, the trabecular bone becomes thickened with the structure of the trabecular bone resembling that of the adjacent cortex, likely a hyperplastic effect of the extant pathology.

TREATMENT AND MANAGEMENT OF REPTILE DERMATITIS

Correcting deficiencies in husbandry practices is paramount to a successful treatment plan. If husbandry is inappropriate, the recovery is temporary, at best, and at worst, the patient may not recover.[57] Specifically this should include, at least temporarily, changing the environment to a solid, absorptive, dry substrate, such as paper towels, cloth layers, or unprinted newspaper; frequent (daily or when soiled, whichever is more frequent) bedding changes; adjusting ambient humidity or improving ventilation; and keeping the animal in the higher end of its preferred optimal temperature zone.[58] Continued feeding of a balanced and appropriate diet should be part of therapy because all animals require a good plane of nutrition to maintain systemic and immune system health; some individuals require nutritional support in the form of assisted feeding to maintain caloric intake.

Semiaquatic and aquatic *Chelonia* can present unique challenges in treatment and recovery. "Dry-docking" is a common and useful adjunct therapy, but keep in mind that these species require anywhere from regular (ie, daily) to constant water exposure to maintain proper hydration in a healthy individual, and often have higher fluid demands when shell or skin disease is present. The general treatment-based husbandry requirements must include regular, thorough water changes; high-efficiency filtration and water disinfection; appropriate amounts of time out of water; regular lesion cleaning and debridement; and regular topical lesion antimicrobial therapy.

Specific treatment of VUND involves a systemic treatment plan and a dermal treatment plan. The first element is antimicrobial therapy, based on results of vesicular fluid, or preferably blood, culture and sensitivities. Histopathologic results and the unique physiology, natural history, and general condition of the specific species being treated must be considered before choosing antibiotic or antifungal therapies. For example, antibiotics that concentrate in the kidneys and have a known potential for causing renal damage should not be used in arid-environment species, nor should medications that require hepatic processing be used in patients that have evidence of hepatic disease.[59] If pathologies are identified in other body systems, part of the treatment plan must include addressing and correcting these issues.

Pain management is paramount to successful recovery. Although there are few studies describing symptoms and markers for pain in reptiles, it is easy to conclude that widespread ulcers, exposed tissue, and damaged bone are all sources of moderate to severe pain. Nonsteroidal anti-inflammatory drugs should be considered, ideally with prior assessment of renal and hepatic function. Although there are mixed reports on the efficacy of opiates in reptiles, so long as there are no contraindications they should be considered in the effort to provide pain relief. A review of analgesic therapies is not within the scope of this article, but readers are referred to a 2011 *Veterinary Clinics of North America, Exotic Animal Practice* for more information.[60]

Topical treatment is an important adjunct in wound healing and improving skin hygiene. This therapy should be designed so that it promotes healing and migration of regenerating tissues and includes flushing and removing all debris from the surface of the wounds followed by cleaning with a disinfectant, such as povidone-iodine or chlorhexidine. It should be performed daily to reduce the degree of superficial infection and to remove any crusts or debris that may build up from material in the enclosure or from exudate produced by the wound. Topical medications are often used, but should be chosen with caution because many commonly available topical antimicrobials (eg, polymyxin, neomycin) may inhibit epithelial migration in mammals[61] and may be cytotoxic in reptiles or inhibit wound healing.[62] Chlorhexidine also should be used with caution, because there have been reports of toxicities involving its topical application in chelonians.[63] Again, the choice of a topical medication not only depends on the wound depth and location, but also the specific physiology of the patient being treated.

Wound dressings and coverings have been found to be beneficial in promoting wound healing. Choice of the bandage material used depends on the clinician's preference, lesions location, and extensiveness of the wounds being covered, and the species or behavior patterns of the patient. This covering should prevent further material from adhering to the wound, prevent additional secondary contamination and infection, and promote healing by stopping desiccation of new tissue. Additionally, these bandage products reduce systemic fluid loss until the impermeable epidermal layers have regenerated. Choices include an adhesive bandage product (eg, Tegaderm and Tegaderm Colloid [3M Corporation, St. Paul, MN]); standard gauze bandaging material; a clear plastic drape[64]; or a liquid "bandage" product (eg, NewSkin [Prestige Brands Holdings, Inc, Tarrytown, NY]). This author uses all of these products interchangeably based on the previously mentioned criteria.

When treating shell wounds in chelonians, lesions must be thoroughly debrided of infected tissue. In severe cases better success has been observed when the necrotic tissue is first debulked at the onset of therapy and subsequent debriding performed after healing and tissue regeneration has proceeded. In most cases of aquatic and semiaquatic turtles, open wound management with careful application of "dry-docking" and topical and systemic therapies produce the best outcomes.

In terrestrial chelonian species, covering the wound after debridement seems to be best for good healing and prevention of further wound contamination. Many options exist, including wet-to-dry bandaging, dry bandaging, vacuum-assist closure techniques, and "replaceable cap" methods. Each patient must be evaluated individually for all these options, depending on the scope of the wounds, the ease of appropriate management, and expense. In any case, the wound covering must be kept accessible for continued therapy because it has been found that sealing chelonian wounds often produces conditions that promote worsening of infections rather than recovery. In comparison, current therapies for treatment of shell fractures have found greater success with fewer complications by providing open stabilization of these wounds in contrast to bridging wounds and lesions with a long-term sealing product (ie, acrylic, fiberglass, epoxy).[65] For this reason, the author uses primarily open wound management in aquatic and semiaquatic turtles, and either open wound management or "replaceable cap" management[66] in land turtles and tortoises.

After the inciting causes have been controlled and recovery begins, in squamates it generally takes several shed cycles for the skin to completely regenerate. Although migration of fibroblasts is a slow, continual process in squamates, the restoration of the α and β layers of the skin is discontinuous and coordinates itself to the rest and regeneration cycles of ecdysis. Therefore, in a properly managed case, each shed exhibits more "normal" skin surrounding the gradually contracting lesions. In nonsquamate reptiles, the amount of time to heal is not determined by shed cycles because the regeneration is more continuous in form and more analogous to mammals except that accommodations must be made for the generally lower reptilian metabolism.

Prognosis for these cases is variable and depends on several factors: severity and chronicity of the condition; compliance of the owner, because these cases require long-term management and care; correction of the husbandry to a more optimal state; and identification and appropriate treatment of additional or underlying health issues.

SUMMARY

VUND cases are not simple skin conditions, but are frequently dermatologic manifestations of systemic disease. A proper and thorough work-up is necessary. The rule-outs are varied and include husbandry, environmental, viral, fungal, and bacterial causes, although at the same time it is not uncommon to find that multiple pathologies and underlying problems compound a diagnosis. A complete evaluation of the patient's history is necessary to determine not only the husbandry factors that may be responsible for the presenting condition, but also to determine possible exposure to pathogens. Beyond that, systemic and organized diagnostic testing is essential to understand the presenting lesions and to form an appropriate treatment plan. Tailoring the specific treatment plan for the patient, based on natural history, physiology, and anatomy, is essential so that targeted pathology is treated successfully and iatrogenic diseases do not develop.

VUND cases in reptiles can be very difficult to treat, but rewarding when managed well. As is commonly said, "Reptiles are slow to ill, and slower to heal," and patience is an important adjunct to any well thought out diagnostic and treatment plan.

REFERENCES

1. Maderson PF, Zucker AH, Roth SI. Epidermal regeneration and percutaneous water loss following cellophane stripping of reptile epidermis. J Exp Zool 1978;204:11–32.
2. Hargis AM. Integumentary system. In: Carlton WW, McGavin MD, editors. Thompson's special veterinary pathology. 2nd edition. St. Louis (MO): Mosby-Year Book; 1995. p. 461–511.
3. Yager JA, Wilcock BP. Color atlas and text of surgical pathology of the dog and cat: dermatopathology and skin tumors. London: Mosby-Year Book; 1994. p. 407–10.
4. Cooper JE. Dermatology. In: Mader DR, editor. Reptile medicine and surgery. 2nd edition. St. Louis (MO): Saunders Elsevier; 2006. p. 196–216.
5. Jacobson ER. Overview of reptile biology, anatomy, and histology. In: Jacobson ER, editor. Infectious diseases and pathology of reptiles: color atlas and text. Boca Raton (FL): CRC Press; 2007. p. 1–130.
6. Vitt LJ, Caldwell JP. Herpetology: an introductory biology of amphibians and reptiles. 3rd edition. Burlington (MA): Elsevier; 2009. p. 35–81.
7. Zangerl R. The turtle shell. In: Gans C, Bellairs A, Parsons TS, editors. Biology of the reptilia, Morphology A, vol. I. New York: Academic Press, Inc; 1969. p. 311–39.
8. Landmann L. Epidermis and dermis. In: Bereiter-Hahn J, Matoltsy AG, Richards S, editors. Biology of the integument, vol. 2. Springer-Verlag; 1986. p. 150–87.
9. Mader D. Treating burns in reptiles. Medford (MA): Tufts Animal Expo; 2002.
10. Fraser MA, Girling SJ. Dermatology. In: Girling SA, Raiti P, editors. BSAVA manual of reptiles. 2nd edition. Gloucester (England): British Small Animal Veterinary Association; 2004. p. 188.
11. Han J, Mo I, Na K. Pemphigus-like immune-mediated dermatosis in a Korean native black bone fowl. Avian Dis 2008;32:714–7.
12. Finnegan M, Munson L, Barrett S, et al. Vesicular skin disease of tapirs [poster]. Proceed Ann Conf AAZV 1993.
13. Rossi JV. Biology and husbandry. In: Mader DR, editor. Reptile medicine and surgery. 2nd edition. St. Louis (MO): Saunders Elsevier; 2006. p. 25–41.
14. Broderson JR, Lindsey JR, Crawford JE. The role of environmental ammonia in respiratory mycoplasmosis of rats. Am J Pathol 1976;85(1):115.

15. DeNardo DF. Reptile thermal biology: a veterinary perspective. Proceed Ann Conf ARAV 2002;157–63.
16. Flint M, Limpus DJ, Limpus CJ, et al. Biochemical and hematological reference intervals for Krefft's turtles *Emydura macquarii krefftii* from the Burnett River Catchment, Australia. Dis Aquat Organ 2011;95(1):43.
17. Harkewicz KA. Dermatology of reptiles: a clinical approach to diagnosis and treatment. Vet Clin North Am Exot Anim Pract 2001;4(2):441–62.
18. Turek MM. Cutaneous paraneoplastic syndromes in dogs and cats: a review of the literature. Vet Dermatol 2003;14(6):279–96.
19. Jacobson ER. Viruses and viral diseases of reptiles. In: Jacobson ER, editor. Infectious diseases and pathology of reptiles: color atlas and text. Boca Raton (FL): CRC Press; 2007. p. 395–460.
20. Marschang R. Viruses infecting reptiles. Viruses 2011;3:2087–126.
21. Stenglein MD, Sanders C, Kistler AL, et al. Identification, characterization, and in vitro culture of highly divergent arenaviruses from boa constrictors and annulated tree boas: candidate etiological agents for snake inclusion body disease. MBio 2012;3(5):e00180, 12.
22. Nevarez JG. Lymphohistiocytic proliferative syndrome of alligators (*Alligator mississippiensis*): a cutaneous manifestation of West Nile virus [PhD Thesis dissertation]. Baton Rouge (LA): Louisiana State University, Veterinary Clinical Sciences; 2007.
23. Gartrell BD, Hare KM. Mycotic dermatitis with digital gangrene and osteomyelitis, and protozoal intestinal parasitism in Marlborough green geckos (*Naultinus manukanus*). N Z Vet J 2005;53(5):363–7.
24. Pare JA, Sigler L, Rypien KL, et al. Survey for the *Chrysosporium* anomorph of *Nannizziopsis vriesii* on the skin of healthy captive squamate reptiles and notes on their cutaneous fungal mycobiota. J Herp Med Surg 2003;13(4): 10–5.
25. Jacobson ER. Nectrotizing mycotic dermatitis in snakes: clinical and pathologic features. J Am Vet Med Assoc 1980;177(9):838–41.
26. Toplon DE, Terrell SP, Sigler L, et al. Dermatitis and cellulitis in Leopard Geckos (*Eublepharis macularius*) caused by the chrysosporium anamorph of nannizziopsis vriesii. Vet Pathol 2013;50(4):585–9.
27. Pare JA, Coyle KA, Sigler L, et al. Pathogenicity of the *Chrysosporium* anamorph of *Nannizziopsis vriesii* for veiled chameleons (*Chamaeleo calyptratus*). Med Mycol 2006;44(1):25–31.
28. Hellebuyck T, Baert K, Pasmans F, et al. Cutaneous hyalohyphomycosis in a girdled lizard (*Cordylus giganteus*) caused by the *Chrysosporium* anamorph of *Nannizziopsis vriesii* and successful treatment with voriconazole. Vet Dermatol 2010;21(4):429–33.
29. Bertelsen MF, Crawshaw GJ, Sigler L, et al. Fatal cutaneous mycosis in tentacled snakes (*Erpeton tentaculatum*) caused by the *Chrysosporium* anamorph of *Nannizziopsis vriesii*. J Zoo Wildl Med 2005;36(1):82–7.
30. Han J, Lee S, Na K. Necrotizing dermatomycosis caused by *Chrysosporium* spp. in three captive green iguanas (*Iguana iguana*) in South Korea. J Ex Pet Med 2010;19(3):240–4.
31. Goodman G. Dermatology of reptiles. In: Paterson S, editor. Skin diseases of exotic pets. Ames (IA): Blackwell Publishing; 2006. p. 89–102.
32. Mihalca AD, Fictum P, Skoric M, et al. Severe granulomatous lesions in several organs from *Eustrongylides* larvae in a free-ranging dice snake, *Natrix tessellata*. Vet Pathol 2007;44(1):103–5.

33. Foreyt WJ, Leathers CW, Whaley S, et al. Surgical removal of pleurocercoids from snakes and subsequent diagnosis of experimentally introduced adult tapeworms in coyotes. Vet Med Small Anim Clin 10:1593–96.

34. Jacobson ER, Greiner EC, Clubb S, et al. Pustular dermatitis caused by subcutaneous dracunculensis in snakes. J Am Vet Med Assoc 1986;189(9):1133–4.

35. Ebani VV, Fratani F. Bacterial zoonoses among domestic reptiles. Annali Med Vet 2005;84:85–91.

36. Raiti P. Acute vesicular dermatitis in a red footed tortoise (*Chelonoidis carbonaria*). Proceed Ann Conf ARAV 2010;62–4.

37. Branch S, Hall L, Blackshear P, et al. Infectious dermatitis in a ball python (*Python regius*) colony. J Zoo Wildl Med 1998;29(4):461–4.

38. Jacobson ER. Bacterial diseases of reptiles. In: Jacobson ER, editor. Infectious diseases and pathology of reptiles: color atlas and text. Boca Raton (FL): CRC Press; 2007. p. 461–526.

39. Wallach JD. The pathogenesis and etiology of ulcerative shell disease in turtles. J Zoo An Med 1975;6:11–3.

40. Wallach JD. The pathogenesis and etiology of ulcerative shell disease in turtles. Aq Mamm 1976;4:1–4.

41. Johnson VM, Guyer C, Shawkey MD, et al. Abundance, identification and prospective participation of bacteria on gopher tortoise shell degredation. J Ala Acad Sci 2008;79(3–4):190–1999.

42. Jacobson ER, Wronski TJ, Schumacher J, et al. Cutaneous dyskeratosis in free-ranging desert tortoises, *Gopherus agassizii*, in the Colorado Desert of southern California. J Zoo Wildl Med 1994;25:68–81.

43. Homer BL, Berry KH, Brown MB, et al. Pathology of diseases in wild desert tortoises from California. J Wildl Dis 1998;34(3):508.

44. Ladyman JM, Kuchling G, Burford D, et al. Skin disease affecting the conservation of the western swamp tortoise (*Pseudemydura umbrina*). Aust Vet J 1998; 76(11):743–5.

45. Garner MM, Herrington R, Howerth EW, et al. Shell disease in river cooters (*Pseudemys concinna*) and yellow-bellied cooters (*Trachemys scripta*) in a Georgia (USA) Lake. J Wildl Dis 1997;33(1):78–86.

46. Obst FJ, Richter K, Jacob U. The completely illustrated atlas of reptiles and amphibians for the terrarium. Neptune City (NJ): TFH Publications; 1988.

47. Available at: www.anapsid.org, www.animalarkshelter.org/cin, www.arav.org, www.devenomized.com. Accessed December, 2012.

48. Chinnadurai SK, DeVoe RS. Selected infectious diseases of reptiles. Vet Clin North Am Exot Anim Pract 2009;12(3):583–96.

49. Smith DA, Barker IK. Healing of cutaneous wounds in the common garter snake (*Thamnophis sirtalis*). Can J Vet Res 1988;52:111–9.

50. Smith DA, Barker IK. The effect of ambient temperature and type of wound in healing of cutaneous wounds in the common garter snake (*Thamnophis sirtalis*). Can J Vet Res 1988;52:120–8.

51. Maderson PF, Baranowitz S, Roth SI. A histological study of the long-term response to trauma of squamate integument. J Morphol 1978;157(2): 121–35.

52. Chiu KW, Lynn WG. The role of the thyroid in skin-shedding in the shovel-nosed snake, *Chionactis occipitalis*. Gen Comp Endocrinol 1970;14:467–74.

53. Chiu KW, Leung MS, Maderson PF. Thyroid and skin-shedding in the rat snake (*Ptyas korros*). J Exp Zool 1983;225:407–10.

54. Chiu KW, Lam KY. Plasma T3 and T4 levels in a snake, *Elaphe taeniura*. Comp Biochem Physiol 1994;107A(1):107–12.
55. Rivera S, Lock B. The reptilian thyroid and parathyroid glands. Vet Clin North Am Exot Anim Pract 2008;11(1):163–75.
56. El-Deib S. Serum catecholamime and hormonal titers in the hibernating snake *Naje haje haje*, with reference to the annual climatic cycle. J Therm Biol 2005; 30:580–7.
57. Hoppmann E, Barron HW. Dermatology in reptiles. J Ex Pet Med 2007;16(4): 210–24.
58. Burns G, Ramos A, Muchlinski A. Fever response in North American snakes. J Herp 1996;30:133–9.
59. Mader DR. Antibiotic therapy in reptiles. Proceedings Central Veterinary Conference, Kansas City, 2008.
60. Mosley C. Pain and nociception in reptiles. Vet Clin North Am Exot Anim Pract 2011;14(1):45.
61. Geronemus RG, Mertz PM, Eaglstein WH. Wound healing: the effects of topical antimicrobial agents. Arch Dermatol 1979;115(11):1311.
62. Smith DA, Barker IK, Allen OB. The effect of certain topical medications on healing of cutaneous wounds in the common garter snake (*Thamnophis sirtalis*). Can J Vet Res 1988;52(1):129.
63. Lloyd ML. Chlorhexidine toxicosis in a part of red-bellied short-necked turtles (*Emudura subglosa*). Bull Rep Amph Vet 1996;6(4):6–7.
64. Cooper JE. Use of a surgical adhesive drape in reptiles. Vet Rec 1981;108:56.
65. Fleming GJ. Clinical technique: chelonian shell repair. J of Ex Pet Med 2008; 17(4):246–58.
66. Maas A. Replaceable cap technique in treatment of chelonian shell disease. In progress.

Ovarian Cysts in the Guinea Pig (*Cavia porcellus*)

Andrew D. Bean, DVM

KEYWORDS

- Ovarian cyst • Ovary • Rete ovarii • Guinea pig • Rodent • Leuprolide • Deslorelin
- Ovariohysterectomy

KEY POINTS

- Most guinea pig sows develop ovarian cysts.
- Ovarian cysts in guinea pigs are frequently, but not always, derived from the rete ovarii. Other possible sources of ovarian cysts are periovarian structures; persistent, unluteinized tertiary follicles; neoplasia; and infection.
- Many clinical signs classically associated with ovarian cysts (including bilateral, nonpruritic alopecia of the flanks) are likely the result of excess sex steroid production by follicular cysts. Rete cysts are not thought to be steroidogenic.
- The most sensitive diagnostic test is abdominal ultrasonography, whereas the most specific is histopathologic analysis of the cysts. Hematology, serum biochemistry, serum hormone levels, radiography, and fluid cytology are neither sensitive nor specific.
- Ovariohysterectomy is the definitive treatment of all ovarian cysts. Ovariectomy without hysterectomy is not recommended, because ovarian cysts have been associated with several uterine diseases.
- Alternative therapies include hormone injections and percutaneous cyst drainage. Treatment with hormone injections may cause resolution of follicular cysts, but is not likely to affect other types of cysts. Cysts often refill with fluid shortly after drainage.

INTRODUCTION

Ovarian cysts are known to develop in many species, including mice, cats, sheep, cows, monkeys, and humans.[1–5] The condition has been reported in guinea pigs (*Cavia porcellus*) since at least the early twentieth century and may be known as ovarian cysts, cystic ovaries, or cystic ovarian disease.[6] In modern exotic companion mammal practice, it is common knowledge that ovarian cysts are a cause of bilateral, nonpruritic alopecia of the flanks in guinea pig sows. Cysts may be derived from

Funding Sources: None.
Conflict of Interest: None.
Pet Care Veterinary Hospital, 5201 Virginia Beach Boulevard, Virginia Beach, VA 23462, USA
E-mail address: adbean@gmail.com

Vet Clin Exot Anim 16 (2013) 757–776
http://dx.doi.org/10.1016/j.cvex.2013.05.008
1094-9194/13/$ – see front matter © 2013 Elsevier Inc. All rights reserved.

vetexotic.theclinics.com

several possible structures, and this origin may profoundly influence treatment recommendations. Ovarian cysts are mentioned in most veterinary texts that cover guinea pigs, but the subject is not usually discussed in depth. This article provides a thorough review of ovarian cysts in the guinea pig.

ANATOMY AND PHYSIOLOGY
Classification

Ovarian cysts are classified by their location of origin in relation to the ovary: periovarian (also called paraovarian or parovarian) or intraovarian.[7] They may also be categorized according to cause: physiologic, infectious, and neoplastic.[8] Most ovarian cysts in guinea pigs are physiologic and intraovarian, derived from the rete ovarii or ovarian follicles.

Rete Ovarii: Anatomy

The rete ovarii is a network of tubules and cords that arises from the mesonephros. It is homologous with the rete testis of male mammals. It is lined by variably ciliated cuboidal to columnar epithelial cells and rests on a basement membrane. The rete ovarii is a normal structure in adult female mammals, with substantial morphologic differences between species.[9,10] Tubules begin in the periovarian tissue, enter the ovary at the hilus, and spread to varying degrees throughout the ovary. The rete ovarii is divided into 3 sections[9,11]:

- Extraovarian rete (ER): the portion in the periovarian tissue; also known as the transverse ductules of the epoöphoron
- Intraovarian rete (IR): the portion within the ovary; also known as the primary sex cords, medullary cords, or ovigerous cords
- Connecting rete (CR): the segments connecting the IR and ER

The ER is generally regarded as a blind-ended structure, although evidence exists in some species for a small communication (ie, the tuboretial connection) with the infundibulum of the fallopian tube.[12] The ER begins as a single wide tubule, branching and becoming more convoluted as it approaches the ovary. Many of the branches of the ER end blindly, but some segments join adjacent to the ovary.[11]

The adjoined ER branches become the compact cell cords of the CR, and are associated with the smooth muscles in the ovarian ligament. The cords pass through the ovarian hilus and into the medulla to become the IR.[13,14]

The extensiveness of the IR depends on the age and species of the individual; in some it may be absent, whereas in others it may branch heavily and even communicate with the ovarian cortex.[9,10,15] The cavian (ie, guinea pig) IR is most developed before birth (at approximately 49 days' gestation), and is largely situated in the hilus and medulla.[16,17] Most of the medullary IR has degenerated by parturition, with only the hilar portion remaining.[16] In contrast, the murine (ie, mouse) IR is extensive, branching throughout the ovarian medulla and into the cortex (**Fig. 1**).[9,18,19]

Rete Ovarii: Physiology

The function of the rete ovarii has not been clearly defined. In adults it is generally regarded as a nonfunctional embryonic remnant.[20] As such, it is not covered by some anatomy/reproductive biology texts.[21,22] The rete ovarii may have a role in folliculogenesis in some species.[9] Serial examinations of neonatal mouse ovaries reveal an extensive IR that extends into the cortex and contains many oocytes (see **Fig. 1**). Over the course of the first 2 weeks of life, murine granulosa cells

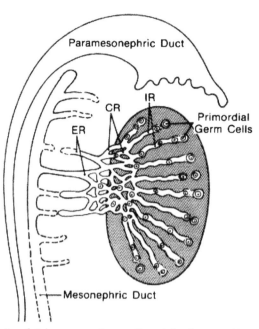

Fig. 1. The developing fetal mouse rete ovarii and its degenerating connection to the mesonephric duct. The IR of the guinea pig is less extensive, existing in the medulla only at its developmental peak. (*From* Wenzel JG, Odend'hal S. The mammalian rete ovarii: a literature review. Cornell Vet 1985;75:415.)

differentiate from the rete cells and surround the oocytes, eventually forming follicles.[19] Experimental grafts of mouse ovaries lacking intact rete ovarii were less likely to develop follicles than those with intact rete ovarii.[23,24] Granulosa cell differentiation from the IR has also been shown in several other species, including macaques, rats, and marmosets.[9] Studies of folliculogenesis in the guinea pig have not shown a role for the rete ovarii; instead, the ovarian surface epithelium is implicated as the catalyst for follicle development.[16,17,25] A recent genetic study of the function of the rete ovarii in sheep did not favor a role in folliculogenesis, but neither did it rule one out.[26]

Whether the cells of the rete ovarii have a secretory function may also be species dependent. There is evidence suggesting that the rete ovarii in mice secretes a meiosis-inducing substance during gonadal development. When fetal mouse ovaries with intact ER were cultured alongside fetal mouse testes that had yet to undergo testicular cord development, testicular germ cells were induced to enter meiosis. Germ cells in testes cultured alone did not enter meiosis.[27] Another study showed induction of germ cell meiosis in fetal hamster ovaries cultured in the presence of ER excised from neonatal hamster ovaries. Germ cells from fetal hamster ovaries cultured alone did not enter meiosis.[28] Histologic studies of the rete ovarii in heifers showed both secretory material and cell debris at various times within the lumina of the rete tubules.[29] Secretions have also been noted in the canine rete ovarii.[30] A report examining the rete ovarii in prenatal and neonatal guinea pigs and rabbits makes no mention of rete cell secretions.[16] Light and electron microscopic studies of rete cysts in Hartley guinea pigs failed to discern the presence of secretory granules within cells lining the cysts.[18,31]

Ovarian Follicles: Anatomy and Physiology

Ovarian follicles consist of an oocyte surrounded by varying types of cells (depending on the stage of development). In most species the follicles reside in the ovarian cortex. Follicles progress through 4 developmental stages[26,32,33]:

- Primordial: an oocyte surrounded by a single layer of simple squamous epithelial cells. Primordial follicles remain in a quiescent state until recruited to develop into primary follicles, or signaled to undergo atresia.
- Primary: an oocyte surrounded by a single layer of cuboidal granulosa cells. Primary follicles remain arrested in prophase I until stimulated to develop by gonadotropins.
- Secondary: an oocyte surrounded by multiple layers of stratified granulosa cells on a basement membrane. Exterior to the basement membrane are theca cells. Interior to the granulosa layer is a glycoprotein coat, the zona pellucida, surrounding the oocyte. Continued development into a tertiary follicle depends on follicle-stimulating hormone secretions from the pituitary gland.
- Tertiary: an oocyte surrounded by the zona pellucida and granulosa cells, located within a fluid known as the antrum. The theca cells have differentiated into theca interna and theca externa layers and have become functional, producing androgens that are converted into estrogens by the granulosa cells. A tertiary follicle that is ready to ovulate is known as a Graafian follicle.

A Graafian follicle is induced to ovulate by a surge of luteinizing hormone (LH) released from the pituitary gland. The oocyte is released and the follicle becomes the corpus luteum. The associated granulosa and theca interna cells differentiate into luteal cells, which produce progesterone for a period of time dependent on whether the animal is pregnant.[32,33]

EPIDEMIOLOGY

Cyst prevalence and influencing factors in guinea pigs are variably reported. None of the cyst varieties discussed is exclusive of the others. A patient presenting for ovarian cysts may possess multiple types of cysts.

Rete Cysts: Prevalence

Cysts originating from the rete ovarii seem to be common in guinea pig sows, regardless of age. Two separate studies of inbred Abyssinian-Hartley cross sows (n = 83 and 71) found rete cysts in ~76% of individuals.[34,35] A survey of 43 pet guinea pigs representing multiple breeds in Denmark reported a rete cyst prevalence of 58%.[36] A study of Hartley strain sows aged 10 weeks to 2 years showed rete cysts in 100% of individuals (n = 12).[18] In another study, necropsies performed on 33 Dunkin-Hartley sows that were 18 months old found an ovarian cyst prevalence of 94%.[37] Some of the variability in cyst prevalence can be attributed to differences in populations examined (inbred laboratory strains vs mixed breed pets), sample size, and diagnostic tests (abdominal ultrasound vs gross necropsy accompanied by histopathology and/or electron microscopy).

Rete Cysts: Influence of Age, Parity, and Duration of Estrus

There seems to be a positive association between animal age, and rete cyst prevalence and size. Neither parity nor duration of estrus has been shown to influence cyst development.[35] The aforementioned Danish survey of pet guinea pigs found that 93% of the subjects more than 2 years of age (n = 14) had at least 1 ovarian cyst, and there were significant positive associations between age and both cyst presence (*P*<.02) and cyst diameter (*P*<.01).[35] Comparison of mean cyst diameter in Abyssinian-Hartley sows showed a direct relationship with age: cysts were not grossly measurable (ie, microscopic) in 1.5-year-old individuals, and steadily increased to 3.58 cm in diameter in 4.5-year-old sows.[35] Another survey of Hartley sows ranging in age from 10 weeks to 2 years (n = 12) found the largest cysts in sows more than 1 year of age.[18] Young and colleagues[38] failed to find an association between cyst prevalence and duration of estrus when the latter was determined subjectively by observation of individuals' behavior.

Follicular Cysts

Follicular cysts are less commonly reported in guinea pigs, and reports on prevalence vary widely. One researcher noted that, "In studying a great many [guinea pig] ovaries for cystic conditions during several years we have never observed a follicular cyst."[39] A study of 85 Hartley sows showed a follicular cyst prevalence of 22.4% when cyst diameter was greater than 0.5 mm. Follicular cysts were most commonly seen during the first half of the estrous cycle.[40] Beregi and colleagues[41] ultrasonographically verified the presence of ovarian cysts in 10 guinea pigs; histopathology later identified 100% of these cysts as follicular. The true prevalence of follicular cysts in guinea pigs remains unknown.

Neoplastic Cysts

Ovarian neoplasia with cystic characteristics may be encountered, but it is rarely reported in the literature. A granulosa cell tumor with a 7-mm cystic area has been described in a 4-year-old American satin sow.[42] Papillary cystadenocarcinoma has been reported in 2 Dunkin-Hartley sows aged 18 months.[37] Ovarian teratomas with multifocal small cystic areas have been reported in 2 sows aged 9 weeks and 1 year (breed was not specified).[43] Ovarian teratomas were reported without mention of cystic components in an approximately 2.5-year-old sow, and an adult sow of unspecified age.[34,35] The prevalence of ovarian teratomas in guinea pigs remains unknown, but they are considered by some to be the species' most common ovarian neoplasm.[44]

Concurrent Diseases

Evidence suggests that numerous uterine diseases are associated with ovarian cysts in guinea pigs. Uterine leiomyoma, mucometra, cystic endometrial hyperplasia, and endometriosis have all been reported in sows with ovarian cysts.[34,35,45] Whether there is a causal relationship between these conditions and ovarian cysts is unknown. Given the high prevalence of ovarian cysts in sows of all ages, it is possible that the association between cyst presence and the aforementioned uterine diseases is coincidental.

PATHOGENESIS
Rete Cysts

The pathogenesis of rete cysts remains controversial, and several possible explanations have been proposed.

Proliferation of rete cyst epithelium has been considered as a cause or accelerator of cyst development.[18] Microscopic surveys of rete cysts in guinea pigs have not consistently shown mitotic figures, so epithelial proliferation is unlikely to play a role in rete cyst formation.[18,40]

In light of evidence that the rete ovarii has a secretory capacity in various species (eg, cat, mink, cow), some have postulated that cysts result from an accumulation of secretions within the lumina of the rete tubules. Secretions would accrue over time in the blind-ended tubules, causing progressive expansion and dilation of the rete system.[4,15,29,30] Although rete epithelial secretions have been noted in other species, none have been shown in the guinea pig.[18,31,46]

Some have speculated that phytoestrogens in pelleted guinea pig feed may contribute to rete cyst formation.[45,47] Phytoestrogens are compounds naturally present in plants (particularly legumes) that bind to estrogen receptors to induce potentially significant effects.[48] Three phytoestrogens (coumestrol, genistein, and daidzein) have been found in research animal diets from a variety of manufacturers.[49,50] The major sources of these compounds are often soybean meal and alfalfa.[49,51] In the past, the primary concern with phytoestrogen content of feed has been whether they influence results in biomedical research settings.[52] A thorough review of the effects of phytoestrogens on rodent health and development is beyond the scope of this article. No investigations of associations between diet and ovarian cysts in guinea pigs have been undertaken.

Permeability of the rete epithelium may influence cyst development. Ultrastructural analysis of guinea pig rete cyst epithelium reveals almost a complete absence of tight junctions, the component of junctional complexes responsible for maintaining the paracellular pathway barrier.[31,53] Permeability studies have shown that these intercellular junctions are permeable to the tracers lanthanum and horseradish peroxidase. No significant intracellular presence of either tracer was noted, and there was no significant difference in permeability of rete tubules in female pups (juveniles) compared with rete cysts of mature sows.[46,54] No further research into these potential associations have been performed in guinea pigs.

The presence of an ion-dependent pump system has been proposed as a cause of rete cysts. The basis for this theory is the presence of numerous caveolae (small invaginations in the plasma membrane) on the cyst epithelium, which resemble the calcium ion pumps present in smooth muscle. No studies into this possible link have been conducted.[54]

Follicular Cysts

The pathogenesis of ovarian follicular cysts has not been definitively described. Although not well studied in the guinea pig, follicular cysts have been extensively researched in cows, because their presence may cause prolonged calving intervals.[40,41,55]

The current consensus is that the cause of bovine follicular cyst development is multifactorial, manifesting as a dysfunction of the hypothalamic-pituitary-ovarian axis in which the LH surge is either premature, absent, or insufficient to cause follicular luteinization.[55] The mature follicle continues to grow and produce steroids, including estradiol, testosterone, and progesterone.[56] The cyst may eventually become nonsteroidogenic, allowing the normal ovulatory cycle to resume. Genetic background, stress, and negative energy balance have all been implicated as predisposing factors for development of follicular cysts.[55] It is possible that similar mechanisms are involved in the formation of follicular cysts in guinea pigs.

Follicular cysts have been experimentally induced in guinea pigs through implantation of estradiol-secreting capsules, as well as immunization against inhibin.[57,58] Because the mechanism(s) of natural follicular cyst formation in the guinea pig are unknown, these experimental induction methods may or may not be relevant.

DIAGNOSIS

Diagnosis of ovarian cysts is usually made using a combination of patient history, physical examination findings, and imaging. Hematology, serum biochemistry, hormone assays, and cytology may or may not be useful. Definitive diagnosis requires histopathologic evaluation of the cysts.

History and Physical Examination

Clinical signs in sows with ovarian cysts vary widely, and depend on the nature, size, and distribution of the cysts. Rete cysts in guinea pigs are not thought to be steroidogenic, whereas follicular cysts may actively produce steroids.[59] This difference may profoundly influence the history and clinical signs (**Table 1**). Historical findings associated with cystic ovaries are as follows[42,60,61]:

- Behavioral changes: depressed attitude or increased aggression
- Gradual increase in abdominal distension as a result of growing cysts
- Decreased appetite
- Weight gain
- Decreased fertility
- Acute collapse (secondary to blood loss from hemorrhagic ovarian neoplasia)
- Decreased defecation

Increased sexual activity has not been shown to be significantly associated with the presence of ovarian cysts in general.[38,62] It is unknown whether such behavior is more common in sows with steroidogenic cysts.

Physical examination findings in sows with cystic ovaries may include any of the following[42,60,63]:

- Abdominal distention (**Fig. 2**)
- Clitoral hypertrophy
- Depression
- Hyperkeratosis and/or hyperpigmentation of the nipples
- Nonpruritic truncal and/or inguinal alopecia (**Figs. 3–5**)
- Pain
- Rounded, fluctuant mass or masses identified on abdominal palpation

Table 1
Comparison of historical findings and clinical signs associated with rete cysts versus follicular cysts

Historical Finding/Clinical Sign	Rete Cyst	Follicular Cyst
Abdominal distention	+	+
Clitoral hypertrophy	−	+
Decreased appetite	+	+
Decreased defecation	+	+
Decreased fertility	+	+
Depression	+	+
Increased aggression	−	+
Nipple hyperkeratosis	−	+
Pain	+	+
Round, intra-abdominal mass	+	+
Tachypnea	+	+
Truncal or inguinal nonpruritic alopecia	−	+
Vaginal bleeding	−	+
Weight gain	+	+

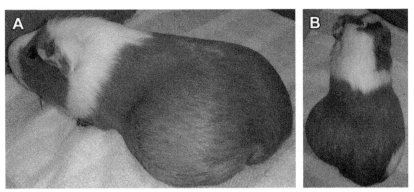

Fig. 2. (*A, B*) Guinea pig sow with abdominal distention secondary to ovarian cysts. (*Courtesy of* Dan H. Johnson, DVM, Dipl ABVP-ECM.)

- Tachypnea
- Vaginal bleeding

The most common guinea pig dermatosis associated with ovarian cysts is nonpruritic alopecia of the lumbosacral, bilateral flank, inguinal, and/or perineal areas.[47,64,65] The hair loss may be progressive or static. It is presumed to result from the catabolic effect of increased levels of estrogen produced by steroidogenic follicular or neoplastic ovarian cysts.[66] The prevalence of nonpruritic alopecia among sows with

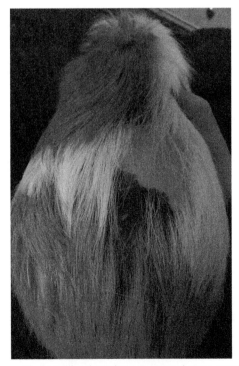

Fig. 3. Guinea pig sow with dorsal lumbar alopecia secondary to ovarian cysts. (*Courtesy of* Peter G. Fisher, DVM, Dipl ABVP-ECM, Virginia Beach, VA.)

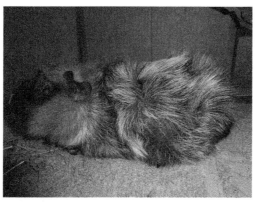

Fig. 4. Guinea pig sow with left flank alopecia (*arrow*) secondary to ovarian cysts. (*Courtesy of* Peter G. Fisher, DVM, Dipl ABVP-ECM, Virginia Beach, VA.)

ovarian cysts is unknown. A study of 10 pet sows with ovarian cysts reported that 60% displayed nonpruritic alopecia.[64] A larger study of 43 pet sows found the prevalence of nonpruritic alopecia to be only 4.7%.[36]

Enlarged, hyperpigmented, and/or hyperkeratotic nipples have also been anecdotally associated with ovarian cysts. Seborrhea and hyperpigmentation of the nonmammary skin are rarely reported. Infectious dermatopathies (eg, dermatophytosis, pyoderma, ectoparasites) and their associated clinical signs may be present concurrently (**Fig. 6**).

Besides ovarian cysts, differential diagnoses for nonpruritic truncal or inguinal alopecia in guinea pigs include the following conditions[47,63,67]:

- Barbering
- Dermatophytosis
- Hereditary predisposition
- Hyperadrenocorticism
- Hyperthyroidism
- Hypovitaminosis C
- Lactation (early)
- Pregnancy (late)
- Stress

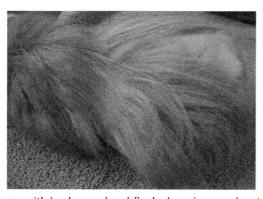

Fig. 5. Guinea pig sow with lumbosacral and flank alopecia secondary to ovarian cysts.

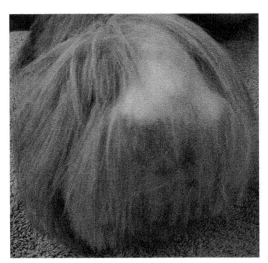

Fig. 6. The same guinea pig sow as shown in **Fig. 5**; a circular area of crusting and erythema is seen on the rump, suggesting concurrent dermatitis.

Hematology, Serum Biochemistry, and Hormone Assays

Evaluation of a complete blood count may be unremarkable, although an increase of Kurloff bodies in lymphocytes may be seen in sows with steroidogenic cysts as a result of increased estrogen levels. Serum biochemical analysis is usually unremarkable.[63] Measurement of endogenous hormone concentrations is not reliable for diagnosis, because the cysts may or may not be steroidogenic.[44] Even if the cyst fluid contains high levels of hormones, serum estrogen and progesterone concentrations may be normal.[42,56] In cows, high levels of serum progesterone are associated with luteinized cysts, and high levels of serum estradiol are associated with follicular cysts.[55] Studies linking hormone levels to ovarian cysts have not been performed in guinea pigs.

Imaging

Imaging is a key component of diagnosis. Abdominal radiography may help to localize clinical signs, but its specificity for detecting ovarian cysts is low: the radiopacity of the cysts is similar to that of trichobezoars and soft tissue abdominal masses. Abdominal ultrasonography is the imaging modality of choice. A 6–12 MHz frequency transducer is recommended. The patient's ventral abdomen should be shaved, and ultrasound gel applied.[64] Ultrasonographic visualization of the ovaries may be impeded by gas in the gastrointestinal tract, especially in patients presented in gastrointestinal stasis, in which severe gas dilatations of the stomach and cecum are common.

Cysts are contiguous with the ovaries and may be visualized dorsal to the kidney. They feature a thin wall containing a variable amount of fluid (**Fig. 7**). Echogenicity of cyst fluid is reported as anechoic, although fluid contained in bovine luteinized cysts has been described as having echogenic spots and weblike structures.[36,55,64,68] Cysts are often multilocular (**Fig. 8**), although unilocular cysts have also been described in guinea pigs.[18,35,54] Neoplastic cysts are likely to be associated with solid masses of varying echogenicity (**Fig. 9**).[42]

Cytology

Fine needle aspiration (FNA) and cytologic analysis of cyst contents may be used to rule out an infectious or neoplastic cause. Samples may be acquired with

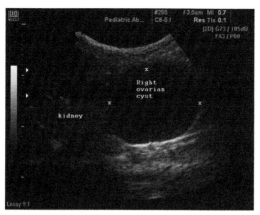

Fig. 7. Ultrasonographic image of a unilocular ovarian cyst in a guinea pig sow. (*Courtesy of* Peter G. Fisher, DVM, Dipl ABVP-ECM, Virginia Beach, VA.)

ultrasonographic guidance, or blindly by stabilizing the cyst against the lateral body wall between the thumb and index finger. The site of needle insertion should be clipped and scrubbed, and aseptic technique should be used.[63] Ultrasonographic evaluation for neoplasia is recommended before FNA.

The cytologic characteristics of rete cyst fluid have been described as serous to proteinaceous with few to no cells present.[69] Fluid from neoplastic cysts may yield neoplastic cells.[42] To the author's knowledge, ovarian abscessation has not been reported in the guinea pig, but aspirates thereof are likely to yield large numbers of degenerate heterophils, with or without infectious agents.

Complications associated with FNA may vary with the type of cyst. Several investigators caution that FNA may cause cyst rupture and/or peritonitis.[47,69] No such occurrences have been reported in the literature. Aspiration of neoplastic cysts carries risks of hemorrhage and tumor cell seeding along the needle tract.

Notes on Sedation

Sedation may be necessary for acquisition of diagnostic images, blood collection, or cyst aspiration. Guinea pigs are easily stressed, and often actively resist restraint. Use

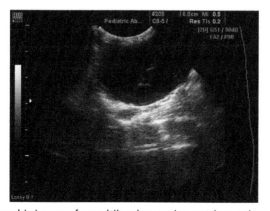

Fig. 8. Ultrasonographic image of a multilocular ovarian cyst in a guinea pig sow.

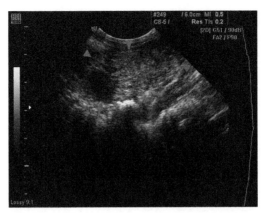

Fig. 9. Ultrasonographic image of an ovarian neoplasm (*arrowheads*) containing cystic areas (*arrow*).

of sedation often ensures a faster, safer procedure that is more likely to yield diagnostically useful results. Midazolam, butorphanol, and ketamine are commonly used in guinea pigs to provide chemical restraint for short procedures. The reader is referred to other works for a detailed discussion of sedation in guinea pigs.[70–72]

Gross Pathology

Rete cysts
Rete cysts are usually centered near the hilus on the cephalic pole of the ovary.[73] Cyst size varies, from microscopic in pups to as large as 7 cm in geriatric sows.[18,35,74] They are commonly present on both ovaries, but when unilateral they are more commonly found on the left ovary.[36] As the cysts grow, they exert increasing pressure on the ovary, causing atrophy and eventually obliteration of the normal ovarian tissue. Fluid within the cyst is clear and serous.[73] Large cysts are often multilocular.[18,54]

Follicular cysts
The gross appearance of follicular cysts in guinea pigs has not been formally described.

Histopathology

Rete cysts
Rete cysts in the guinea pig are lined with low cuboidal to columnar epithelium.[18] In large cysts the epithelial cells may appear compressed.[43] The cells rest on a basal lamina, and a junctional complex connects the cells at their apices. The junctional complexes are composed mainly of zonulae adherentes and maculae adherentes; no tight junctions are present.[31,54] Most cells have a single, long cilium, whereas others have tufts of numerous small cilia; some have no cilia. The cilia are always located on the luminal surface.[18] Cells with tufts of small cilia also possess microvilli around and between the cilia, and basal bodies are seen underlying the cilia.[31] Numerous caveolae may be present on the lateral and basal surfaces.[46] The cytoplasm is variably basophilic. Nuclei may be irregularly shaped with deep clefts, and may be located centrally or basally. A single nucleolus is present.[18] Cysts with a diameter of less than 0.5 mm may connect to each other, forming a network of cysts.[18,75]

Follicular cysts

The histologic appearance of follicular cysts in guinea pigs has been sparsely reported. The cysts are lined by 1 to 2 layers of granulosa cells, with an inner vacuolated thecal layer that may be in disarray.[58] The cysts may contain an oocyte.[40]

TREATMENT
Surgery

Surgical treatment is by ovariohysterectomy, and is considered the treatment of choice (**Figs. 10** and **11**).[59,61] Ovariectomy is not recommended, because ovarian cysts are associated with multiple uterine diseases (discussed earlier).[61,68] Adhesions may be present between the ovaries and the peritoneum or other abdominal viscera. Cyst fluid may be drained by aspiration before surgery if cyst size poses an impediment to efficient removal.[61] Potential complications of surgery include hemorrhage, infection, cyst rupture (with secondary sterile peritonitis), ureteral injury, cecal laceration (with secondary septic peritonitis), and death.[42,76] Postoperative complications may include gastrointestinal stasis, suture dehiscence, occult hemorrhage, ovarian remnant syndrome, and death.

Percutaneous Drainage

Percutaneous drainage of cyst fluid may be performed. The effects are temporary, because fluid usually reaccumulates within the cyst. Rate of fluid reaccumulation is variable, anecdotally occurring in only a few days.[59] One important indication for cyst drainage is patient stabilization; large cysts may impede respiration, digestion, and/or tissue perfusion.[68,74] Technique for drainage is similar to that used for FNA (discussed earlier). If the syringe is to be disconnected from the needle before the needle is withdrawn, use of a 3-way stopcock is advised to avoid introducing air and/or pathogens into the abdomen.

Hormone Therapy

Medical therapy with hormone injections has variable success, and likely depends on the nature of the cyst(s). Rete cysts and neoplasms are unlikely to respond to hormone therapy, whereas follicular cysts and their associated clinical signs may regress (**Fig. 12**).[59,61] The following treatments have been used in guinea pigs:

- Gonadotropin-releasing hormone (GnRH) (Cystorelin, Merial, Duluth, GA): 25 μg/ animal intramuscularly (IM); 2 treatments, 14 days apart.[77]

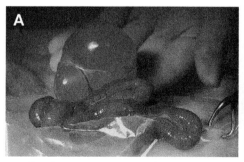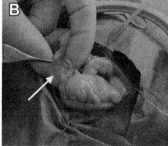

Fig. 10. (*A, B*) Ovarian cysts identified during ovariohysterectomy of 2 guinea pig sows. The *arrow* in (*B*) indicates the ovarian cyst. (*Courtesy of* Peter G. Fisher, DVM, Dipl ABVP-ECM, Virginia Beach, VA.)

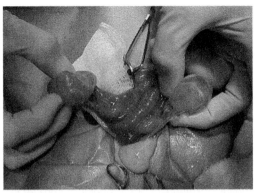

Fig. 11. Bilateral ovarian cysts identified during ovariohysterectomy of a guinea pig sow. (*Courtesy of* Dan H. Johnson, DVM, Dipl ABVP-ECM, Raleigh, NC.)

- Leuprolide acetate depot (Lupron Depot, TAP Pharmaceuticals, Lake Forest, IL): 100–300 μg/kg subcutaneously (SC) or IM every 3 to 4 weeks as needed to control clinical signs.[63,78]
- Deslorelin acetate implant (Suprelorin F, Virbac Animal Health, Fort Worth, TX): one 4.7-mg implant SC. Few reports of deslorelin use in guinea pigs exist, and most are anecdotal. Treatment failures have been reported, and the effective life of a single implant in guinea pigs is unknown. Use of Suprelorin F in the United States is limited to ferrets; extralabel use is prohibited by the US Food and Drug Administration.[79,80]
- Human chorionic gonadotropin (hCG; Chorulon, Merck Animal Health, Summit, NJ): 1000 USP units/animal IM; 2 treatments, 7 to 10 days apart. hCG has been associated with hypersensitivity reactions in humans. Development of

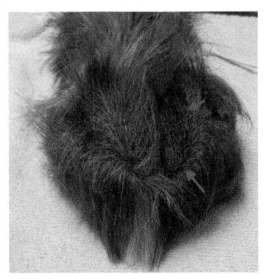

Fig. 12. Guinea pig sow with ovarian cyst–induced alopecia showing hair regrowth (*arrows*) after treatment with gonadotropin-releasing hormone. (*Courtesy of* Peter G. Fisher, DVM, Dipl ABVP-ECM, Virginia Beach, VA.)

antibodies to hCG may reduce the effectiveness of repeated doses. The volume required may be large (eg, 1 mL), causing substantial pain.[77,78]

GnRH, hCG, and GnRH agonists (eg, leuprolide, deslorelin) have been used to treat follicular cysts in cows. All three treatments work by causing luteinization of the cyst(s) and possibly luteinization or ovulation any mature follicles, which in turn develop into corpora lutea. There is a consequent increase in serum progesterone, causing negative feedback on LH secretions and resensitizing the pituitary to estradiol.[55,81]

Guinea pigs are known to have a unique form of GnRH (guinea pig GnRH [gpGnRH]), featuring 2 amino acid substitutions relative to the GnRH of other mammals (mammalian GnRH [mGnRH]).[82] This difference is reflected in their respective receptors, with the gpGnRH receptor having several amino acid substitutions compared with receptors for GnRH.[83] Current evidence suggests that the gpGnRH receptor has a higher affinity for mGnRH than gpGnRH, resulting in a more efficient release of LH.[84,85] However, it is unknown how gpGnRH conformational differences affect the pharmacodynamics of mGnRH agonists (eg, leuprolide or deslorelin).

In the event of medical treatment failure, several scenarios are possible:

- Cysts are not the cause of the patient's clinical signs
- Some or all of the cysts are not follicular
- The drug dosage was insufficient to increase LH levels enough to cause luteinization of any follicular cysts
- The patient may have a defect in its hypothalamic-pituitary-ovarian axis, predisposing it to repeated cyst development

PROGNOSIS

The general prognosis for guinea pigs with clinical disease caused by ovarian cysts is good with ovariohysterectomy.[44,79] Prognosis for patients with neoplastic cysts varies with the neoplastic cell type, degree of malignancy, and presence of metastasis. Complicating factors, including hemorrhage, gastrointestinal stasis, and uterine disease, may worsen the prognosis.

Dermatologic signs associated with ovarian cysts resolve gradually after treatment. Hair regrowth is reported to be complete within 3 months after ovariohysterectomy.[61,86] There are no reports of time frames for resolution of dermatologic signs after treatment with hormone injections.

SUMMARY

Ovarian cysts are common in guinea pig sows, with prevalence estimates ranging from 58% to 100%. The cysts most commonly, but not exclusively, develop from the rete ovarii, a remnant of the fetal mesonephric duct that may have a role in folliculogenesis in some species. Ovarian follicles are also known to transform into cysts, and ovarian neoplasia may include cystic components. The pathogenesis of ovarian cysts is unknown, and numerous hypotheses have been proposed. Diagnosis is made primarily from history, clinical signs, abdominal ultrasonography, and histopathology. The primary dermatologic sign of ovarian cysts in guinea pigs is nonpruritic alopecia of the lumbosacral, flank, inguinal, and/or perineal areas. This is thought to be caused by excessive estrogen produced by follicular cysts or functional ovarian tumors. The definitive treatment is ovariohysterectomy. Hormone injections are thought to affect only follicular cysts, and their efficacy is variable. Both cyst drainage and hormone injections are not reliable long-term solutions, because relapses are common.

REFERENCES

1. Franks S. Animal models and the developmental origins of polycystic ovary syndrome: increasing evidence for the role of androgens in programming reproductive and metabolic dysfunction. Endocrinology 2012;153(6):2536–8.
2. Xu N, Kwon S, Abbott DH, et al. Epigenetic mechanism underlying the development of polycystic ovary syndrome (PCOS)-like phenotypes in prenatally androgenized rhesus monkeys. PLoS One 2011;6(11):e27286.
3. Veiga-Lopez A, Lee JS, Padmanabhan V. Developmental programming: insulin sensitizer treatment improves reproductive function in prenatal testosterone-treated female sheep. Endocrinology 2010;151(8):4007–17.
4. Gelberg HB, McEntee K, Heath EH. Feline cystic rete ovarii. Vet Pathol 1984; 21(3):304–7.
5. Probo M, Comin A, Cairoli F, et al. Selected metabolic and hormonal profiles during maintenance of spontaneous ovarian cysts in dairy cows. Reprod Domest Anim 2011;46(3):448–54.
6. Detlefsen JA. The fecundity of the female hybrids. In: Detlefsen JA, editor. Genetic studies on a cavy species cross. Washington, DC: Carnegie Institution of Washington; 1914. p. 100–1.
7. Foster RA. Female reproductive system and mammary gland. In: Zachary JF, McGavin MD, editors. Pathologic basis of veterinary disease. 5th edition. St Louis (MO): Mosby; 2011. p. 1085–126.
8. BMJ Group. Ovarian cysts - basics - classification. Best Pract 2012. Available at: http://bestpractice.bmj.com/best-practice/monograph/660/basics/classification. html. Accessed December 12, 2012.
9. Wenzel JG, Odend'hal S. The mammalian rete ovarii: a literature review. Cornell Vet 1985;75(3):411–25.
10. Wilkerson WV. The rete ovarii as a normal structure of the adult mammalian ovary. Anat Rec 1923;26(1):75–7.
11. Byskov AG. The anatomy and ultrastructure of the rete system in the fetal mouse ovary. Biol Reprod 1978;19(4):720–35.
12. Odend'hal S, Wenzel JG, Player EC. The rete ovarii of cattle and deer communicates with the uterine tube. Anat Rec 1986;216(1):40–3.
13. Lee SH, Ichii O, Otsuka S, et al. Ovarian cysts in MRL / MpJ mice are derived from the extraovarian rete: a developmental study. J Anat 2011;219(6):743–55.
14. Long GG. Apparent mesonephric duct (rete anlage) origin for cysts and proliferative epithelial lesions in the mouse ovary. Toxicol Pathol 2002;30(5):592–8.
15. Byskov AG. The role of the rete ovarii in meiosis and follicle formation in the cat, mink and ferret. J Reprod Fertil 1975;45(2):201–9.
16. Deanesly R. Follicle formation in guinea-pigs and rabbits: a comparative study with notes on the rete ovarii. J Reprod Fertil 1975;45(2):371–4.
17. Bookhout CG. The development of the guinea pig ovary from sexual differentiation to maturity. J Morphol 1945;77(2):233–63.
18. Quattropani SL. Serous cysts of the aging guinea pig ovary. I. Light microscopy and origin. Anat Rec 1977;188(3):351–60.
19. Byskov AG, Lintern-Moore S. Follicle formation in the immature mouse ovary: the role of the rete ovarii. J Anat 1973;116(Pt 2):207–17.
20. Mossman HW, Duke KL. Comparative morphology of the mammalian ovary. Madison (WI): University of Wisconsin Press; 1973.
21. Kumar M. The urogenital system. In: Kumar M, editor. Clinically oriented anatomy of the dog and cat. Ronkonkoma (NY): Linus Publications; 2012. p. 1423–92.

22. Schatten H, Constantinescu GM, editors. Comparative reproductive biology. Ames (IA): Blackwell Publishing; 2007.
23. Byskov AG. Does the rete ovarii act as a trigger for the onset of meiosis? Nature 1974;252(5482):396–7.
24. Byskov AG, Skakkebaek NE, Stafanger G, et al. Influence of ovarian surface epithelium and rete ovarii on follicle formation. J Anat 1977;123(Pt 1):77.
25. Jeppesen T. The ultrastructure of follicle cells in fetal guinea-pig ovaries. Anat Rec 1977;189(4):649–67.
26. Smith PR. Development of the rete ovarii in the sheep ovary (thesis, Master of Science). Dunedin (New Zealand): University of Otago; 2012. Available at: http://hdl.handle.net/10523/2153. Accessed December 19, 2012.
27. Byskov AG, Saxén L. Induction of meiosis in fetal mouse testis in vitro. Dev Biol 1976;52(2):193–200.
28. Fajer AB, Schneider J, McCall D, et al. The induction of meiosis by ovaries of newborn hamsters and its relation to the action of the extra ovarian structures in the mesovarium (rete ovarii). Ann Biol Anim Biochim Biophys 1979;19(4B): 1273–8.
29. Archbald LF, Schultz RH, Fahning ML, et al. Rete ovarii in heifers: a preliminary study. J Reprod Fertil 1971;26(3):413–4.
30. O'Shea JD. Histochemical observations on mucin secretion by subsurface epithelial structures in the canine ovary. J Morphol 1966;120(4):347–58.
31. Quattropani SL. Serous cysts of the aging guinea pig ovary. II. Scanning and transmission electron microscopy. Anat Rec 1978;190(2):285–98.
32. Rosenfeld CS, Schatten H. Overview of female reproductive organs. In: Schatten H, Constantinescu GM, editors. Comparative reproductive biology. Ames (IA): Blackwell Publishing; 2007. p. 99–109.
33. Walters EM. Comparative reproductive physiology of domestic animals. In: Schatten H, Constantinescu GM, editors. Comparative reproductive biology. Ames (IA): Blackwell Publishing; 2007. p. 117–31.
34. Field KJ, Griffith JW, Lang CM. Spontaneous reproductive tract leiomyomas in aged guinea-pigs. J Comp Pathol 1989;101(3):287–94.
35. Keller LS, Griffith JW, Lang CM. Reproductive failure associated with cystic rete ovarii in guinea pigs. Vet Pathol 1987;24(4):335–9.
36. Nielsen TD, Holt S, Rueløkke ML, et al. Ovarian cysts in guinea pigs: influence of age and reproductive status on prevalence and size. J Small Anim Pract 2003; 44(6):257–60.
37. Hong CC. Spontaneous papillary cystadenocarcinoma of the ovary in Dunkin-Hartley guineapigs. Lab Anim 1980;14(1):39–40.
38. Young WC, Dempsey EW, Myers HI, et al. The ovarian condition and sexual behavior in the female guinea pig. Am J Anat 1938;63(3):457–87.
39. Papanicolaou GN, Stockard CR. Morphology of cystic growths in the ovary and uterus of the guinea pig. Proc Soc Exp Biol 1922;19(8):401–2.
40. Shi F, Petroff BK, Herath CB, et al. Serous cysts are a benign component of the cyclic ovary in the guinea pig with an incidence dependent upon inhibin bioactivity. J Vet Med Sci 2002;64(2):129–35.
41. Beregi A, Molnár V, Perge E, et al. Radiography and ultrasonography in the diagnosis and treatment of abdominal enlargements in five guinea pigs. J Small Anim Pract 2001;42(9):459–63.
42. Burns RP, Paul-Murphy J, Sicard GK. Granulosa cell tumor in a guinea pig. J Am Vet Med Assoc 2001;218(5):726–8.
43. Willis RA. Ovarian teratomas in guinea-pigs. J Pathol Bacteriol 1962;84(1):237–9.

44. Greenacre CB. Spontaneous tumors of small mammals. Veterinary Clin North Am Exot Anim Pract 2004;7(3):627–51.
45. Preetha S, Thangapandiyan M, Selvaraj J, et al. Cystic ovarian disease in a laboratory guinea pig–a case report. Indian J Anim Res 2011;45(3):228–9.
46. Quattropani SL. Serous cysts of the aging guinea pig ovary. III. Permeability of the cyst epithelium to lanthanum and horseradish peroxidase. Anat Rec 1980; 197(2):213–9.
47. Meredith A. Skin diseases and treatment of guinea pigs. In: Paterson S, editor. Skin diseases of exotic pets. Oxford: Blackwell Science; 2008. p. 232–50.
48. Retana-Márquez S, Aguirre FG, Alcántara M, et al. Mesquite pod extract modifies the reproductive physiology and behavior of the female rat. Horm Behav 2012;61(4):549–58.
49. Degen GH, Janning P, Diel P, et al. Estrogenic isoflavones in rodent diets. Toxicol Lett 2002;128(1–3):145–57.
50. Heindel JJ, Saal vom FS. Meeting report: batch-to-batch variability in estrogenic activity in commercial animal diets – importance and approaches for laboratory animal research. Environ Health Perspect 2008;116(3):389–93.
51. Kato H, Iwata T, Katsu Y, et al. Evaluation of estrogenic activity in diets for experimental animals using in vitro assay. J Agric Food Chem 2004;52(5):1410–4.
52. Brown NM, Setchell KD. Animal models impacted by phytoestrogens in commercial chow: implications for pathways influenced by hormones. Lab Invest 2001;81(5):735–47.
53. Kierszenbaum AL, Tres LL. Epithelium. In: Histology and cell biology: an introduction to pathology. Philadelphia: Saunders; 2011. p. 1–58.
54. Quattropani SL. Serous cystadenoma formation in guinea pig ovaries. J Submicrosc Cytol 1981;13(3):337–45.
55. Vanholder T, Opsomer G, de Kruif A. Aetiology and pathogenesis of cystic ovarian follicles in dairy cattle: a review. Reprod Nutr Dev 2006;46(2): 105–19.
56. Hernandez-Ledezma JJ, Garverick HA, Elmore RG, et al. Gonadotropin releasing hormone treatment of dairy cows with ovarian cysts. III. Steroids in ovarian follicular fluid and ovarian cyst fluid. Theriogenology 1982;17(6): 697–707.
57. Shi F, Ozawa M, Komura H, et al. Secretion of ovarian inhibin and its physiologic roles in the regulation of follicle-stimulating hormone secretion during the estrous cycle of the female guinea pig. Biol Reprod 1999;60(1):78–84.
58. Quandt LM, Hutz RJ. Induction by estradiol-17 beta of polycystic ovaries in the guinea pig. Biol Reprod 1993;48(5):1088–94.
59. Hawkins MG, Bishop CR. Disease problems of guinea pigs. In: Quesenberry KE, Carpenter JW, editors. Ferrets, rabbits and rodents: clinical medicine and surgery. 3rd edition. St Louis (MO): Elsevier; 2012. p. 295–310.
60. Bacsich P, Wyburn GM. Masculinizing influence of cystic ovaries in female guinea pigs. Nature 1946;157:588.
61. Bennett RA. Soft tissue surgery: guinea pigs, chinchillas, and degus. In: Quesenberry KE, Carpenter JW, editors. Ferrets, rabbits and rodents: clinical medicine and surgery. 3rd edition. St Louis (MO): Elsevier; 2012. p. 326–38.
62. Young WC, Dempsey EW, Hagquist CW, et al. Sexual behavior and sexual receptivity in the female guinea pig. J Comp Psychol 1939;27(1):49.
63. Paul-Murphy JR. Guinea pigs: ovarian cysts. In: Oglesbee BL, editor. Blackwell's five-minute veterinary consult: small mammal. 2nd edition. Ames (IA): Wiley-Blackwell; 2011. p. 301–2.

64. Beregi A, Zorn S, Felkai F. Ultrasonic diagnosis of ovarian cysts in ten guinea pigs. Vet Radiol Ultrasound 1999;40(1):74–6.

65. Johnson-Delaney CA. Endocrine system and diseases of exotic companion mammals. In: American Board of Veterinary Practitioners Symposium. 2009. Available at: http://www.vin.com/members/proceedings/proceedings.plx?CID=ABVP2009 &PID=26736&O=VIN&id=3944802. Accessed February 22, 2013.

66. Miller WH. Sex hormone dermatoses. In: World Small Animal Veterinary Association World Congress 2004 Proceedings. Available at: http://www.vin.com/members/ proceedings/proceedings.plx?CID=WSAVA2004&PID=8630&O=VIN&id= 3852179. Accessed February 22, 2013.

67. Mans C. Small mammals: guinea pigs – skin diseases. In: Mayer J, Donnelly TM, editors. Clinical veterinary advisor: birds and exotic pets. St Louis (MO): Saunders; 2013. p. 278–80.

68. Rueløkke ML, McEvoy FJ, Nielsen TD, et al. Cystic ovaries in guinea pigs. Exotic DVM 2003;5(5):33–6.

69. Garner MM. Cytologic diagnosis of diseases of rabbits, guinea pigs, and rodents. Veterinary Clin North Am Exot Anim Pract 2007;10(1):25–49.

70. Lennox AM. Sedation of exotic companion mammals [session 188]. In: Proceedings of the 31st Annual AAV Conference and Expo with AEMV. San Diego (CA); 2011. p. 117–20.

71. Longley LA. Rodent anaesthesia. In: Longley LA, editor. Anaesthesia of exotic pets. Edinburgh (United Kingdom): Saunders; 2008. p. 59–84.

72. Hawkins MG, Pascoe PJ. Anesthesia, analgesia, and sedation of small mammals. In: Quesenberry KE, Carpenter JW, editors. Ferrets, rabbits and rodents: clinical medicine and surgery. 3rd edition. St Louis (MO): Elsevier; 2012. p. 429–51.

73. Percy DH, Barthold SW. Guinea pig. In: Percy DH, Barthold SW, editors. Pathology of laboratory rodents and rabbits. 3rd edition. Ames (IA): Wiley-Blackwell; 2008. p. 248–9.

74. Jenkins JR. Diseases of geriatric guinea pigs and chinchillas. Veterinary Clin North Am Exot Anim Pract 2010;13(1):85–93.

75. Tan OL, Hurst PR, Fleming JS. Location of inclusion cysts in mouse ovaries in relation to age, pregnancy, and total ovulation number: implications for ovarian cancer? J Pathol 2005;205(4):483–90.

76. Adin CA. Complications of ovariohysterectomy and orchiectomy in companion animals. Vet Clin North Am Small Anim Pract 2011;41(5):1023–39.

77. Mayer J. The use of GnRH to treat cystic ovaries in a guinea pig. Exotic DVM 2003;5(5):36.

78. Mayer J. Rodents. In: Carpenter JW, Marion CJ, editors. Exotic animal formulary. 4th edition. St Louis (MO): Elsevier; 2012. p. 498–9.

79. Donnelly TM, Richardson VC. Small mammals: guinea pigs – ovarian cysts. In: Mans C, editor. Clinical veterinary advisor. St Louis (MO): Saunders; 2013. p. 269–71.

80. Virbac Animal Health. Suprelorin F [package insert]. 2012. Available at: http://www.virbacferretsusa.com/assets/pdfs/L-2000-F-US-1_Suprelorin_Insert. pdf. Accessed February 25, 2013.

81. Parkinson TJ. Infertility in the cow: structural abnormalities, management deficiencies, and non-specific infections. In: Noakes DE, Parkinson TJ, England GC, editors. Veterinary reproduction & obstetrics. Edinburgh (United Kingdom): Saunders-Elsevier; 2009. p. 439–48.

82. Gao CQ, van den Saffele J, Giri M, et al. Guinea-pig gonadotropin-releasing hormone: immunoreactivity and biological activity. J Neuroendocrinol 2000; 12(4):355–9.

83. Fujii Y, Enomoto M, Ikemoto T, et al. Molecular cloning and characterization of a gonadotropin-releasing hormone receptor in the guinea pig, *Cavia porcellus*. Gen Comp Endocrinol 2004;136(2):208–16.
84. Gao CQ, Kaufman JM, Eertmans F, et al. Difference in receptor-binding contributes to difference in biological activity between the unique guinea pig GnRH and mammalian GnRH. Neurosci Lett 2012;507(2):124–6.
85. Grove-Strawser D, Sower SA, Ronsheim PM, et al. Guinea pig GnRH: localization and physiological activity reveal that it, not mammalian GnRH, is the major neuroendocrine form in guinea pigs. Endocrinology 2002;143(5):1602–12.
86. Rosenthal KL. Small mammals. In: Rosenthal KL, Forbes NA, Frye FL, et al, editors. Rapid review of small exotic animal medicine & husbandry: pet mammals, birds, reptiles, amphibians, and fish. London: Manson Publishing; 2008. p. 57.

Dermatological Conditions Affecting the Beak, Claws, and Feet of Captive Avian Species

Amy Beth Worell, DVM, ABVP-Avian

KEYWORDS

- Beak • Claws and feet • Beak trauma • Beak growth abnormalities • Pododermatitis
- Self-mutilation of the feet

KEY POINTS

- Dermatologic involvement of the beak, claws, and feet are common presentations in a veterinary clinic.
- These dermatologic presentations are often part of the presentation rather than the sole reason for the presentation.
- Three general categories encompass the array of presentations: those of environmental and nutritional causes, those with infectious causes, and those with potentially idiopathic causes.
- Resolution, when possible, of these dermatologic conditions is as varied as the conditions themselves.

INTRODUCTION

Dermatologic problems that are present or reflected in the beak, claws, and feet of captive avian species are common presentations to veterinary facilities. Most of the birds presented for concerns that involve these anatomic areas may have a generalized condition whereby involvement of the beak, claws, and/or feet are *part* of the condition rather than the sole reason for the presentation. Of course, this may not be immediately apparent to the avian caretaker who may perceive that the problem is localized rather than generalized. Such would be the case, for example, with a budgie (*Melopsittacus undulates*) that is presented for an abnormal beak, which on closer inspection has an infestation with the *Knemidokoptes* mite that is affecting not only the beak but also the skin around the vent as well as the legs and feet.

Dermatologic conditions involving the beak, claws, and feet can collectively be organized in several categories that are often overlapping. These categories are suggested to reflect the general nature of the condition rather than the specific cause. The

Disclosures: The author has nothing to disclose.
Avian Veterinary Services, PO Box 4907, West Hills, CA 91308, USA
E-mail address: Yourpets7606@gmail.com

Vet Clin Exot Anim 16 (2013) 777–799
http://dx.doi.org/10.1016/j.cvex.2013.05.005
1094-9194/13/$ – see front matter © 2013 Elsevier Inc. All rights reserved.

general categories are environmental and nutritional causes, infectious agent causes, and potentially idiopathic causes.

- Environmental and nutritional causes include trauma of all types, leg-band injuries, thermal and frost injuries, fractures, pododermatitis, avascular necrosis of distal extremities, and possibly beak growth abnormalities.
- Infectious agent causes includes parasitic, viral, fungal, and bacterial agents that produce physical changes in the beak, claws, or feet.
- Potentially idiopathic causes include neoplasia, self-mutilation of the legs and feet in Amazon parrots and other species, articular gout, and overgrowth of the beak.

ANATOMY: FORM AND FUNCTION OF THE BEAK, CLAWS, AND FEET

There are currently more than 10 000 living avian species in the world. With such a large number of bird species that exist from the Arctic to the Antarctic, there is no one description that can encompass all this diversity. Hence, in the following brief anatomic review, the discussion is general rather than specific because the evolutionary modifications can be quite varied.

The Beak or Bill

- The terms *beak* and *bill* are often used interchangeably when discussing birds. This use is generally considered to be correct. Some distinction can be made; for example, a beak refers to a wide range of animals, including birds, turtles, some fish, some insects, and other mammals, whereas a bill is usually applied only to birds and the duck-billed platypus.
- It consists of the bones of the *maxillary and mandibular jaws* and their horny covering, the *rhamphotheca*. There are no teeth or lips present.[1]
- The rhamphotheca is a thick, modified integument that is hard and heavily cornified in most birds but may be soft at the tip in some species. It resembles skin and is comprised of a dermis and modified epidermis. It is continuously growing.[2]
- The *maxillary rhamphotheca* is also known as the *rhinotheca*, and the *mandibular rhamphotheca* is also known as the *gnathotheca*.[2]
- The dermis of the rhamphotheca consists of somatosensory receptors that aid in feeding and environmental interactions.[3]
- The beak is continually growing and is worn down through environmental interactions.
- The edges of the bill (*tomia*) are modified according to the bird's feeding preferences.[2]
- The nares are located within the basal one-third of the upper bill in most birds.
- The *cere* is a modification of the rhamphotheca located at the base of the upper beak in some birds. It is sometimes soft and thickened.[1,3]
- The beak functions as a tool for feeding, courtship, object manipulation, defense, nest building and preening.

The Claws

- Avian claws are coverings of heavily cornified integument over the bone of the terminal phalanx of each digit.[2,3]
- The toe claw is comprised of plates containing beta-keratin and calcium salts.[2]
- Toe claws vary in length, curvature, and pointedness in relation to their usage and the environment in which the bird lives.[3]
- All birds have toe claws, and some birds have wing claws (eg, in adult loons and owls).

- The claws are continually growing and are worn down through environmental interactions.

The Feet

- Most birds have 4 toes on each foot. Some birds only have 3 toes.
- Feet types can be divided into 3 main types:
  1. *The grasping foot*: The foot is adapted to hold prey or for perching.
  2. *The walking and wading foot*: The foot is modified often with webbing, or the toes may be greatly elongated to facilitate movement.
  3. *The swimming foot:* The foot is modified with webbing to facilitate swimming.[2]
- The *podotheca*, the integument covering the feet, is comprised of layers of scales.

The scales are highly keratinized epidermis, which vary with the part of the foot and species.[3] The extent of feathers covering the legs varies, being replaced at various points by scales.

DERMATOLOGIC CONDITIONS OF THE BEAK, CLAWS, AND FEET

Conditions involving the beak, claws, and feet may occur jointly or separately. They may additionally occur as separate entities but more commonly as part of a generalized cause.

Environmental and Possible Nutritional Causes

Environmental and possible nutritional causes (**Table 1**) and suggested treatment protocols:

Table 1
Environmental and possible nutritional causes

Category	Beak Involvement	Claw Involvement	Feet Involvement
Trauma	XX	XX	XX
Leg-band injuries	—	—	XX
Thermal injuries	—	—	XX
Frostbite injuries	—	XX	XX
Fractures	XX	XX	XX
Pododermatitis	—	—	XX
Avascular necrosis of distal extremities	—	XX	XX
Beak growth abnormalities	XX	—	—

1. Trauma: Common causes of beak, claw, and/or feet trauma include the following:
   - Attacks by other birds, including cage mates and other pets or aviary birds, as well as attacks from a noncontained bird, such as a hawk
   - Attacks from other pet animals, including dog and cat bites
   - Attacks from wild animals, including raccoon bites
   - Collision with a solid surface, such as a window or wall; can lead to severe beak injuries, especially if the underlying nutritional level is subpar or if metabolic bone disease (nutritional secondary hyperparathyroidism) is present (**Fig. 1**)
   - Lacerations caused by a variety of situations, including those obtained while in an enclosure or cage and those obtained while free in a house or outdoors

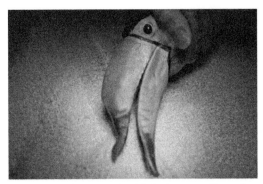

Fig. 1. Sulfur-breasted toucan, also called keel-billed toucan (*Ramphastos sulfuratus*), with metabolic bone disease that traumatically impacted the enclosure resulting in a malleable beak.

- Unknown trauma resulting in beak damage and toe or claw amputations (**Fig. 2**)
- Damage resulting from human intervention, such as accidents occurring during handling, grooming, or restraint
- Treatment for trauma
  - External assessment of patients for extent of injuries and general condition
  - Stabilization of patients as needed with fluid therapy and medications, such as analgesics and antibiotics
  - Brief wound cleansing if patients are not yet stable
  - When stabilized, specific treatment of the particular lesion, which might include cleaning bite wounds, surgical repair if needed, and bandaging damaged or affected toes and claws
2. Leg-band injuries: Two main types involve the feet and claws. The bands may be open or closed.
   - Constriction and tissue destruction caused by compression of underlying tissue by the leg band (**Fig. 3**)
     - Occurs with open and closed bands
     - Can occur when the leg or foot is bandaged
     - Can occur with tissue swelling, such as from trauma or a leg or foot fracture
     - Can occur with presence of the *Knemidokoptes* mites under the band resulting in excessive keratin production and mild to severe tissue destruction of the foot or leg

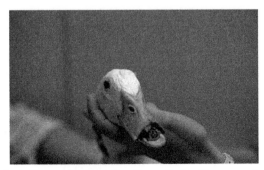

Fig. 2. Pet Pekin duck (*Anas platyrhynchos domestica*) with severe trauma of unknown cause to the distal upper bill.

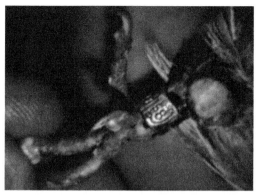

Fig. 3. Leg-band injury to the foot and leg of a budgerigar (*Melopsittacus undulatus*). There is a tremendous amount of tissue swelling and inflammation. Gout nodules are also visible just distal to the open band.

- Injury resulting from catching the leg band on another inanimate object
  ○ Most commonly occurs with open bands
  ○ Can result in soft tissue damage, fractures, loss of blood supply to the leg or foot, and even death if the bird severely struggles or hangs from the leg for a prolonged time period
- Treatment for leg-band injuries
  ○ Stabilize patients.
  ○ Remove the band if possible; if the band is very tight, fractures and additional trauma can result when band removal is attempted.
  ○ Surgery and bandaging may be indicated depending on the specific presentation.
3. Thermal injuries: These injuries most commonly involve the feet and claws.
   - Exposure to hot surfaces, such as a stove, hot liquids, or a heater, resulting in tissue damage to the feet and claws
   - Treatment for thermal injuries
     ○ If the tissue is still overheated, cooling of the affected tissue with cool water may be helpful.
     ○ Topical and systemic antiinflammatory and antibacterial medications should be used.
     ○ Use of silver sulfadiazine cream should be considered.[4]
4. Frostbite injuries: These injuries can occur in northern climates with freezing or less-than-freezing temperatures (**Fig. 4**).
   - These injuries can occur when the feet and claws are exposed to prolonged low temperatures resulting in shunting of blood away from peripheral tissues with freezing and death of affected tissue; the affected toes and claws may eventually fall off, and death can also occur.
   - Treatment for frostbite injuries includes the following:
     ○ Supportive care may include heat, fluid, and antiinflammatory and antibacterial medications applied both topically and systemically.
     ○ Surgery, including amputation, may be indicated in some instances.[4]
5. Fractures: Fractures can occur to the beak, claws, or feet.
   - Fractures can occur because of trauma or metabolic abnormalities.
   - Beak fractures can be classified into 4 types: *simple fractures, depressed fractures, fractures with bone defects, and avulsion fractures.* Simple fractures

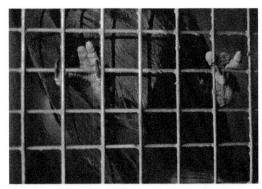

Fig. 4. Frostbite resulting in loss of digits and claws on the feet of a female vosmaeri eclectus (*Eclectus roratus vosmaeri*). This bird had both indoor and outdoor aviaries and chose to remain outside in freezing temperatures resulting in her frostbite injuries.

may involve the least damage to the beak, may be easiest to resolve, and may involve a split mandible, which tends to split at the midline. The 2 halves rarely can be reunited (**Fig. 5**).
- ○ Depressed fractures may occur with a bite injury to the beak from another bird or household pet (**Fig. 6**).
- ○ Fractures with bone defects may occur with a bite injury to the beak (**Fig. 7**).
- • Avulsion fractures most commonly occur from the bite of another bird, tearing off the beak at its base. Reattachment is generally unsuccessful (**Fig. 8**).[5] Toe, foot, and claw fractures can also occur.
- • Treatment for fractures
  - ○ *Beak fractures* may range from displacement and loss of the mandibular tip to extensive fractures involving tissue of the maxillary and mandibular jaws and the rhamphotheca.
  - ○ For a fracture of the mandibular tip, a topical anticoagulant and systemic pain medication may be all that is indicated.
  - ○ For more involved beak fractures, surgical repair may or may not be possible. Use of adhesives, such as polymethyl methacrylate, epoxy, or dental

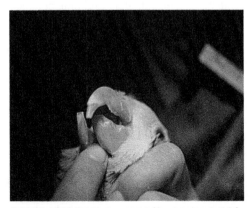

Fig. 5. This double yellow-headed Amazon parrot (Amazona oratrix) presented with a split mandible. This injury occurred many years prior, and the pet required intermittent beak trims.

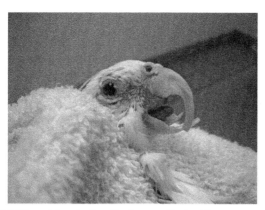

Fig. 6. This cockatiel (*Nymphicus hollandicus*) was attacked by a larger parrot. Permanent injuries included a split mandible and damage to the growth plates of the maxillary beak producing abnormal beak growth.

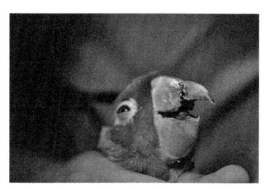

Fig. 7. This red-masked parakeet or cherry-headed conure (*Aratinga erythrogenys*) was attacked by a macaw resulting in a severe fracture to the maxillary beak.

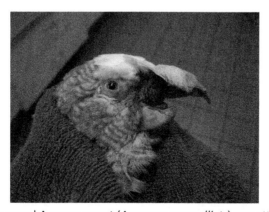

Fig. 8. This yellow-naped Amazon parrot (*Amazona auropalliata*) was attacked by another bird resulting in an avulsion fracture of the maxillary beak. The bird presented with the beak fragment taped in place.

composites, may be used as well as orthopedic wires and pins, modified external skeletal devices, and bone plates and screws, in some instances. Prosthetic beak replacements may be used in some situations.

○ Beak repairs are not always possible. Many birds with extensive beak injuries can learn to eat and survive on soft food. These birds may require initial supportive care, including tube feeding during their adjustment phase after the beak injury/fracture.

○ *Claw and foot fractures* often require fracture stabilization by external coaptation, which should immobilize the fracture site. This stabilization may involve a simple support bandage or a more complex bandage with wires or pins.

○ Bandaging options vary with the fracture and patient but may include bandaging a fractured toe to an adjacent toe and the use of syringe cases for fracture support in a bandage.

○ Ball bandages that allow the feet and toes to heal may be used in some cases. The toes are wrapped around padding in a ball shape and then covered with materials, such as elastic gauze, to hold the toes and foot immobile.

○ Snowshoe splints can be constructed from materials such as tongue depressors and used to hold the toes in a specific position to allow healing to occur (**Fig. 9**).[4]

○ Toe and foot fractures often heal rapidly, many times in periods of less than 3 weeks.

6. Pododermatitis: This condition is also called bumblefoot.

   • This term is used for a degenerative and inflammatory condition affecting the weight-bearing surface of the foot, in this case, in captive birds. The species commonly affected are birds of prey, parrots, waterfowl, and poultry.

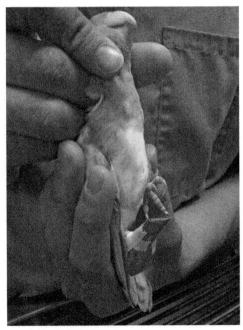

Fig. 9. This rosy- or peach-faced lovebird (*Agapornis roseicollis*) was fitted with a snowshoe splint to aid in the healing of fractured toes.

- The causes of pododermatitis are multifactorial and primarily involve trauma to the plantar surface of the foot or toes. The blood supply to the foot may be compromised, the bird may be in an immune-challenged state, and infection may secondarily become an issue.
- Common specific contributing factors may include perches of an inappropriate size, shape, or texture; inactivity; obesity; puncture wounds to the foot; and malnutrition.
- Various classification systems grade the foot lesions into categories (often up to 7), which divide the lesions from mild inflammation to severe changes, including osteomyelitis.[4,6,7]
- Treatment of pododermatitis or bumblefoot includes the following:
  - Treatment, which depends on the severity of the lesions, may be prolonged, complex, and involved. It generally involves changes in management and nutrition and treatment of the feet lesions.
  - Treatment may involve topical and systemic medications, bandaging, and surgery of the foot (**Fig. 10**). Details of more specific treatment protocols are addressed in another article within this issue of *Veterinary Clinics of North America: Exotic Animal Practice*.
7. Avascular necrosis of distal extremities: This condition is also known as constricted toe syndrome.
   - This condition can be caused by heat, cold, low humidity, foreign-body constriction, aflatoxins, and unknown causes such that a foot or, more commonly, a digit demonstrates constriction with a resulting avascular necrosis of the distal tissue.
   - It may be seen more commonly in young growing birds but can occur in birds of any age (**Fig. 11**).
   - It can occur in many species, including macaws, eclectus parrots, passerines, and toucans (**Fig. 12**).[1,8]
   - Treatment of avascular necrosis of distal extremities includes the following:
     - If a foreign body, such as a string or a piece of nesting material, is present, careful removal of the constricting foreign body is needed.
     - Consider diet change if a foreign body causing the constriction is not identified.
     - Topical massage and the application of medications, such as dimethyl sulfoxide, can be used.
     - Surgical intervention with the use of linear relief incisions perpendicular and through the band of constricted tissue may be curative. This incision is left

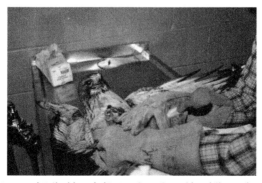

Fig. 10. This immature red-tailed hawk (*Buteo jamaicensis*), while undergoing treatment of pododermatitis, had the feet wrapped with ball bandages during the prolonged treatment.

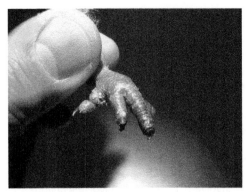

Fig. 11. Avascular necrosis in a young psittacine. Note the area of constriction in digit number one as well as the missing nails on the other digits. (*Courtesy of* Thomas Tully, DVM, Baton Rouge, LA.)

open but protected and covered with a bandage. An alternate surgical technique involves the use of superficial circumferential skin incisions just proximal and distal to the affected constricted tissue. The affected tissue is carefully removed, and the skin edges are closed with 4-0 to 6-0 monofilament sutures in a simple interrupted pattern.[9]
   ○ Amputation of distal affected tissue may also be indicated in some situations.
8. Beak growth abnormalities: These abnormalities most commonly occur in young cockatoos and macaws that are being hand-fed.
   • The 2 common types are *scissor beak deformity* and *mandibular prognathism.*
   • Scissor beak deformity occurs primarily in young macaws. This condition is characterized by a lateral deviation of the premaxilla/maxilla and rhinotheca to the right or left. The mandible and gnathotheca overgrow in the opposing direction. A scissor-type movement is produced (**Fig. 13**).
   • Mandibular prognathism primarily occurs in young cockatoos. The normal beak configuration is such that the maxilla is longer in length and extends over the mandible. In mandibular prognathism, there is an abnormal protrusion of the mandible. The maxilla is often of normal length, whereas the length of the mandible is excessive resulting in its extension over the maxilla (**Fig. 14**).

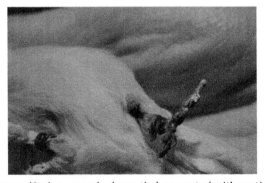

Fig. 12. This pet canary (*Serinus canaria domestica*) presented with nesting material tightly wrapped around the distal leg, resulting in avascular necrosis of the foot and digits.

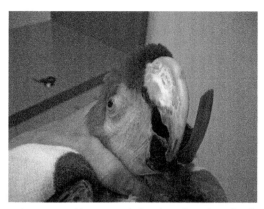

Fig. 13. Adult pet scarlet macaw (*Ara macao*) developed a scissor beak when younger that was not treated when the bird had a malleable beak. A permanent scissor beak deformity resulted that requires intermittent trimming.

- The causes of scissor beak deformity and mandibular prognathism are unknown. Possible causes include incubation issues, such as malposition of the chick in the egg; hand-feeding practices, such as syringe feeding the young bird on only one side of the beak; genetic influences; and infectious and possibly unapparent sinusitis infections.[5,10,11]
- It may also be associated with subpar or inappropriate nutritional levels, with vitamin and/or mineral imbalances or inadequate or excessive dietary protein theorized. With a resulting softening of the growing beak occurring, mild to severe bending of the beak may occur.
- Treatment of beak growth abnormalities includes the following:
  - *Physical therapy* for beak growth abnormalities can sometimes be successful if started early before significant changes in the beak have occurred and the bone is still pliable. This therapy involves applying digital pressure to the beak multiple times daily to encourage growth in the correct plane and direction.
  - If physical therapy fails in the young growing bird for either of the common deformities, there are 2 technique groupings that are generally successful in

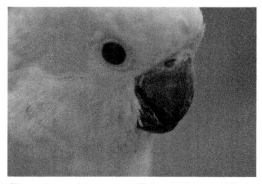

Fig. 14. A young Goffin cockatoo (*Cacatua goffiniana*) with mandibular prognathism. Note that the maxilla sits inside of the mandible rather than extending over it. (*Courtesy of Stephen Fronefield, DVM, Sugar Land, TX.*)

correcting the condition. These techniques are the *acrylic ramp and the pin/ rubber band techniques.* A description of these techniques can be found in the literature (**Fig. 15**).[5,10,11]

○ Treatment of these conditions is usually unsuccessful in adult birds with non-pliable beaks.

Infectious Agent Causes and Suggested Treatment Protocols

Infectious agent causes and suggested treatment protocols			
Infectious Agent Causes			
Category	Beak Involvement	Claw Involvement	Feet Involvement
Parasitic agents	XX	—	XX
Viral agents	XX	—	XX
Fungal agents	XX	XX	XX
Bacterial agents	XX	XX	XX

1. Parasitic agents
   - The most commonly encountered parasite affecting the feet and beak of captive birds is the *Knemidokoptes* mite, *Knemidokoptes pilae.* This mite is often referred to as the *scaly face and leg mite.*
   - It is the definitive cause of scaly face/leg mite in budgerigars and tassel foot in canaries. Other avian species are occasionally affected with this mite.
   - The mite spends its life cycle on birds and is transmitted by direct contact or fomite transmission (such as on a wood perch) to other birds. It is postulated that immunosuppressive and genetic factors may be factors in producing clinical signs.[12]
   - Invasion with large number of this microscopic mite can result in characteristic proliferative honeycomb appearing lesions on the unfeathered areas of the bird, in particular on the face, beak, feet, legs and around the cloaca.[8,13,14] It can cause severe deformity of the beak (**Figs. 16 and 17**).

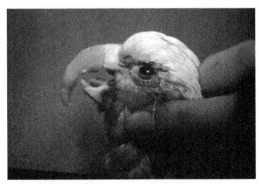

Fig. 15. A young rose-breasted cockatoo or Galah (*Eolophus roseicapilla*) that has had an acrylic beak placed on the maxillary beak for repair of mandibular prognathism. These synthetic beaks made of acyclic or other composite substances will eventually slough off resulting in the underlying maxillary beak projecting over the mandible.

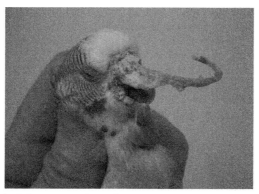

Fig. 16. Severe beak deformity resulting from infestation with the Knemidokoptes pilae mite in this budgerigar (*Melopsittacus undulatus*).

- Diagnosis of *Knemidokoptes pilae* includes the following:
    - Diagnosis is frequently obtained by direct visual examination of the nonfeathered areas of the body for the presence of the characteristic honeycombed proliferation of tissue. Characteristic holes will commonly be readily evident in the proliferated tissue. These holes can usually be visualized by the unaided eye, or a magnifying optic (such as a loupe or magnifying glass) can be used.
    - An additional diagnostic step involves microscopic identification of the mites following a skin scraping of affected tissue.
- Treatment of *Knemidokoptes pilae* includes the following:
    - Ivermectin applied either topically, orally, or injected for 1 to 3 treatments is generally curative.
2. Viral agents
    - The most frequently encountered viral disease affecting the beak and claws of captive birds is *psittacine beak and feather disease* (PBFD), which is caused by a psittacine circovirus. This viral disease is sometimes referred to as *psittacine circovirus* or *PCV*.
    - The virus most commonly affects young birds, less than 2 years of age.
    - Exposure resulting in infection with the development of disease is unlikely to occur in immunologically mature birds (after bursal involution). The age of virus

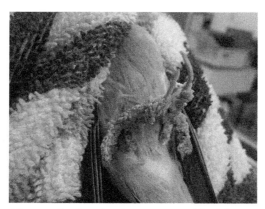

Fig. 17. A budgie with extensive foot involvement caused by infestation of the *Knemidokoptes pilae* mite. (*Courtesy of* Yoko Tamura, DVM, Tarzana, CA.)

involution has not been well studied to date but may range from 4 to 8 months depending on the species of parrot involved (David Phalen, DVM, PhD, ABVP [Avian], Wildlife Health and Conservation Center, University of Sydney, New South Wales, Australia, personal communication, 2013).

- The virus is most commonly encountered in Old World birds, including cockatoos, eclectus parrots, African gray parrots, and lovebirds. More than 40 species have been affected with the virus (**Fig. 18**).
- The virus is spread by both inhalation and ingestion of aerosols as well as through fomite transmission.[15]
- The disease can affect the beak and claws as well as the feathers and the immune system. Affected beaks may show overgrowth and growth abnormalities, and the nails may demonstrate abnormal growth because keratin production seems to be disrupted (**Fig. 19**).[15,16]
- Diagnosis of PBFD includes the following:
  - The diagnosis of PBFD has changed through the years, and the current diagnostic methods involve the use of DNA polymerase chain reaction (PCR) testing and in situ hybridization of tissues.
  - Commonly submitted samples include heparinized whole blood and/or swab samples.
  - DNA PCR samples test birds for the presence of psittacine circoviral nucleic acid. The virus assay uses viral-specific nucleic acid primers and a probe to detect as few as 10 copies of a small segment of viral-specific DNA in white blood cells, swabs of feather pulp, or swabs of samples from the environment.[17]
  - Test results are reported as either positive or negative, and the interpretation of the results are far from definitive. The presence or absence of feather

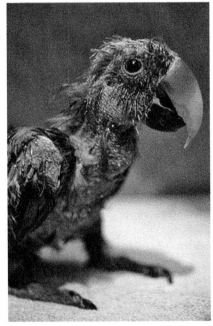

Fig. 18. PBFD in this male eclectus parrot (*Eclectus* species) with feather and beak abnormalities.

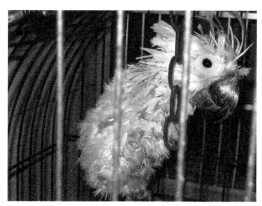

Fig. 19. PBFD resulting in beak and feather abnormalities in this 50-year-old plus imported Moluccan cockatoo (*Cacatua moluccensis*).

abnormalities is suggested to be significant. False-positive and negative results can occur, sometimes because of environmental contamination.

- Treatment of PBFD includes the following:
  - There is no specific treatment of PBFD. Care is supportive. Isolation and DNA PCR testing of affected and exposed individuals should be strongly considered.
- In addition to PBFD, captive avian species may be affected by cutaneous papillomas of virus origin. The etiologic agent responsible for the cutaneous papillomas in African gray parrots and Cuban Amazon parrots is a papillomavirus. In contrast, the cutaneous papillomas that are found in cockatoos and macaws seem to be caused by a herpesvirus (Darrel K. Styles, DVM, PhD, National Center for Animal Health Emergency Management, USDA APHIS Veterinary Services, Riverdale, MD, personal communication, 2013).[18] These benign growths appear as wartlike lesions on the feet. The affected birds tend to be clinically normal otherwise.
- Diagnosis of papillomas includes the following:
  - Diagnosis of cutaneous papillomas involves submission of affected tissue for histopathology. The laboratory may elect to pursue further diagnostic testing if indicated.
- Treatment of papillomas of the feet includes the following:
  - Treatment options include removal by laser, cryosurgery or surgical excision, and simple benign neglect (leaving the lesion alone without treatment).
    A third but less commonly encountered viral disease affecting the beak commissures and toes of captive birds is *avian poxvirus* caused by the *Avipoxvirus*. This presentation represents the cutaneous form of the virus. These viruses seem to be species specific.
  - Although more common in psittacines in the past, canaries may currently be the most common bird presented with papillomas of the feet.
  - Transmission is through insect vectors, such as mosquitoes and mites, which infect a host through an area of traumatized or damaged skin. Infections tend to be most common during the late summer and autumn when mosquitoes are more common.
  - The incubation period is less than 1 week, and the morbidity and mortality rate can approach 100%. Young birds are most frequently affected.
  - Clinically, affected birds with epithelial lesions are infected with the cutaneous form of the virus (also known as dry pox).

- ○ Papular lesions develop initially that progress into vesicles that eventually open resulting in dry, crusty lesions.[8,15,19]
- The diagnosis of *Avipoxvirus* includes the following:
  - ○ Definitive diagnosis of avian pox is through histopathology with the demonstration of eosinophilic intracytoplasmic inclusion bodies (Bollinger bodies) in the tissue.
- Treatment and prevention of *Avipoxvirus* includes the following:
  - ○ Treatment can vary from topical application of a variety of medications, including topical povidone-iodine solution, to benign neglect. Because clients often seem happier with some medication, consideration of a topical solution might be considered.
  - ○ Protection of birds from vectors, such as mosquitoes, should also be considered as a preventive measure.
  - ○ Further preventative measures include vaccinating unaffected canaries with a canary pox vaccine.
3. Fungal agents
   - Chronic infection with the fungus *Aspergillus* in the sinus of birds can result in a sinusitis/rhinitis that may produce drainage onto the beak from the nares. This drainage, in time, may lead to permanent changes and defects in the beak such that a troughlike indentation is formed in the beak.
   - Diagnosis of *Aspergillus* includes the following:
     - ○ Diagnostic tests include fungal culture, DNA PCR, Elisa antibody testing, galactomannan assay for a specific *Aspergillus* antigen, protein electrophoresis, radiology, endoscopy with sample collection, and complete blood count results. A collaboration of diagnostic tests may be beneficial in arriving at a diagnosis of *Aspergillosis*.
     - ○ Diagnosis of Aspergillosis is controversial and can be difficult.
     - ○ Response to antifungal therapy can also be considered as a potential diagnostic modality.
   - Interpretation of diagnostic test results may be subject to error. False-negative and positive test results are possible.
   - Treatment for *Aspergillus* includes the following:
     - ○ Long-term treatment with antifungal agents is required. The fungus may cause permanent enlargement of the nares because of the destruction of the sinus and a permanent trough in the beak.
     - ○ Because fungal diseases are generally a secondary problem, identifying the primary immunosuppressive factors may be helpful in resolving or controlling the fungal infection.
4. Bacterial agents
   - Various bacteria can invade the sinus of a bird resulting in destruction of the sinus and chronic drainage onto the beak. The drainage resulting from the sinusitis/rhinitis may, in time, lead to permanent changes and defects in the beak, including formation of a troughlike indentation extending from the affected nostril.
   - Deep bacterial infection of the beak rhamphotheca and underlying bone secondary to trauma has been reported (Peter G. Fisher, DVM, Pet Care Veterinary Hospital, Virginia Beach, VA, personal communication, 2012) (**Fig. 20**).
   - Diagnosis of bacterial agents is through bacterial culture and possibly cytology.
   - Treatment of bacterial sinusitis includes the following:
     - ○ Identification, if possible, of the pathogenic bacteria resulting in the sinusitis/rhinitis. Treatment with antibacterial both systemically and topically most likely will be indicated.

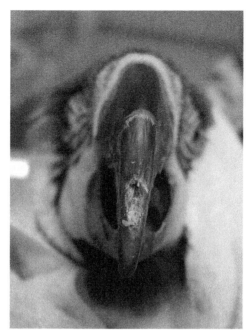

Fig. 20. Beak necrosis with a secondary bacterial infection in the maxilla of this blue and gold macaw (*Ara ararauna*). (*Courtesy of* Peter Fisher, DVM, Virginia Beach, VA.)

○ Correction of possible nutritional deficiencies, such as vitamin A deficiency and overall nutritional plane, is also extremely important.

Potentially Idiopathic Causes and Suggested Treatment Protocols

Potentially idiopathic causes and suggested treatment protocols			
	Potentially Idiopathic Causes		
Category	**Beak Involvement**	**Claw Involvement**	**Feet Involvement**
Neoplasia	XX	XX	XX
Self-mutilation of the feet	—	XX	XX
Articular gout	—	—	XX
Beak overgrowth	XX	—	—
Brown hypertrophy of cere	XX	—	—

1. Neoplasia
   • Neoplasia is not a common presentation on the beak or feet of captive avian species, but it does occasionally occur. It has been reported in budgerigars and other psittacines. Passerines can also be affected.
   • Tumor types vary but include squamous cell carcinoma of the rhamphotheca and phalanges (**Fig. 21**).[20,21]
   • The author has seen many red raised, rapidly growing tumors on the feet of canaries. Owners declined biopsies after surgical removal (**Fig. 22**).

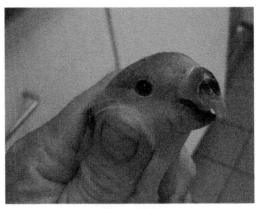

Fig. 21. A peach-faced lovebird (*Agapornis roseicollis*) with a large tumor of the beak.

- Treatment of neoplasia on the beak or feet includes the following:
  - Surgical removal of the mass, if possible, and consideration of radiation or chemotherapy if indicated based on histologic diagnosis.
2. Self-mutilation of the feet (If Amazons are affected, it may be called *Amazon foot necrosis* or *syndrome*.)
   - Captive birds commonly affected are Amazon parrots, particularly yellow-naped Amazons (*Amazona auropalliata*) and double yellow-headed Amazons (*Amazona oratrix*) (**Fig. 23**).[8,21]
   - It can also occur in other species, including some conures and Quaker or monk parakeets (*Myiopsitta monachus*)
   - Affected birds chew and bite at their feet and sometimes their legs. The skin becomes dry, flakey, and reddened from the persistent trauma. Bleeding and possible secondary infections are not uncommon.
   - The severity of the skin lesions may wax and wane and may be noted to be most severe in the springtime. Reasons for this are unknown but may possibly be related to inhalant or contact allergens.
   - The cause is unknown, but suggested theories include allergic, immune-mediated, bacterial, fungal, or reproductive-related causes (Dr Drury Reavill, DVM, ABVP [Avian], Zoo and Exotic Pathology Service, West Sacramento, CA, personal communication, 2013).[21,22]

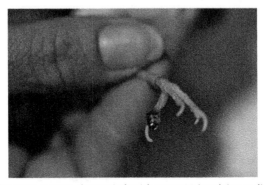

Fig. 22. A canary (*Serinus canaria domestica*) with a tumor involving a distal digit and claw.

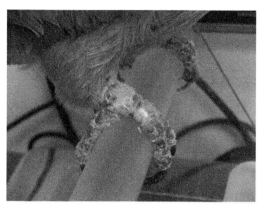

Fig. 23. Amazon foot necrosis in an older yellow-naped Amazon parrot (*Amazona auropalliata*). Note the peeling skin resulting in multiple layers of tissue exposure. These feet tend to peel, crack, bleed, and ooze, which is exacerbated by the bird's apparent intermittent irritation with its feet.

- Treatment of self-mutilation of the feet includes the following:
  - A variety of treatment protocols have resulted in only mild improvement of lesions. Topical therapy with a spray containing an antibiotic and antiinflammatory has shown to be helpful in some cases.
3. Articular gout
  - Articular gout is the deposition of uric acid crystals in the joints. The accumulation of uric acid deposits is called *tophi*. The condition itself is a form of arthritis that causes pain and swelling in the joints.

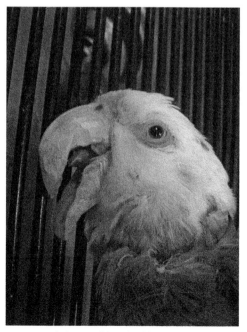

Fig. 24. Severe beak overgrowth in an older double yellow-headed Amazon parrot (*Amazona oratrix*).

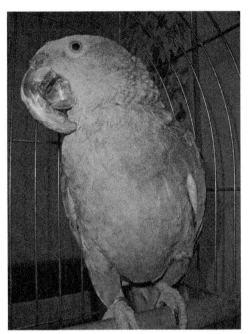

Fig. 25. Severely overgrown maxillary beak in an overweight yellow-naped Amazon parrot (*Amazona auropalliata*). Intermittent trimming is required for this bird to eat.

- These tophi tend to accumulate in the phalanges of the feet. The feet become painful, and the bird is reluctant to place weight on its feet.[8,23]
- Nodules can be visibly noted on the phalanges. They may appear white because of the tophi formation.
- It is noted with some frequency in older budgerigars.
- The cause may be multifactorial, yet is essentially undetermined and poorly understood. In some cases, it may be related to elevated uric acid levels, diet, and genetics, among other factors.

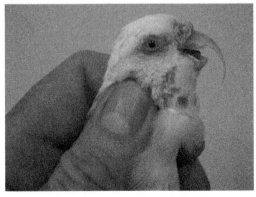

Fig. 26. A common presentation in pet budgerigars (*Melopsittacus undulates*) whereby the maxillary beak overgrows. Growth rates seem to vary with individual birds.

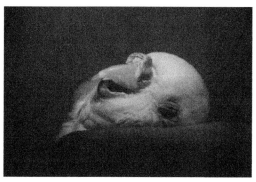

Fig. 27. Brown hypertrophy of the cere in a female budgerigar (*Melopsittacus undulatus*). Note the characteristic prominent layered look to the cere.

- Treatment of articular gout includes the following:
  - Treatment of articular gout aims to alleviate pain and prevent the long-term accumulation of uric acid crystals.
  - Treatment is not curative, and the outlook is very guarded; surgery is not recommended.
  - Medications often used for the treatment of articular gout include allopurinol, colchicines, probenecid, and nonsteroidal antiinflammatories, which can be used both topically and orally.
4. Beak overgrowth
   - Overgrowth of the beak, particularly the maxillary beak and rhamphotheca, is a fairly common presentation in captive avian species (**Figs. 24–26**).
   - It seems to most commonly occur in psittacines but is also seen in Columbiformes, passerines, and pet poultry.
   - The cause probably varies with the individual but may include previous damage to the growth areas of the beak, underlying metabolic problems, and nutritional components.
   - Treatment of an overgrown beak includes the following:
     - Intermittently trim the beak.
     - Increased use of abrasive structures in the environment does not seem to have a significant influence on the abnormal growth of the beak.
5. Brown hypertrophy of the cere
   - This condition is characterized by a visually apparent layered thickening of the cere of both sexes of budgerigars (*Melopsittacus undulatus*).[1]
   - Clinically, the condition is characterized by hyperplasia and keratinization of the cornified layer of the cere and tends to occur most commonly in older females.[8]
   - It is thought to occur when reproductive hormones (most likely estrogen) are elevated, although the cause and significance of the changes in the cere is not known.[1]
   - Treatment of brown hypertrophy of the cere is not indicated because the condition is considered to be normal (**Fig. 27**).

SUMMARY

When one considers the subject of dermatology, a common first thought is that of the skin covering the body's core, even though, in the case of a bird, the skin additionally extends over the beak, feet, and claws. These ancillary structures, the beak, claws and feet, are often involved in dermatologic conditions that affect the entire bird as well as discrete entities themselves. It is hoped that this article will open your eyes as to the possible other dermatologic presentations that involve the beak, feet, and claws (the second skin covering the bird's body).

REFERENCES

1. Cooper JE, Harrison GJ. Dermatology. In: Ritchie BW, Harrison GJ, Harrison LR, editors. Avian medicine: principles and application. Lake Worth (FL): Wingers Publishing; 1994. p. 607–39.
2. King AS, McLelland J. Integument. In: King AS, McLelland J, editors. Birds: their structure and function. 2nd edition. London: Pitman Press; 1984. p. 23–42.
3. Stettenheim PR. The integumentary morphology of modern birds-an overview. Am Zool 2000;40:461–77.
4. Degeres LA. Trauma medicine. In: Ritchie BW, Harrison GJ, Harrison LR, editors. Avian medicine: principles and application. Lake Worth (FL): Wingers Publishing; 1994. p. 417–33.
5. Bennett RA. Surgery of the avian beak. In: Proceedings of the Association of Avian Veterinarians, 32nd Annual Conference. Seattle (WA): 2011. p. 191–5.
6. Redig PT, Cruz-Martinez L. Raptors. In: Tully TN, Dorrestein GM, Jones AK, editors. Handbook of avian medicine. 2nd edition. Edinburgh (United Kingdom): Saunders Elsevier; 2009. p. 209–42.
7. Molina R. The birds of prey in the practice. In: Proceedings of the SEVC. 2008. Available at: www.ivis.org. Accessed October 23, 2012.
8. Gill JH. Avian skin diseases. In: Schmidt R, editor. The VCNA exotic animal practice: dermatology. Philadelphia: WB Saunders; 2001. p. 463–92.
9. Doolen M. Avian soft tissue surgery. Proceedings Association of Avian Veterinarians Annual Conference. 1997. p. 499–506.
10. Speer B. Surgery of the head and beak. In: Proceedings of the NAVC. Orlando (FL): 2005. p. 1214–8.
11. Speer B. Surgical procedures of the psittacine skull. In: Proceedings of the AAV, 33rd Annual Conference. Louisville (KY): 2012. p. 181–91.
12. Doneley RJ. Bacterial and parasitic diseases of parrots. In: Wade L, editor. VCNA exotic animal practice: bacterial and parasitic diseases. Philadelphia: Elsevier; 2009. p. 417–32.
13. Greiner EC, Ritchie BW. Parasites. In: Ritchie BW, Harrison GJ, Harrison LR, editors. Avian medicine: principles and application. Lake Worth (FL): Wingers Publishing; 1994. p. 1007–29.
14. Jimenez J. Avian dermatology: more than feather picking. In: Proceedings of SEVC. Barcelona. 2008. Available at: www.ivis.org. Accessed October 23, 2012.
15. Gerlach H. Viruses. In: Ritchie BW, Harrison GJ, Harrison LR, editors. Avian medicine: principles and application. Lake Worth (FL): Wingers Publishing; 1994. p. 862–948.
16. Harcourt-Brown NH. Psittacine birds. In: Tully TN, Dorrestein GM, Jones AK, editors. Handbook of avian medicine. 2nd edition. Edinburgh (United Kingdom): Saunders Elsevier; 2009. p. 138–68.
17. University of Georgia infectious disease laboratory tests and interpretation. Available at: www.vet.uga.edu/idl/. Accessed January 22, 2013.
18. Styles DK, Tomaszewski EK, Jaeger LA, et al. Psittacid herpesviruses associated with mucosal papillomas in neotropical parrots. Virology 2004;325:24–35.
19. Powers LV. Veterinary care of passerines (songbirds). AAV Proceedings. 2011. 135–47.

20. Lightfoot TL. Overview of tumors. Section I: clinical avian neoplasia and oncology. In: Harrison GJ, Lightfoot TL, editors. Clinical avian medicine. Available at: www.ivis.org. Accessed October 23, 2012.
21. Koski MA. Dermatological diseases in psittacine birds: an investigational approach. Seminars in Avian and exotic Pet Medicine 2002;11(3):105–24.
22. Johnson M. Avian medicine: integument. ABVP Proceedings. 2011.
23. Macwhirter P. Malnutrition. In: Ritchie BW, Harrison GJ, Harrison LR, editors. Avian medicine: principles and application. Lake Worth (FL): Wingers Publishing; 1994. p. 842–61.

Behavioral Dermatopathies in Small Mammals

Valarie V. Tynes, DVM, Diplomate ACVB

KEYWORDS

- Behavior • Dermatology • Small mammals • Stereotypies
- Impulse control disorders • Stress

KEY POINTS

- Behavioral dermatopathies may represent maladaptive behaviors that develop secondary to the stress of an inadequate environment.
- Some of the dermatologic conditions of small mammals may reflect these maladaptive behaviors but much more research is needed to better understand their causes.
- Barbering in mice may represent a psychological disorder similar to trichotillomania in humans.
- Pain, discomfort, or altered sensation should never be ignored as a possible underlying cause for self-inflicted alopecia or injury.

INTRODUCTION

The skin is the largest organ in the body and throughout the life of the individual it plays an important role in communication on several levels. Although there is no way of knowing whether animals experience psychological distress (ie, embarrassment) caused by disfiguring skin conditions as people may, their fur does plays an important role in body homeostasis, and whiskers in particular may be critical to rodents' ability to explore their environment in a normal, effective way.

The behavioral dermatopathies include those dermatologic conditions in which the mind or emotions play a major role in the development of and/or maintenance of the skin disorder. In human medicine, the term psychodermatology is used to refer to the discipline that integrates dermatology and psychiatry, and it has been estimated that in as many as one-third of human patients with skin disease the problem is complicated by significant psychosocial and psychiatric morbidity.[1] Connecting these two disciplines is a complex interplay between the neuroendocrine and immune systems that has been described as the neuroimmunocutaneous system.[2] The close relationship between the skin and the central nervous system (CNS) has been recognized for some time and likely exists because of their common ectodermal origins. The skin and

Disclosures: The author has nothing to disclose.
Premier Veterinary Behavior Consulting, PO Box 1413, Sweetwater, TX 79556, USA
E-mail address: pigvet@hughes.net

CNS share many hormones, neuropeptides, and receptors.[3] The complex overlap between psychiatric and dermatologic disease has led to an awareness of the need for a multidisciplinary approach to many skin disorders. A biopsychosocial approach in humans is often critical to successful treatment of these conditions.[4]

There are several different systems for categorizing the psychocutaneous disorders in human medicine and there may be much overlap between these categories. One common system separates the disorders into 3 categories: the psychophysiologic disorders (in which stress plays an important role in the symptoms), the cutaneous sensory disorders, and primary psychiatric disorders resulting in cutaneous signs.[4] Although some empirical data exist on the behavioral dermatopathies of certain species, such as nonhuman primates and mice, little is known about some of the behavioral skin conditions of other species, such as the sugar glider and the chinchilla, making it difficult to apply these categories to small mammals. Many of the conditions that are described in this article likely represent true psychopathologies that result in skin lesions. Others may represent maladaptive behaviors that occur as an individual attempts to cope with an environment that it did not evolve to deal with. It is also possible that stress of varying degrees, and that occurs at varying periods during development, plays an important role in many behavioral dermatopathies, resulting in some overlap of causation. To further complicate matters, the nonverbal characteristic of veterinary patients means that it is impossible to know what they are experiencing, thus cutaneous sensory disorders may never be well understood and the potential for pain, discomfort, or other forms of altered sensation to be the driving cause behind a skin lesion must never be underestimated. Future research into the genetics of behavior and the role of temperament should continue to shed light on why some animals develop these problems.

Stress and boredom are words frequently used to describe causes for the development of these conditions. However, these terms are used in a nonspecific way and greatly oversimplify what are complex, multifactorial conditions. The role that stress plays in the development of skin disorders in humans is only now beginning to be elucidated and has been determined to play an important role both in the development of and maintenance of many common skin conditions.

In addition, in animals, some of the behavioral dermatopathies may be in the category of abnormal repetitive behaviors. Abnormal repetitive behaviors are a heterogeneous set of behaviors that include skin picking, feather picking, hair plucking or chewing, as well as pacing, somersaulting, tongue rolling, and bar chewing. For many years in the veterinary literature, the terms stereotypies and compulsive disorders have been used interchangeably when describing these behaviors but recent research is pointing to the likelihood that many of these behaviors have differing neurobiological underpinnings and caution must be used when applying these labels. The current research is suggesting that stereotypies and impulsive/compulsive disorders represent dysfunction arising from 2 different systems within the brain and represent 2 different classes of repetitive behavior.[5] It is important to be aware of these likely differences in order to understand the potential causes of these behaviors and ultimately discover how to either prevent or treat them.

PSYCHOPHYSIOLOGIC DISORDERS

The psychophysiologic disorders are skin disorders that can be precipitated by stress. Several chronic dermatoses in human patients have been identified that fit these criteria. They include acne, psoriasis, and atopic dermatitis.[6] In small mammals, it is possible that fur plucking or chewing in chinchillas and guinea pigs may be in this category but the cause of most of the behavioral dermatopathies in animals remains unclear. With the increasing amount of information supporting barbering in mice as a model for human trichotillomania (hair plucking), the possibility that all of the other conditions listed earlier instead represent true psychopathologies cannot be ignored. Nevertheless, if confronted with any skin condition in which pruritus seems to be playing a role, then the contribution of stress to the itch-scratch-itch cycle must be considered as well. To further complicate attempts at categorizing these conditions, stress often contributes to the development of many of the psychopathologies, such as stereotypies and impulse control disorders as well as a variety of other medical conditions.

Stress and the Skin

The reaction of the skin to stress includes increased sweat gland activity and increases in skin conductance. In humans, skin conductance is considered to be a direct measure of general sympathetic nervous system arousal.[7] The skin is directly affected by stress, especially when the individual's ability to cope is overwhelmed. The skin is richly innervated and has bilateral communication with the CNS where it is involved in regulating affect and coping with intense emotional states. Sympathetic hyperarousal is a feature of several psychopathological states in humans including the self-induced dermatoses, such as trichotillomania.[7] The skin is both a target and a source of key stress mediators. As a result of stress, the skin experiences enhanced immune function and increased intracutaneous migration of immune competent cells. With time, chronic stress leads to suppressed cutaneous immunity.[7]

The stress response begins when the body perceives a threat to homeostasis. It does not matter whether the threat is real or not, only how the animal perceives it.[8] Stress can be defined as the neuroendocrine response of the organism to a threat, which often requires an adaptation of function as the organism attempts to cope with adverse effects of the environment and management.[9] If the subsequent reaction is damaging to the individual, leading to associated changes in behavior, physiology, and disease susceptibility, then the individual may be said to be experiencing distress.[10]

To further review, the first recognized stress axis is the sympathetic axis (SA). Under acute stress, activation of the SA results in rapid redistribution of the cells of the immune system into target organs. One of the most significant effects is the activation of natural killer cells and the enhancement of neutrophil function and cellular immunity.[9]

The second stress axis is the hypothalamic pituitary axis (HPA). Depending on the secretion mode and amounts, the neuropeptide and endocrine mediators released by the activation of this axis produce a large number of immunologic effects.[9] These mediators act systemically and locally to produce a response ideally suited to adapt to either acute or chronic challenges. Under chronic stress, the mediators released by the HPA have been implicated as the prime mechanism for the stress-induced induction and aggravation of allergic and autoimmune disease.[11]

More recently a third stress axis has been postulated, mediated by neurotrophins and neuropeptides, such as substance P, nerve growth factor (NGF), and brain-derived neurotrophin factor (BDNF).[9] These neuropeptide mediators activate neurogenic inflammation, which leads to the degranulation of mast cells, enhanced endothelial permeability, plasma extravasation, and infiltration of affected tissue. This neuroimmune response has been shown to aggravate virtually all of the chronic inflammatory diseases of the skin studied thus far.[9] More importantly, substance P supports acute inflammatory cellular immune responses. NGF is produced in peripheral tissues in response to perceived or mechanical stress and it has been shown to play a key role in aggravating humeral, allergic, and hyperproliferative cutaneous inflammation. BDNF has been shown to play an important role in stress biology and neuroimmune regulation and may prove to be a useful marker for acute stress and cellular immunity.[9]

Furthermore, the skin is equipped with an abundant supply of nerve fibers that travel in close contact with keratinocytes, Schwann cells, fibroblasts, endothelial cells, mast cells, and other immune cells. These cell populations produce neurotrophins and plasticity of peripheral innervation that leads to contact between nerve fibers and cells of the immune system.[11] These changes facilitate neurogenic inflammation and promote cutaneous inflammation in healthy as well as diseased skin. The neurotrophins, neuropeptides, and cytokines derived from the skin subsequently have an effect on the central stress axis. Thus, the peripheral immune response and the central stress axis are intimately interconnected in a bidirectional manner.[9]

Stress can contribute to the worsening of many pruritic skin conditions, as well. Psychological stress lowers the itch threshold or aggravates itch sensitivity.[12] Stress leads to the release of histamines, vasoactive neuropeptides, and inflammatory mediators, as well as contributing to stress-related hemodynamic changes (changes in skin temperature, blood flow, and sweat responses), all of which contribute to the itch-scratch-itch cycle.[13]

In addition, stress can also interfere with normal hair growth. When stressed, the nerve fibers associated with hair follicles result in the release of substance P and neurotrophins as well as mast cell activation that can block normal hair growth in mice, whether or not they have a genetic predisposition to alopecia.[14,15] These effects suggest how stress may play a role in the alopecia seen in small rodents such as breeding female guinea pigs.

PRIMARY PSYCHIATRIC DISORDERS WITH CUTANEOUS SIGNS

In humans, this category includes trichotillomania, delusional parasitosis, and body dysmorphic disorder (a condition characterized by a person's preoccupation with a perceived defect or an excessive concern with a slight physical abnormality).[4] Much research into barbering in mice has led to the recent theory that barbering in mice may share a similar phenomenology to trichotillomania in humans, and the mouse may serve as an excellent model for this condition.[16]

Abnormal Repetitive Behaviors

Because of a history of confusing terminology, the term abnormal repetitive behaviors is often used in an attempt to simplify a group of conditions about which much remains to be learned. Stereotypies, obsessive-compulsive disorders, compulsive disorders, and impulse control disorders can all be included under this heading. Although these conditions all share some similarities, research is continuing to reveal some important differences between them.

The term stereotypy is used to refer to a behavior that is repetitive, invariant, and seems to serve no function. One of the most intriguing aspects of stereotypies is the huge variety of forms that they can take between and within species. Thus tigers pace; elephants sway; rodents back flip, bar bite, and spin; and calves tongue roll. The feature that most of these unusual behaviors seem to have in common is that of frustration; frustration that seems to arise because of the thwarting of highly motivated behaviors (**Box 1**).[17,18] These behaviors have not been documented in noncaptive animals so they are generally thought to be associated with a captive and suboptimal environment. Stereotypies have been suggested to develop as a result of an animal's attempts to cope with a stressful environment but no research has been able to

---

Box 1
Some important definitions

Conflict occurs when an individual is motivated to perform 2 opposing behaviors at the same time.

Frustration occurs when an individual is motivated to perform a particular behavior but is somehow prevented from doing so.

- If conflict and frustration are constant, the result is stress.

- The resulting stress often leads to the development of one or both of the following:

  Displacement behavior is a normal behavior shown at an inappropriate time or out of context for the situation.

  Grooming behaviors are commonly displayed as displacement behaviors.

  Redirected behavior is a behavior that is directed away from the principle target and toward another less appropriate target.

  Aggressive behaviors are commonly seen as redirected behaviors.

---

confirm that all stereotypies succeed in helping animals cope. They may even represent psychological disorders secondary to the inability to carry out highly motivated normal species-typical behaviors. They are thus thought to reflect poor welfare.

Many abnormal repetitive behaviors, including most of the behavioral dermatopathies, are not as unvarying in their repetition and more likely represent impulse control disorders. Impulse control disorders lie within the spectrum of obsessive-compulsive disorders and research is now suggesting that many of the abnormal repetitive behaviors seen in animals (in particular, some of the behavioral dermatopathies such as barbering in mice and feather picking in psittacines) are likely to be in this category. Malfunction in the circuitry involving the basal ganglia and the prefrontal cortex has been shown to lead to the perseveration of behavior (the inappropriate repetition of behavior), and an inability to shift goals that is typical of the impulsive/compulsive disorders.[5] This finding may represent the neurophysiology underlying these unusual behaviors but still does not answer why many animals develop these problems. Not all animals living in captive environments develop repetitive behaviors.

It is theorized by some that an individual's genetic makeup predisposes it to develop abnormal repetitive behaviors when exposed to certain environmental experiences. In animals, these experiences may be associated with inappropriate environment, early or abrupt weaning, or other forms of stress during development. In addition, it has been shown that developing in an impoverished environment leads to permanent changes within the CNS. Animals forced to live in a barren environment during the early weeks, months, or years of their development have been shown to have fewer neurons in their brain, decreased dendritic branching and spine density, and reduced synaptic connectivity, plus a higher incidence of abnormal repetitive behaviors.[19,20] This finding further points to the complex, multifactorial basis of these problems, why they may be so difficult to prevent and treat, and why boredom alone does not help explain the development of the abnormal repetitive behaviors.

Self-injurious Behaviors (Self-mutilation)

Pathologic self-mutilating behavior has been studied in humans for more than 75 years, but little is understood about the psychological function of this behavior or its cause.[21]

Pathologic self-injury is not necessarily related to cognitive impairment and, in the human literature, is differentiated from the self-injurious stereotypical behavior seen in mentally retarded or autistic children. Self-mutilation is repetitive but is not considered a stereotypy. In humans, it is often referred to as self-cutting, self-mutilation, self-harm, or self-injurious behavior (SIB), and cutting the arms or legs using knives or razor blades is the most commonly seen form of the behavior. Most patients seen in psychiatric clinics for SIB are single female adolescents or young adults.[21,22] The precipitating event is often a real or perceived interpersonal loss. However, more recent research has shown that these patients are more likely to come from families of divorce, neglect, or parental deprivation. A history of physical or sexual abuse is also often associated with the condition,[21–23] again highlighting the important role stress may play in all aspects of health. Most commonly, SIB is associated with another psychological disorder such as a personality disorder. However, other conditions such as major or minor depressive disorders, schizophrenia, obsessive-compulsive disorders, substance abuse, and eating disorders have also been associated with SIB. Some researchers argue that rather than being a symptom of another condition, SIB should be the primary criterion for a separate diagnosis of self-harm and suggest that it is an impulse disorder.[22,24]

Individuals generally report feeling tense, anxious, angry, or fearful before self-injury. They also generally report no pain when cutting and state that the feelings of anxiety, anger, or fear disappear afterward.[25] They also often report feeling a sense of release, relief, satisfaction, or calm after cutting. These reports have led to one of the popular models for explaining the function of SIB; the affect regulation model, in which it is postulated that the behavior functions to help the individual gain some control over an overwhelming emotional state.[23] In support of this model, researchers have found that self-injury is often associated with a decrease in physiologic arousal as measured by finger blood volume, heart and respiratory rates, and skin resistance levels.[26]

In animals, SIB has been most studied in nonhuman primates and is phenomenologically similar to SIB in humans in many ways. Rather than seeing it as a symptom of a psychopathological problem, it is thought by some to represent a maladaptive coping mechanism, similar to many of the other abnormal repetitive behaviors of captive animals.[23] In animals, SIBs are typically included under the broader context of stereotypic or abnormal repetitive behaviors. In primates, the term SIB also usually includes self-injury as well as hair plucking.

A common factor linking most cases of SIB is rearing in a suboptimal environment. Social isolation is considered an important risk factor[23] and the provision of social companionship has been shown to stop SIB in some cases.[27,28] Stressors such as relocation have also been shown to increase the severity of SIB in rhesus macaques.[29] However, it is also clear that not all animals that experience suboptimal environments, or other stressors, display SIB so, again, a genetic predisposition may exist that leads to this type of response to a stressful environment.

To further complicate matters, self-injury can also occur as a result of increased pain sensitivity or dysesthesia, so careful attention to appropriate use of analgesics and antiinflammatories may be necessary when managing any self-inflicted injury in an animal.

CUTANEOUS SENSORY DISORDERS

Cutaneous sensory disorders in humans are not associated with any identifiable organic cause, but because of the subjective nature of the individual's experience, these can be challenging problems to deal with. In humans, sensations of burning, crawling, stinging, and pruritus may be described. Neuropathic itch can occur as a result of multiple sclerosis or spinal tumors. Psychogenic itch can be associated with depression, obsessive-compulsive disorders, and psychotic illness.[4]

Cutaneous sensory disorders in animals homologous to those in humans have not been clearly defined. However, much evidence exists pertaining to animals self-traumatizing in association with pain, paresthesia, or dysesthesia.[30,31] Rodents self-mutilate a limb that has been denervated.[30] SIB has been seen in humans with neuropathic pain[32] and self-mutilation has been described in rodents and rabbits after intramuscular injection of anesthetic agents resulting in nerve damage.[33,34] In these cases, the self-mutilation can occur as much as 7 to 14 days after the injection.[33,34]

When presented with any animal that is self-traumatizing either by scratching or biting, the clinician should not be too quick to determine that the problem is purely behavioral. If in doubt, it is more humane to err on the side of assuming that the animal is experiencing some uncomfortable sensation than to focus on behavioral remedies such as environmental enrichment while leaving the animal to suffer. A trial of analgesics or antiinflammatories may be useful in getting to the cause of the problem.

SOME BEHAVIORAL DERMATOPATHIES OF SMALL MAMMALS
Alopecia

Alopecia can be a nonspecific sign in many animals. Infectious, parasitic, and metabolic conditions must all be ruled out. In addition, rough hair coats may also be a nonspecific sign of a medical problem and may be associated with dehydration, malnutrition, or general malaise leading to inadequate or ineffective grooming behavior.

Some alopecia, such as bald noses on small rodents, is a result of behavior but does not necessarily represent a psychological disorder. Rubbing the nose against rough cage edges or between bars of block feeders can result in hair loss around the nose and face. Correcting these conditions simply requires finding and repairing rough edges and changing feeding methods whenever possible.

Hair pulling is a behavior that occurs in humans and may be seen in some animals when confined in a captive environment. In humans, the condition is called trichotillomania and is seen more often in female patients. It commonly manifests in contexts of depression, anxiety, frustration, and boredom.[35] In nonhuman primates, it is usually directed toward a subordinate but occasionally is self-directed. However, one study found that in a group of rhesus macaques, most group members both plucked and were recipients of plucking, which detracts from the theory that it is associated with dominance behvaiors.[36] In primates, hair plucking is associated with moderate to intense crowding conditions that result in social stress. In single caged primates, it is the most common behavioral disorder with some primates plucking until they are almost bald. Others focus plucking to 1 area of the body, leading to focalized areas of alopecia and in some cases bleeding skin. Promoting more species-typical behavior patterns has been reported to be helpful in decreasing the severity of hair plucking behavior.[35] Hair loss among nonhuman primates is a complex problem and one study in rhesus macaques found it to be affected by multiple factors including substrate, reproductive condition, rank, season, and age. The lack of foraging opportunities coupled with social stressors resulted in worse hair loss in lower ranking monkeys.[37]

Barbering (hair pulling) has been described in gerbils housed in large groups.[38] Hair loss has been described on the crown of the head and the base of the tail,[38] as well the ventral areas, legs, neck, flank, and thorax.[39] Some investigators recommend reducing population density, as well as removing the dominant animal and improving husbandry.[38]

One retrospective study of pet degus presented to one animal hospital described alopecia caused by fur chewing and found it to be the second most common condition for which degus were presented.[40] Hair loss was most notable on forepaws and medial aspects of the thighs. Both self-barbering and barbering of cage mates was described. Barbering of cage mates was ascribed to dominance behavior and lack of foraging opportunities was claimed to be the cause of self-barbering even though no description of how these determinations were made was included in the report.[40] Another author has suggested that degus may develop stereotypies and self-mutilation behaviors when foraging opportunities are lacking.[41]

Rabbit fur pulling has also been described by at least one researcher who found it in both singly housed and group housed individuals of both sexes.[35] However, it was suggested that it occurred more often in singly housed than group housed individuals. The provision of species-typical foraging opportunities may prevent the problem but no empirical data were given to support either of these contentions. It is normal for female rabbits to remove some of their hair when nesting and this should not be confused with a psychological disorder.

Pet prairie dogs and rats have also been noted to pull hair or barber or excessively groom one another, resulting in alopecia.[38] Literature on barbering in rats seems to be scarce. More research on barbering or hair pulling in rodents other than mice is needed before it is possible to determine that these are homologous conditions that share similar causes or functions.

Barbering in Mice

Barbering (fur/whisker trimming, the Dalila effect) is a common spontaneously occurring abnormal behavior of mice in which mice chew, pluck, and remove the whiskers and fur of their cage mates (**Figs. 1** and **2**).[16] Some mice spend time manipulating and chewing on the hair after removal and eventually consume the hair. Barbering seems to be painful for the mouse being plucked, and the barber mouse often holds its cage mate down to pluck hair from it.[42] Barbering mice have even been known to pluck hair

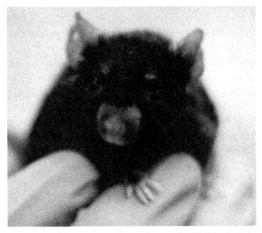

Fig. 1. Barbering in a mouse. (*Courtesy of* Tom Donnelly, DVM, Ossining, NY.)

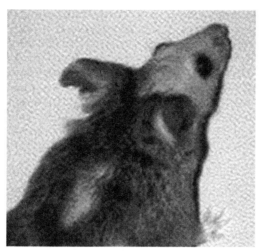

Fig. 2. Barbering in a mouse. (*Courtesy of* Tom Donnelly, DVM, Ossining, NY.)

from other species (eg, rats) if confined with them.[43] The skin of barbered mice is typically not erythematous and barbered mice show no indication of pruritus. Scratches, scabs, or ulcerated lesions should not be present in a barbered mouse. When barbering is suspected, bacterial infections, dermatophytes, and ectoparasites must be ruled out as possible causes for the hair loss.

Barbering shares many similarities to trichotillomania in humans and it has recently been shown that barbering also shares neurophysiologic biomarkers with trichotillomania, suggesting that it is a highly specific animal model for trichotillomania with neurobiological underpinnings that are unique from obsessive-compulsive disorders and stereotypies.[44] Barbering mice predominantly remove hair from around the eyes, the top of the head, and the genitals of other mice, similarly to patients with trichotillomania. Genetics plays an important role in barbering, with marked differences in frequencies between different strains of mice.[43,45] Trichotillomania has also been shown to have a heritable component in people. Epidemiologic studies have shown that barbering is more common in female mice than male mice, and that it typically begins at or around the time of sexual maturation.[16] Female breeding mice also show barbering behavior at a higher rate than nonbreeding mice. This finding also parallels trichotillomania in humans with many women reporting worsening severity of signs associated with pregnancy. The reasons behind these differences have not been elucidated but are suspected to be associated with changes in oxytocin levels associated with the reproductive cycle. Oxytocin is also known to play a role in grooming behavior of rodents.[16]

In the past, several husbandry factors (eg, diet, weaning age and enrichment, overcrowding)[46,47] have been suspected of affecting barbering and it has been hypothesized that barbering occurs as result of stress.[48,49] The evidence on the role of population density in barbering mice is equivocal[50] but one study found higher concentrations of fecal corticosterone metabolites in mice confined to higher density housing, lending some support to the role of stress caused by overcrowding in barbering.[51]

Another study showed that mice were more likely to barber if housed in stainless rather than plastic caging and if housed with siblings rather than nonsiblings.[50] Barbering was more severe in mice that lived in plastic cages located on higher shelves, whereas the lower the steel cage, the less severe the barbering. This finding suggests that, for the mouse, an animal that is typically cover seeking, the housing situation that leaves it the most exposed may lead to the higher level of stress.[50] It can be postulated that barbering was more severe among siblings because of their inability to disperse from their natal territory as they normally would in the wild. Being forced into confinement and unable to disperse may lead to social stress. The same study also found that there may be some social transmission of barbering behavior. Whether this is caused by learning or stimulus enhancement has yet to be clarified. Barbering mice were also noted to remove idiosyncratic patterns of hair from other mice, and these patterns were more similar within barbers in a cage compared with barbers in other cages.[50]

Contrary to popular belief, the evidence is mounting that barbering is not a dominance behavior. Barbering has been shown to develop in both dominant and subordinate mice.[16] Another study showed that barbering mice were not all dominant to nonbarbering mice.[50] In addition, studies have shown that some mice self-barber, further eroding the theory that dominance is involved in the behavior. Self-barbering individuals confine their barbering to their ventrum and the ventral surfaces of their forelegs. This distribution of hair removal may have been easily overlooked in the past, thus allowing the misconception that barbering mice only barbered their cage mates. However, other studies have documented a negative correlation between aggression and barbering, suggesting that barbering may substitute for aggression and does play some role in the establishment of a hierarchy within a group of mice.[49]

Environmental enrichment has been shown to delay onset and reduce the overall prevalence of barbering in a predisposed strain of mice. The enrichment in this particular study was in the form of larger cages and the provision of manipulable items that were rotated on a biweekly basis.[52]

What should not be in dispute is that barbering is associated with poor welfare. Whiskers play an important role in the behavioral repertoire of the mouse and their removal must be significant to the mouse. In addition, the frequency with which stressful environments are associated with hair pulling in all documented species supports the need for further study into the welfare implications of barbering and other hair pulling or hair chewing behaviors.

In addition, barbering has been associated with mandibulofacial and maxillofacial abscesses in mice. It is suspected that the mastication and fragmentation of hair allows it to be trapped in the gingival sulcus. The hair acts as a foreign body, resulting in ulceration and inflammation, and allows commensal bacteria to be carried deep into the submucosa, leading to abscesses and, in some cases, osteomyelitis.[53]

Fur Chewing in Chinchillas

Fur chewing, or fur-biting, is a problem found in chinchillas in which fur is chewed, primarily from the sides and hips, flanks, ventral neck, legs, paws, and thorax, resulting in patchy alopecia and broken hair shafts.[38,39] Some investigators have also referred to this as barbering.[38] The head often remains unaffected, which suggests that in many cases the individual is removing its own hair. Some investigators have reported the chewing of hair by cage mates, and occasional secondary cutaneous ulcers have also been reported.[39] There is no evidence that fur chewing chinchillas ingest hair, and one study failed to show any hair within the gastrointestinal tract at necropsy.[54]

Reports of fur chewing associated with dental disease have also been published,[55,56] which suggests that, in some cases, fur chewing may be associated with chronic pain or stress and emphasizes the need for further research in this area to prevent needless suffering.

This incidence of fur chewing in farm-raised chinchillas has been shown to range from 4% to 30%.[57,58] Most information published on the problem has been performed using farm-raised chinchillas so the incidence of the problem in pet chinchillas that are not housed under intensive rearing conditions has not been documented. In the past, fur chewing has been suspected of being associated with dietary deficiencies, endocrine imbalance, dermatophytes, and stressors such as overcrowding.[57] Research has found correlations between increased thyroid activity, increased adrenal activity, and reduced body temperature in fur chewing chinchillas.[59] However, it has been suggested that the changes in thyroid activity and body temperature are secondary to the hair loss, not the cause of it. More recent studies suggest that fur chewing is likely stress related. One study found higher urinary cortisol metabolites as well as increased anxietylike behaviors in female chinchillas that expressed high levels of fur chewing.[60] Another study showed histopathologic changes in the skin and adrenal glands of fur chewing chinchilla that were typical of Cushing syndrome.[54] Although it is unlikely that a simple cause-and-effect relationship exists between hyperadrenocorticism and fur chewing in the chinchilla, the data from this study suggest that fur chewing chinchillas are particularly sensitive to the effects of stress.[54] It has been suggested that the condition has a heritable component[38,39] and that an inability for some individuals to cope with the stress of captivity could be genetically transmitted.

A survey of fur chewing in commercially raised chinchillas[58] attempted to identify any management and/or environmental factors that influenced the occurrence of fur chewing. The study found several risk factors for fur chewing in the chinchillas. There was a lower incidence of fur chewing in farms where the breeder had 3 or more years of experience, wood shavings were changed more frequently each week, and the volume of the facility was larger. Contrary to what might be expected, this study found a lower incidence of fur chewing in more densely populated facilities. These farmed chinchillas were housed singly in identically sized cages. What varied by facility was the numbers of chinchillas placed within each room within the facility. Because the chinchillas had olfactory, auditory, and visual contact with one another, the perception of being crowded may remain high, regardless of the population density.[58] If the social organization of the chinchilla in the wild is taken into consideration, these results might seem less surprising. Chinchillas in the wild live in large colonies of several hundred animals that may range over a territory of 1.5 to 113.5 ha (3.75–285 acres).[61] It is possible that the presence of higher numbers of conspecifics gives animals the perception of increased protection from predators, thus resulting in decreased fur chewing and supporting the suggestion that fur chewing occurs secondary to a stressful environment. Although some reports have found that high stocking density in rodent habitats leads to behavioral and physiologic changes, others have found no effect. The role of stocking density in rodent housing needs further study.

The frequency of dust baths did not predict fur chewing. However, there was a tendency for more dust baths to be associated with lower incidence of fur chewing. The trend was not statistically significant. The study also examined the presence or absence of loud noises in the area of the farm and found a slight tendency for higher noise levels and fur chewing to be associated. The chinchilla has excellent auditory capabilities and the potential for loud noises to be uncomfortable is high, but the correlation in this study only approached significance.[58]

Although the term barbering has occasionally been used to describe the problem, to date no research has confirmed that it is homologous to barbering in mice, although it shares some similarities. For example, one study documented a higher incidence in females[58] and another suggested that fur chewing first appears around the time of puberty.[54] Both of these features are common to barbering in mice and trichotillomania in humans.

Guinea Pig Alopecia

The alopecia commonly seen in guinea pigs has also been referred to as barbering and trichophagia.[39,62] Few controlled studies have been performed in an attempt to further elucidate the causes behind noninfectious hair loss in the guinea pig. Hair growth may stop when a female pig is bred, frequently resulting in varying degrees of alopecia. Female guinea pigs with cystic ovaries also show bilateral symmetric hair loss over their flanks and rumps (**Fig. 3**). The hair loss associated with pregnancy in guinea pigs is referred to as effluvium postpartum and is likely caused by high levels of estrogen.[62,63] Under the influence of estrogen, hairs enter the telogen phase and stop growing. Six weeks later, new hairs begin growing and the old, dead hairs are brittle and easily epilated. It has been hypothesized that trichophagia may be easiest and least painful for the guinea pig at this time.[62]

Trichophagia, or barbering, behavior has been noted in guinea pigs of all ages and genders and has not been observed to cause distress in the pig being barbered.[62] The resulting patchy alopecia usually presents as broken hair shafts without any apparent inflammation. Self-barbering also has been described that occurs on the dorsal lumbar and flank areas.[38] Barbering of cage mates results in hair loss on the rump, back, ears, and around the eyes, and has been attributed by some investigators to dominance.[39,63] Barbering of the young around the eyes and ears and chewing of the sow's hair by young has also been reported.[63] Particularly severe chewing has been described among males caused by competition associated with food, water, toys, or space, and also been attributed to dominant-submissive relationships.[63]

Different investigators have suggested that guinea pig barbering may develop because of boredom, stress, or overcrowding, as has been suggested with other rodents.[39,63,64] The behavior has also been hypothesized to occur during the development of social hierarchies.[64] Suggestions for the prevention of barbering and hair chewing have included reducing environmental stressors, enriching the environment, increasing roughage, provision of chew toys, weaning early, and separation of boars into individual cages.[38,63] However, no empirical evidence has been published to confirm the efficacy of these methods or to show any information about the neurobiological underpinnings of this condition.

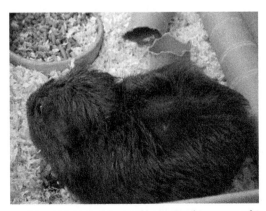

Fig. 3. Hair loss in a guinea pig caused by cystic ovaries. (*Courtesy of* Peter G Fisher, DVM, Virginia Beach, VA.)

One study examined the role of diet in guinea pig alopecia and found that a high-protein, low-fiber diet resulted in thinning hair in breeding animals.[62] When fiber was increased, hair growth noticeably improved. The data from this study suggest that, although proper nutrition in the form of a high-fiber diet is important, the presence of additional hay in the environment is also important. This finding may be a result of the opportunity for foraging it provides, especially because spreading hay throughout the habitat resulted in less alopecia than when hay was placed in a single, central location. The study did not attempt to document or quantify the amount of trichophagia that occurred or which animals engaged in trichophagia (or their position in the hierarchy) so it is still unclear how the role of nutrition and behavior interact in this condition.

Hair loss progressing to ulcers has also been described in the guinea pig and the possible suggested causes include physical trauma from rough caging or bedding, trauma from fighting, dietary deficiency, and stress.[65]

Self-mutilation in Sugar Gliders

Self-mutilation in sugar gliders has been mentioned by several investigators but no empirical research has been published documenting incidence, cause, or potential treatments for the problem. Pacing and mutilation of feet, tails, and scrotum have all been described. It has been anecdotally described as being stress related and being more likely in solitarily housed animals.[38,66] Because inappropriate husbandry and nutrition have historically been the cause of most health problems of sugar gliders in captivity, the behavior may be a form of SIB similar to the SIB that occurs in nonhuman primates.

However, sugar gliders are also known to mutilate surgical sites so the possibility that these behaviors are associated with pain or neurasthenia should not be ignored (**Fig. 4**). One case report of self-mutilation in a sugar glider described the mutilation of a pericloacal mass that was associated with transitional cell carcinoma.[67] These incidences should remind the clinician that self-mutilation in any species may be related to sensations of pain or discomfort that animal patients cannot describe and that the more commonly available diagnostics cannot identify.

Treatment of self-mutilating sugar gliders with fluoxetine at 0.5 to 1 mg/kg by mouth daily has been recommended[38] but no data exist as to its efficacy for this condition. The selective serotonin reuptake inhibitors (SSRIs) such as fluoxetine or paroxetine have typically been used to treat stereotypic behaviors and impulsive/compulsive behaviors in animals. However, the tricyclic antidepressant, clomipramine, has also been used, all with varying degrees of efficacy. In nonhuman primates, the evidence suggests that SIB is linked to malfunctions in both the norepinephrine and serotonin neurotransmitter systems, suggesting that tricyclic antidepressant such as clomipramine might be the more appropriate choice for treatment.[68] Research into which neurotransmitter systems are involved in these types of behavior, and therefore which medications may be appropriate, are ongoing and more knowledge is needed before clinicians can choose any medication and be confident of its safety and efficacy in the treatment of any of the behavioral dermatopathies.

Ulcerative Dermatitis

Ulcerative dermatitis (UD) is a severe inflammatory skin disorder of unknown cause. It is most prevalent in C57BL/6 and related strains of inbred mice.[69] UD lesions typically begin as superficial excoriations that progress to deep, necrotic ulcerations with serocellular crusts.[69,70] They are characterized by profound inflammation, and mice with UD frequently have to be euthanized for humane reasons. UD lesions have been

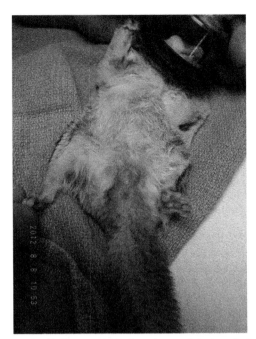

Fig. 4. This sugar glider was licking excessively at its caudal ventral abdomen as the result of an infected pericloacal gland abscess. Once treated with analgesics and antibiotics this excessive grooming behavior stopped. (*Courtesy of* Cindy Fulton, DVM, VCA, Portsmouth, NH.)

determined to be self-inflicted because of severe pruritus and recent research has determined that the lesions are typical wounds that are subject to normal wound healing.[71] The lesions usually present on the dorsal scapula but torso, shoulder, head, and facial lesions are also seen.[69,70] Lesions may be single or multifocal in distribution. Disease prevalence peaks at 10 to 16 months of age but the pathogenesis is poorly understood and the epidemiology is complex. Numerous environmental factors, including temperature, humidity, and nutrition have been hypothesized to play a role. Other possible associated causes considered have been age, gender,[69,70] immune complex vasculitis,[70] and primary follicular dystrophy.[72] Some suggest that hypersensitivity to *Staphylococcus aureus* may play a role in the pathogenesis.[73] In one study, calorie restriction strongly reduced the incidence of ulcerative dermatitis in C57BL/6 wild-type mice,[74] and another study increased the incidence of UD in the same strain of mice with a high-fat diet.[75] Numerous treatments have been studied, including maropitant citrate,[76] cyclosporine,[73] vitamin E,[77] Caladryl lotion,[78] and toenail trimming.[79] Although these interventions have all reduced the severity of lesions, none are curative.[76] However, more recently, one study found that prophylactically feeding young mice higher levels of vitamin E led to the development of UD earlier than in mice that did not receive supplementary vitamin E.[80] All of this evidence supports the theory that UD is primarily an inflammatory condition and the lesions self-inflicted because of extreme pain or pruritus. However, the cause of the inflammation remains a mystery.

One study found a significant association between UD and hair-induced inflammatory lesions of the oronasal cavities.[81] Marked periodontal alveolar bone resorption and new bone formation were associated with most of the inflammatory lesions, suggesting that the pain and discomfort associated with the severe inflammation leads to excessive scratching, self-trauma, and ulceration of the skin. The cascade of local inflammatory mediators that follows results in the itch-scratch-itch cycle being further perpetuated.[81] Severe cases of chronic human periodontitis have been associated with vasoconstriction and free radical production, which stimulate scratching behavior. Severe pain associated with the inflammation has also been reported.[81] However, other investigators have noted that severe foreign body periodontitis such as that described in the Duarte-Vogel study is common in many strains of mice that do not show barbering or UD. Further research is needed to determine whether the correlation is causal.

To further complicate matters, newer evidence suggests that UD may also be a behavioral disorder. Increasing brain serotonin through a diet high in tryptophan increased the severity of UD in a population of C57BL/6 mice.[82] In humans, compulsive skin picking has also been induced by serotonergic agents. This research suggests that UD may share some phenomenological similarities with other body-focused repetitive disorders (BFRD) in humans, such as skin picking.[82] However, this study further shows how much is yet to be learned about these conditions because serotonergic agents have also shown efficacy in treating some patients with BRFDs.

UD has also been described in rats as being caused by self-trauma secondary to staphylococcus infections.[38] These lesions appear as irregular circumscribed ulcers over the head, shoulders, rib cage, neck, and ears. It has also been stated that the problem is more common in males but minimal empirical evidence has been published, leaving many questions about the cause of this condition and the possibility that it represents a psychological disorder.[38]

TREATMENT OF THE BEHAVIORAL DERMATOPATHIES

Because so little information exists about the cause of the behavioral dermatopathies treatment can only be discussed in generalities. Until the neurobiological basis of the conditions can be better understood, treatment with psychotropic medications will be challenging and should not be attempted until all husbandry and environmental needs have been met. Whenever possible, attention must be given to the normal social structure of the species and attempts made to provide the animal with the appropriate social milieu. Providing appropriate social companions has been found to aid in the treatment of SIB in primates.[27]

The recommendation to enrich the environment is commonly made but minimal data exist that show exactly what form enrichment should take with every species or how effective it is. The most important criteria for environmental enrichment must be that it is biologically relevant for the species. To provide the needed environmental enrichment, the question that should first be asked and answered concerns what the animal would be doing if it were in the wild. For example, if dealing with a species that spends 75% of its time foraging, then opportunities for foraging must be increased as much as possible. If the species spends most of its time under cover, then the habitat must provide adequate cover so that the animal feels secure.

Enrichment should provide the animal with opportunities to perform species-typical behaviors and give the animal some control over its environment wherever possible. Being able to control certain aspects of the environment (for example, nest building for thermoregulation) has been shown to decrease the stress of the captive environment for many species.

In addition, every effort must be made to improve on aspects of the environment that the animal finds stressful, remembering that each individual's perception of stress varies depending on many factors including genetics, early experiences, and the predictability of the stressor.[10] Environments that offer unpredictable stressors and a lack of control may be the most stressful of all.

SUMMARY

Although knowledge of the behavioral dermatopathies is growing rapidly, much remains to be learned. Primary issues that should be kept in mind include the role that stress plays in skin disease as well as abnormal repetitive behaviors. In addition, a growing body of evidence suggests that some of these conditions, barbering in particular, may represent psychological disorders. Most of the psychological disorders associated with skin conditions in animals are in the broad category of abnormal repetitive behaviors and may be similar to some of the body-focused repetitive behaviors in humans, such as trichotillomania. There is mounting evidence to suggest that these conditions are impulse control disorders distinct from stereotypies and that, just as in humans, a mixture of genetic and environmental mechanisms is involved in their development.

REFERENCES

1. Wessely SC, Lewis GH. The classification of psychiatric morbidity in attenders at a dermatology clinic. Br J Psychiatry 1989;155:686–91.
2. Basavaraj KH, Nawa MA, Rashmi R. Relevance of psychiatry in dermatology: present concepts. Indian J Psychiatry 2010;52(3):270–5.
3. Van Noorden S, Polak JM, Negri L, et al. Common peptides in the brain, intestine and skin: embryology, evolution and significance. J Endocrinol 1997;75:33–4.
4. Lawrence-Smith G. Psychodermatology. Psychiatry 2009;8(6):223–7.
5. Garner JP. Perseveration and stereotypy - systems level insights from clinical psychology. In: Mason G, Rushen J, editors. Stereotypic animal behavior, fundamentals and applications to welfare. 2nd edition. Oxfordshire (United Kingdom): CAB International; 2006. p. 121–53.
6. Tausk F, Elenkov I, Moynihan J. Psychoneuroimmunology. Dermatol Ther 2008; 21:22–31.
7. Gupta MA. Commentary: psychodermatology. Clin Dermatol 2013;31:1–2.
8. Moberg GP. Biological response to stress: implications for animal welfare. In: Moberg GP, Mench JA, editors. The biology of animal stress. Oxfordshire (United Kingdom): CAB International; 2000. p. 1–22.
9. Peters EM, Liezmann CB, Klapp BF, et al. The neuroimmune connection interferes with tissue regeneration and chronic inflammatory disease in the skin. Ann N Y Acad Sci 2012;1262:118–26.
10. Panconesi E, Hautmann G. Psychophysiology of stress in dermatology. Dermatol Clin 1996;14(3):399–422.
11. Liezmann CB, Klapp BF, Peters EM. Stress, atopy and allergy: a re-evaluation from a psychoneuroimmunologic perspective. Dermatoendocrinol 2011;3: 37–40.
12. Koblenzer CS. Stress and the skin: significance of emotional factors in dermatology. Stress Med 1988;4:21–6.
13. Koblenzer CS. Psychological and psychiatric aspects of itching. In: Bernhard JD, editor. Itch: mechanisms and management of pruritus. New York: McGraw-Hill; 1994. p. 347–56.

14. Peters EM, Arck PC, Paus R. Hair growth inhibition by psychoemotional stress: a mouse model for neural mechanisms in hair growth control. Exp Dermatol 2006; 15:1–13.

15. Siebenhaar F, Sharov AA, Peters EM, et al. Substance P as an immunomodulatory neuropeptide in a mouse model for autoimmune hair loss (alopecia areata). J Invest Dermatol 2007;127:1489–97.

16. Garner JP, Weisker SM, Dufour B, et al. Barbering (fur and whisker trimming) by mice as a laboratory model of human trichotillomania and obsessive compulsive spectrum disorders. Comp Med 2004;54(2):216–24.

17. Rushen J, Mason G. A decade-or-more's progress in understanding stereotypic behavior. In: Mason G, Rushen J, editors. Stereotypic animal behavior, fundamentals and applications to welfare. 2nd edition. Oxfordshire (United Kingdom): CAB International; 2006. p. 1–19.

18. Clubb R, Vickery S. Locomotor stereotypies in carnivores; does pacing stem from hunting, ranging or frustrated escape?. In: Mason G, Rushen J, editors. Stereotypic animal behavior, fundamentals and applications to welfare. 2nd edition. Oxfordshire (United Kingdom): CAB International; 2006. p. 58–86.

19. Cabib S. The neurobiology of stereotypy II: the role of stress. In: Mason G, Rushen J, editors. Stereotypic animal behavior, fundamentals and applications to welfare. 2nd edition. Oxfordshire (United Kingdom): CAB International; 2006. p. 227–55.

20. Lewis MH, Presti MF, Lewis JB, et al. The neurobiology of stereotypy I: environmental complexity. In: Mason G, Rushen J, editors. Stereotypic animal behavior, fundamentals and applications to welfare. 2nd edition. Oxfordshire (United Kingdom): CAB International; 2006. p. 190–226.

21. Suyemoto KL. The functions of self-mutilation. Clin Psychol Rev 1998;18(5): 531–54.

22. Messer JM, Fremouw WJ. A critical review of explanatory models for self-mutilating behaviors in adolescents. Clin Psychol Rev 2008;28:162–78.

23. Dellinger-Ness LA, Handler L. Self-injurious behavior in human and non-human primates. Clin Psychol Rev 2006;26:503–14.

24. Favazza AR. Self-mutilation. In: Jacobs DG, editor. The Harvard Medical School guide to suicide assessment and intervention. Cambridge (United Kingdom): Wiley Company; 1999. p. 124–45.

25. Nock MN. Self-Injury. Annu Rev Clin Psychol 2010;6:339–63.

26. Haines J, Williams CL, Brian KL, et al. The psychophysiology of self-mutilation. J Abnorm Psychol 1995;104:471–89.

27. DeVilliers C, Seier JV. Stopping self-injurious behavior of a young male chacma baboon (*Papio ursinus*). ATW 2010;9(2):77–80.

28. Reinhardt V. Pair-housing overcomes self-biting behaviour in macaques. Laboratory Primate Newsletters 1999;38(1):4.

29. Davenport MD, Lutz CK, Tiefenbacher S, et al. A rhesus monkey model of self-injury: effects of relocation stress on behavior and neuroendocrine function. Biol Psychiatry 2008;63:990–6.

30. Minert A, Gabay E, Dominguez C, et al. Spontaneous pain following spinal nerve injury in mice. Exp Neurol 2007;206:220–30.

31. Rahimi-Movaghar V, Yazdi A, Sadaat S. Saturated picric acid prevents autophagia and self-mutilation in laboratory rats. Acta Med Iran 2008;46(4):283–6.

32. Malais A. Compulsive targeted self-injurious behaviour in humans with neuropathic pain: a counterpart of animal autotomy? Four case reports and literature review. Pain 1996;64:569–78.

33. Beyers TM, Richardson JA, Prince MD. Axonal degeneration and self-mutilation as a complication of the intramuscular use of ketamine and xylazine in rabbits. Lab Anim Sci 1991;41:519–20.
34. Vachon P. Self-mutilation in rabbits following intramuscular ketamine-xylazine-acepromazine injections. Can Vet J 1999;40:581–2.
35. Reinhardt V. Hair pulling; a review. Lab Anim 2005;39(4):361–9.
36. Reinhardt V, Reinhardt A, Houser WD. Hair pulling-and-eating in captive rhesus monkeys. Folia Primatol (Basel) 1986;47:158–64.
37. Beisner BA, Isbell LA. Factors influencing hair loss among female captive rhesus macaques (*Macaca mulatta*). Appl Anim Behav Sci 2009;119:91–100.
38. Ellis C, Mori M. Skin diseases of rodents and small exotic mammals. Vet Clin North Am Exot Anim Pract 2001;4:493–542.
39. Hoppman E, Barron HW. Rodent dermatology. J Exot Pet Med 2007;16(4): 238–55.
40. Jekl V, Hauptman K, Knotek Z. Diseases in pet degus: a retrospective study in 300 animals. J Small Anim Pract 2011;52:107–12.
41. Longley L. Rodents: dermatoses. In: Keeble M, Meredtih MA, editors. BSAVA manual of rodents and ferrets. 2nd edition. Gloucester (United Kingdom): BSAVA; 2009. p. 107–22.
42. Sarna JR, Dyck RH, Whishaw IQ. The Dalila effect: C57BL6 mice barber whiskers by plucking. Behav Brain Res 2000;108:39–45.
43. Hauschka TS. Whisker-eating mice. J Hered 1952;43:77–80.
44. Garner JP, Thogerson CM, Dufour BD, et al. Reverse-translational biomarker validation of abnormal repetitive behaviors in mice: an illustration of the 4P's modeling approach. Behav Brain Res 2011;219:189–96.
45. Kalueff AV, Keisala T, Minasyan A, et al. Influence of paternal genotypes on F1 behaviors: lessons from several mouse strains. Behav Brain Res 2007;177:45–50.
46. Myers DD. C57BL/6J update-C57BL/6J skin lesion problem eliminated. JAX Mice Animal Health Archives, Health Bulletins Aug 14, 1997. Available at: http://web.archive.org/web/20020416162136/http://jaxmice.jax.org/html/archives/animalhealthreport.shtml. Accessed June 13, 2013
47. De Luca AM. Environmental enrichment: does it reduce barbering in mice? AWIC Newslett 1997;8:7–8.
48. Van den Broek FA, Omzight CM, Beynen AC. Whisker trimming behaviour in A2G mice is not prevented by offering means of withdrawal from it. Lab Anim 1993;27:270–2.
49. Kalueff AV, Minasyan A, Keisala T, et al. Hair barbering in mice: implications for neurobehavioural research. Behav Processes 2006;71:8–15.
50. Garner JP, Dufour B, Gregg LE, et al. Social and husbandry factors affecting the prevalence and severity of barbering (whisker trimming) by laboratory mice. Appl Anim Behav Sci 2004;89:263–82.
51. Nicholson A, Malcolm RD, Russ PL, et al. The response of C57BL/6J and BALB/cJ mice to increased housing density. J Am Assoc Lab Anim Sci 2009; 48(6):740–53.
52. Bechard A, Meagher R, Mason G. Environmental enrichment reduces the likelihood of alopecia in adult C57BL/6J mice. J Am Assoc Lab Anim Sci 2011;50(2): 171–4.
53. Lawson GW. Etiopathogenesis of mandibulofacial and maxillofacial abscesses in mice. J Am Assoc Lab Anim Sci 2010;60(3):200–4.
54. Tišljar M, Janić D, Grabarević Z, et al. Stress induced Cushing's syndrome in fur chewing chinchillas. Acta Vet Hung 2002;50(2):133–42.

55. Crossley DA. Dental disease in chinchilla in the UK. J Small Anim Pract 2001; 42(1):12–9.

56. Jekl V, Hauptmann K, Knotek Z. Quantitative and qualitative assessments of intraoral lesions in 180 small herbivorous mammals. Vet Rec 2008;162:442–9.

57. Rees RG. Some conditions of the skin and fur of *Chinchilla lanigera*. J Small Anim Pract 1962;4:213–25.

58. Ponzio MF, Busso JM, Ruiz RD, et al. A survey assessment of the incidence of fur-chewing in commercial chinchilla (*Chinchilla lanigera*) farms. Anim Welf 2007;16:471–9.

59. Vanjonack WJ, Johnson HD. Relationship of thyroid and adrenal function to "fur chewing" in the chinchilla. Comp Biochem Physiol 1973;45A:115–20.

60. Ponzio MF, Monfort SL, Busso JM, et al. Adrenal activity and anxiety-like behavior in fur-chewing chinchillas (*Chinchilla lanigera*). Horm Behav 2012;61:758–62.

61. Jimenez JE. Conservation of the last wild chinchilla archipelago: a meta-population approach. Vida Silvestre Neotropical 1995;4:89–97.

62. Gerold S, Huisinga E, Iglauer F, et al. Influence of feeding hay on the alopecia of breeding guinea pigs. J Vet Med A Physiol Pathol Clin Med 1997;44:341–8.

63. Harkness JE, Murray KA, Wagner JE. Biology and diseases of guinea pigs. In: Fox JG, Anderson LC, Loew FM, et al, editors. Laboratory animal medicine. 2nd edition. San Diego (CA), London: Academic Press; 2002. p. 203–46.

64. Donnelly TM, Brown CJ. Guinea pig and chinchilla care and husbandry. Vet Clin North Am Exot Anim Pract 2004;7:351–73.

65. Huerkamp MJ, Murray KA, Orosz SE. Guinea pigs. In: Laber-Laird K, Swindle MM, Flecknell PA, editors. Handbook of rodent and rabbit medicine. Exeter (United Kingdom): Pergamon Press; 1996.

66. Hernandez-Divers SM. Principles of wound management of small mammals: hedgehogs, prairie dogs, and sugar gliders. Vet Clin North Am Exot Anim Pract 2004;7:1–18.

67. Marrow JC, Carpenter JW, Lloyd A, et al. A transitional cell carcinoma with squamous differentiation in a pericloacal mass in a sugar glider (*Petaurus breviceps*). J Exot Pet Med 2010;19(1):92–5.

68. Kraemer GW, Clarke AS. The behavioral neurobiology of self-injurious behavior in rhesus monkeys. Progr Neuro Psychopharmacol Biol Psychiatr 1990;14: S141–68.

69. Kastenmayer RJ, Fain MA, Perdue KA. A retrospective study of idiopathic ulcerative dermatitis in mice with a C57BL/6 background. J Am Assoc Lab Anim Sci 2006;45:8–12.

70. Andrews AG, Dysko RC, Spilman SC, et al. Immune complex vasculitis with secondary ulcerative dermatitis in aged C57BL/6NNia mice. Vet Pathol 1994;31(3): 293–300.

71. Williams LK, Csaki LS, Cantor RM, et al. Ulcerative dermatitis in C57BL/6 mice exhibits an oxidative stress response consistent with normal wound healing. Comp Med 2012;62(3):166–71.

72. Sundberg JP, Taylor D, Lorch G, et al. Primary follicular dystrophy with scarring dermatitis in C57BL/6 mouse substrains resembles central centrifugal cicatricial alopecia in humans. Vet Pathol 2011;48:513–24.

73. Feldman S, McVay L, Kessler MJ. Resolution of ulcerative dermatitis of mice by treatment with topical 0.2% cyclosporine. J Am Assoc Lab Anim Sci 2006;45:92–3.

74. Perkins SN, Hursting SD, Phang JM, et al. Calorie restriction educes ulcerative dermatitis and infection related mortality in p-53 deficient and wild-type mice. J Invest Dermatol 1998;111(2):292–6.

75. Neuhaus B, Niessen CM, Mesaros A, et al. Experimental analysis of risk factors for ulcerative dermatitis in mice. Exp Dermatol 2012;21:712–3.

76. Williams-Fritz MJ, Scholz JA, Zeiss C, et al. Maropitant citrate for treatment of ulcerative dermatitis in mice with a C57BL/6 background. J Am Assoc Lab Anim Sci 2011;50(2):221–6.

77. Lawson GW, Sato A, Fairbanks LA, et al. Vitamin E as a treatment for ulcerative dermatitis in C57BL/6 mice and strains with a C57BL/6 background. Contemp Top Lab Anim Sci 2005;44:18–21.

78. Crowley M, Delano ML, Kirchain SM. Successful treatment of C57BL/6 ulcerative dermatitis with caladryl lotion. J Am Assoc Lab Anim Sci 2008;47:109–10.

79. Mufford T, Richardson L. Nail trims versus the previous standard of care for treatment of mice with ulcerative dermatitis. J Am Assoc Lab Anim Sci 2009; 48:546.

80. Mader JR, Mason MA, Bale LK, et al. The association of early dietary supplementation with vitamin E with the incidence of ulcerative dermatitis in mice on a C57BL/6 background. Scand J Lab Anim Sci 2010;37(4):253–9.

81. Duarte-Vogel SM, Lawson GW. Association between hair induced oronasal inflammation and ulcerative dermatitis in C57BL/6 mice. Comp Med 2011; 61(1):13–9.

82. Dufour BD, Adeola O, Cheng H, et al. Nutritional up-regulation of serotonin paradoxically induces compulsive behavior. Nutr Neurosci 2010;13(6):256–64.

Index

Note: Page numbers of article titles are in **boldface** type.

A

Abdominal distention, with ovarian cysts, in guinea pig, 763–764
Abscesses, with dermatologic diseases, in chinchillas, 574
    in guinea pigs, 557
    in mice, barbering associated with, 810
    in rabbits, subcutaneous, 554
    in reptiles, 527
    pododermatitis-related, 717
Abuse, self-injurious behaviors related to, 806
Acaricide drugs, for ectoparasites, in small mammals, 641
Acrylic ramp and the pin, for beak growth abnormalities, in avians, 788
Acupuncture, for pododermatitis, 732
Adhesives, for avian fractures, 782, 784
Adrenal disease. See *Hyperadrenocorticism.*
Adrenal panel, for erythema multiforme, in ferrets, 603–604
Aesthetics, of fish dermatology, viral infections and, 688–689
Age, ovarian cysts related to, in guinea pig, 760–761
Aggression, barbering and, 810
Alopecia, as behavioral dermatopathy, 807–808
    in guinea pigs, 812–813
  stress impact on, 804, 809
  with ovarian cysts, in guinea pig, 763–765, 770, 812
    differential diagnosis of, 765
Alternative therapies, for pododermatitis, 731–732
    acupuncture as, 732
    natural remedies as, 731–732
    therapeutic laser as, 731–732
Amphibian dermatology, chytridiomycosis in, **669–685**
    B. dendrobatidis life cycle, 670. See also *Batrachochytrium dendrobatidis (Bd).*
    cause of death from, 671
    clinical signs of, 671–672
    diagnosis of, 672–675
    introduction to, 669–670
    normal skin physiology and, 670
    pathophysiology of, 670–671
    skin physiology in, 670
    summary overview of, 682
    treatment of, 675–682
        chemicals in, 679–680
            benzalkonium chloride as, 680
            formalin as, 679
            malachite green as, 679

Vet Clin Exot Anim 16 (2013) 821–862
http://dx.doi.org/10.1016/S1094-9194(13)00065-0
1094-9194/13/$ – see front matter © 2013 Elsevier Inc. All rights reserved.

vetexotic.theclinics.com

Printed and bound by CPI Group (UK) Ltd, Croydon, CR0 4YY

03/10/2024

01040410-0006